MW01015091

MEDICS AT WAR

Military Medicine
from Colonial Times
to the 21st Century

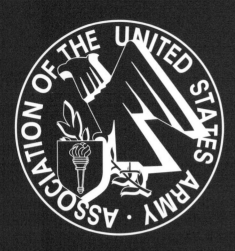

Since 1950, the Association of the United States Army (AUSA) has worked to support all aspects of national security while advancing the interests of America's Army and the men and women who serve the nation.

AUSA is a private, non-profit educational organization that supports America's Army—Active, National Guard, Reserve, Civilians, Retirees, and family members.

Association of the United States Army (AUSA)
2425 Wilson Blvd.
Arlington, VA 22201
703-841-4300
800-336-4570
www.ausa.org

APPRECIATION

The Association of the United States Army wishes to express its profound appreciation to The Henry M. Jackson Foundation for the Advancement of Military Medicine, Inc. (HJF™) and the Uniformed Services University of the Health Sciences (USU) for their generous support in the creation of *Medics at War*.

HJF was named after the late Senator Henry M. "Scoop" Jackson (D-WA), who had a long-standing commitment to military medicine and public health. The Foundation supports medical research and education at the USU and throughout military medicine. HJF also manages and supports more than 600 research projects on military medicine around the globe.

The USU is a fully accredited federal school of medicine and graduate school of nursing, located in Bethesda, Maryland.

The affiliation between HJF and USU provides access to cutting-edge science and technology, and promotes cross-disciplinary collaboration in advancing military medical research and education.

HJF™ is a registered trademark of The Henry M. Jackson Foundation for the Advancement of Military Medicine, Inc.

Its headquarters are located at:
1401 Rockville Pike, Suite 600
Rockville, MD 20852
301-424-0800
www.hjf.org

MEDICS AT WAR

Military Medicine from Colonial Times to the 21st Century

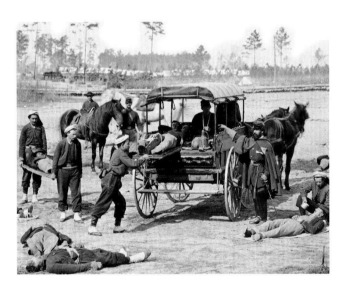
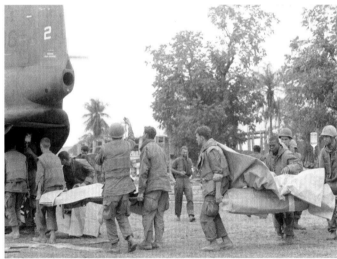

John T. Greenwood, Ph.D.
F. Clifton Berry, Jr.

Presented by the

Association of the United States Army

Naval Institute Press
Annapolis, Maryland

Copyright © 2005 by the Association of the United States Army

All rights reserved. No part of this book may be reproduced, stored in a retrieval system, or transmitted in any form or by any means without permission in writing from the Association of the United States Army.

Design by Hinge, Inc. www.pivotalbrands.com. Liz Weaver, head designer; Greg Spraker, art director.
Editor: Nina D. Seebeck.
Indexer: Amy B. Thompson.
Coordination and liaison: Simone B. Hammarstrand.
Photo research: Cyndy Gilley, Mike Gilley, Michael Dolan.

Naval Institute Press
291 Wood Road
Annapolis, Maryland 21402
www.usni.org

Library of Congress Cataloging-in-Publication Data

Greenwood, John T.
  Medics at war : military medicine from colonial times to the 21st century /
John T. Greenwood, F. Clifton Berry Jr.
     p. ; cm.
"Presented by the Association of the United States Army."
Includes bibliographical references and index.
  ISBN 1-59114-344-6 (alk. paper)
  1. Medicine, Military--United States--History. 2. United States--Armed Forces--Medical care--History.
  [DNLM: 1. Military Medicine--history--United States. 2. History, Modern
1601---United States.] I. Berry, F. Clifton. II. Association of the United States Army. III. Title.
  UH223.G78 2005
  355.3'45'0973--dc22
                          2005007218

Dedication

To the medics of the armed services of the
United States of America: past, present, and future.
Their skills and commitment conserve the fighting strength.

Contents

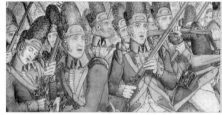
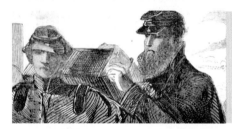
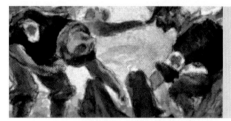
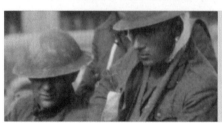
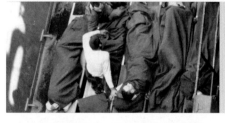
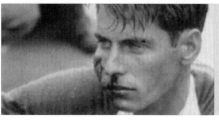

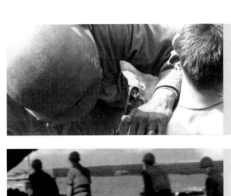
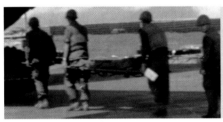
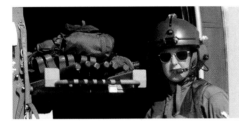
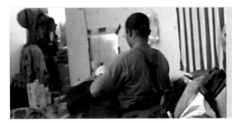
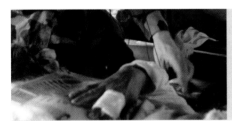

Foreword

The roles and challenges of the medic are as diverse as the military operations they support. Today's military operations not only involve traditional military conflict, but also extend to humanitarian relief, disaster assistance, and nation-building. Military medics are the physicians, dentists, nurses, physician assistants, medical administrators, logisticians, and first responders (those dedicated enlisted medics and corpsmen who provide critical frontline care). Each of these professionals must be armed with specialized knowledge and expertise in preventive and emergency medicine, health promotion, trauma, infectious disease, psychological stress, and extreme physical environments.

Napoleon observed that an army's power and effectiveness is dependent upon its morale, for "the morale is to the material as three to one." Providing the very best medical support to our troops is essential to morale because it sends four very powerful messages. It sends to the American people the message that our nation's leaders are committed to protecting their sons and daughters, their fathers and mothers, their brothers and sisters who have been sent into harm's way. It sends to our military commanders the message that their fighting strength will be supported. It sends to our adversaries the message that we have the requisite medical resources to maintain the will to fight and to win. Most importantly, it sends to our troops the message that their nation honors its covenant to care for them.

A former Navy Surgeon General, Lamont Pugh, wrote of the military medic, "...he can perform no more worthy mission than that of protecting and restoring the most priceless element, that of health, in our most precious national resource, the men and women who comprise the Armed Forces." This book portrays the chronology of those remarkable medics who practiced good medicine in bad places during our nation's conflicts ... from the Revolution to the wars of the 21st century.

The Navy traditionally salutes exceptional performance by proclaiming, "Well done!" through deployment of its signal code, "Bravo-Zulu." I extend a hearty "Bravo-Zulu" to the leadership and staff of AUSA for conceiving and publishing *Medics at War*—a well-deserved and overdue tribute to the men and women who are committed to caring for those the nation sends into harm's way.

James A. Zimble
Vice Admiral, MC
U.S. Navy, Ret.

Preface

We use the title of "medic" in this book as shorthand for the men and women in the medical departments of the U.S. armed forces. They include medics from the active forces plus reserves and National Guard, as well as their civilian colleagues.

Recurring themes appear in the evolution of military medicine in the armed forces of the United States. In this book we present the reader with examples of the themes in words and pictures.

Medics strive to reduce the time from first wounding to definitive care. After lack of progress in the 19th century, significant improvements were achieved in the 20th century and continue in the 21st.

Medics are dedicated to providing the best care for their patients in the immediate situation. They often risk their lives, and many have given their lives, to ensure that their fellow service members receive care.

The medical departments experience cycles of expansion in time of peril and shrinkage when the fighting is finished. Like the nation, the medics must scramble and improvise to meet new challenges and new threats.

The military medics also innovate. The book presents examples that show how the armed forces and society have benefited from the ingenuity of the medics. Casualties and the sick receive better and faster care as a result of the medics' initiative and innovation.

Over the centuries from the Revolution to 2005, military medics have remained true to a fundamental principle: to care for those who face the perils of service to the nation. This is true whether the harm comes from enemy action or debilitating diseases. Their dedication is constant, unvarying, and effective.

In the preparation of this book, we received able authoritative assistance from four experts.

Messrs. Jan K. Herman and André B. Sobocinski contributed the materials on the U.S. Navy. Mr. Herman is Historian of the Navy Medical Department, Curator of the old U.S. Naval Observatory, and Editor of *Navy Medicine*, the bimonthly journal of the Navy Medical Department. His books include *Battle Station Sick Bay: Navy Medicine in World War II* and the forthcoming *Frozen in Memory: Navy Medicine and Korea 1950-1953*. André Sobocinski has worked for the Navy Medical Department's Office of the Historian and *Navy Medicine* magazine since 2001, and has published and contributed to more than 20 articles on military medicine.

James S. Nanney, Ph.D., historian at the Air Force Medical Service, prepared the coverage of Air Force medicine. Dr. Nanney entered federal service in 1980 as an historian for the U.S. Army Center of Military History. In 1989, he transferred to the U.S. Air Force history program and in 1992 became the chief historian for the Air Force Surgeon General.

Dale C. Smith, Ph.D., Chairman of the Department of History at the Uniformed Services University of the Health Sciences, contributed the section on the origin and roles of that institution.

Finally, we are most grateful to Vice Admiral James A. Zimble, MC, USN, Ret., for contributing the Foreword. His distinguished career included service as the 30th Surgeon General of the U.S. Navy. He retired from that post to become president of the Uniformed Services University in 1991, leading the institution for 13 years until 2004.

We are grateful to those contributors, and also to the dozens of other persons who assisted us in preparation of the book. Their assistance improved the product.

Northern Virginia
Spring 2005

John T. Greenwood, Ph.D.
F. Clifton Berry Jr.

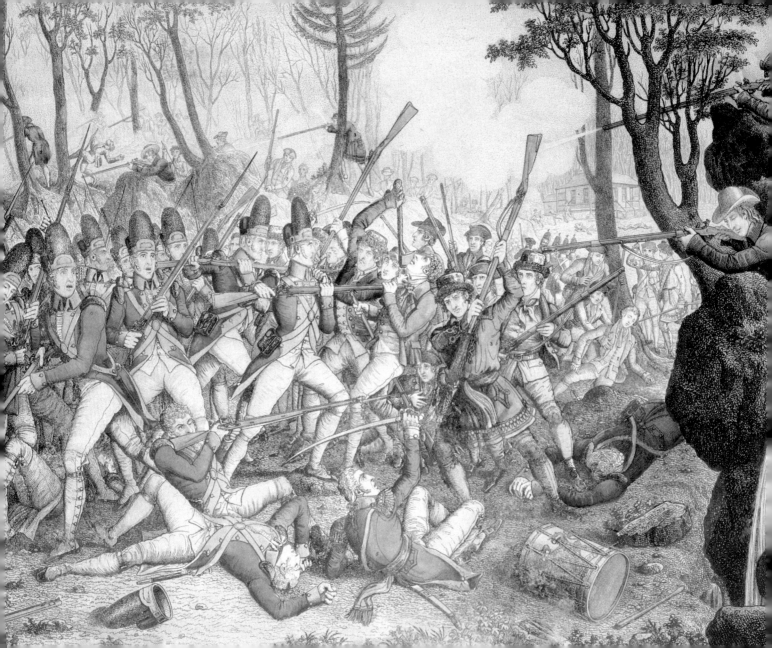

Chapter 1

From Revolutionary War to the Civil War, 1775–1861

left
Battle of Lexington, April 19, 1775. Colonial Minutemen inflicted more than 700 casualties on British troops at the battles of Lexington and Concord and the British retreat to Boston. Minutemen casualties included 49 dead, 39 wounded, and five missing. *National Archives.*

right
Battle of Breed's (Bunker) Hill, June 17, 1775. (Wounded British Redcoats appear at left front.) The attacking British forces suffered more than 1,040 casualties to the Americans' 453. *Library of Congress.*

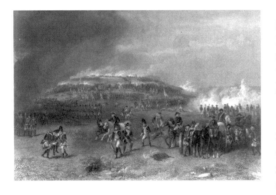

ARMY MEDICINE: BEGINNING AND DEVELOPMENT

REVOLUTIONARY WAR, 1775-83
Fighting between Colonial American militias and British regulars at Lexington and Concord near Boston, Massachusetts, on April 19, 1775, ignited the Revolutionary War. The subsequent siege of British forces in Boston led the Continental Congress to establish the Continental Army under General George Washington on June 14, 1775. The ensuing Battle of Breed's (Bunker) Hill on June 17 resulted in an American defeat and numerous casualties.

On July 20, Washington asked the Continental Congress in Philadelphia to create a military medical organization to care for his sick and wounded soldiers. On July 27, the Continental Congress created a "Hospital for the Army," in essence a hospital or medical department, under the supervision of a Chief Physician and Director General. Thus, the predecessor of today's U.S. Army Medical Department came into being to serve the needs of the American soldier even before the new nation declared its independence from the Crown.

George Washington's leading role in the creation of the Army's new Hospital Department reflected his deep interest in military medicine and concern for the soldiers' welfare. He understood the fundamental responsibility of the commander to care for the health of his troops. He also knew that disease was as much his enemy as the Redcoats.

Like their British counterparts, American regular and militia regiments had a surgeon and surgeon's mates to care for the officers and men in camp and on the battlefield. Regimental surgeons had many jobs—physician, surgeon, nurse, and apothecary. Regiments had their own hospitals; usually a log cabin, barn, or tent in the field, but a surgeon could also send seriously ill or wounded soldiers to a general hospital in the rear. "Flying" hospitals served regiments on the move and bridged the gap between the regimental and general hospitals. Thus, an echeloning of evacuation and medical care that would become fundamental to American military medicine was already emerging—battlefield and camp care at the regimental level, special mobile hospitals to accompany the Army on campaigns, and general hospitals at the rear to provide more definitive care for the sick, wounded, and disabled soldiers.

American medical officers patterned their organizations, procedures, and medical and surgical treatments on the British and European medical and military practices with which they were most familiar. From the British, they also adopted the tradition of preventive medicine based on the work of Sir John Pringle and Dr. Richard Brocklesby during the mid-century wars in Europe. While 18th century military physicians knew nothing of germs and how contagious diseases spread, they were astute and trained observers. They saw soldiers in camp fall sick and die from overcrowded living conditions, poor food, unhealthy water, inadequate clothing, filthy personal hygiene, and bad sanitary practices.

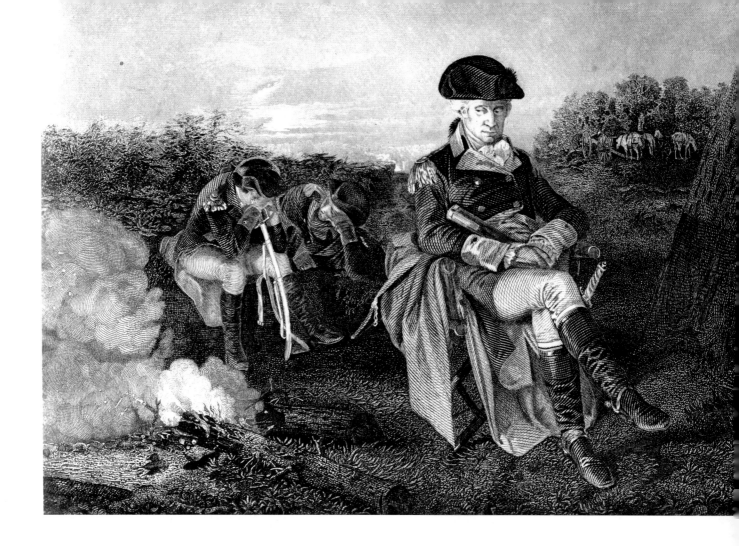

Military physicians believed that it was far better to prevent diseases from occurring in the first place than to treat their victims afterward. While they recommended corrective actions to remedy these problems, the line officers often disregarded the advice because they, like most of the enlisted men, had little or no respect for physicians as a group.

The Continental Army also adopted from the British the artificial division between regimental or troop surgeons and hospital surgeons as well as the practice of denying surgeons military rank. Unfortunately, these flaws in the Continental Army's medical organization not only prevented the development of a strong, centralized Hospital Department, but remained embedded serious weaknesses in the Army's medical tradition for some decades to come. The often formidable skills of the individual physicians, many of them the leading physicians in the Colonies, were largely wasted within an unsound organization.

Neither the Continental Army nor the British Army had any standardized practice for removing the wounded from the battlefield. Regimental surgeons set their own evacuation policies and usually designated infantrymen to carry or use wheelbarrows and other means to transport the wounded to the regiment's surgical area. Many surgeons understood that the lives of the wounded soldiers often depended on the swiftness of treatment, so the time it took for the wounded to reach life-saving medical attention dictated the location of the surgeon on the battlefield. Time was the real enemy, and the military surgeon's greatest challenge was to reduce the length of time the wounded soldier went without medical attention.

General George Washington after the Battle of Monmouth, New Jersey, June 28, 1778. By this time, the entire Continental Army had received smallpox inoculations. Washington himself weathered a case of smallpox at the age of 19. *Library of Congress.*

Dr. John Cochran, Director General of the Army Hospital Department from January 1781. Cochran had served as a surgeon's mate during the French and Indian War. *National Library of Medicine.*

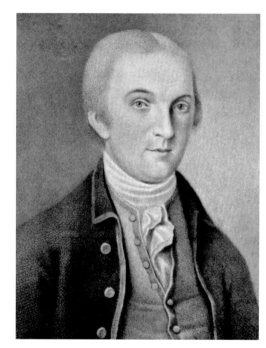

American military surgeons were inexperienced compared to their British counterparts. They relied heavily on standard handbooks of the time, such as Dr. John Jones's *Plain, Concise, and Practical Remarks on the Treatment of Wounds and Fractures to Which is Added an Appendix on Camps and Military Hospitals Principally Designed for the Use of Young Military and Naval Surgeons of North America* (Philadelphia, 1776). Military surgeons closely followed such handbooks and used rudimentary techniques for treating wounds and illness. Thoracic and abdominal wounds were usually fatal. Amputation was the principal surgical technique used to treat serious limb wounds. Infections were a potential threat with any surgery, and many patients died of gangrene.

Diseases, especially the dreaded smallpox, typhus, and typhoid fever, were ever-present dangers in the tightly packed camps. At Boston in 1775–76, Washington suffered a constant drain of soldiers to disease. After an American expedition to Canada was largely destroyed by smallpox, and a New York campaign in 1776 faced equal devastation, Washington took action. In an unprecedented step, he ordered the Hospital Department to undertake the mass inoculation of the Continental Army using variolation, a now obsolete method whereby soldiers were exposed to small amounts of the smallpox virus to develop an immunity to the disease. The mass inoculation programs in the winter camps of 1777 and 1778 were successful and made the Continental Army largely immune from this scourge for the remainder of the war. Washington's calculated risk may well have saved the American cause. He also established a basic principle of preventive medicine that the U.S. Army has followed to this day—the mandatory immunization of all soldiers to protect against the threat of contagious diseases.

Malaria also was a persistent foe and major health threat as far north as New York City. Although not a major killer like smallpox and typhus, malaria incapacitated large numbers of troops for considerable periods of time. Its victims were weakened and more vulnerable to deadly attacks of fatal diseases. Army physicians' main weapon against malaria was the reliable cinchona bark (quinine), which was used with marked success against malaria and other diseases, and remained a staple antimalarial medication for centuries.

From the very outset, the leadership of the Hospital Department was compromised. The first Chief Physician and Director General, Dr. Benjamin Church of Boston, served barely three months before being court-martialed for treason and stripped of his office. The Director Generals who followed Church, John Morgan and William Shippen, Jr., both leading physicians and medical educators, spent more time criticizing each other than organizing the Hospital Department. Only with Shippen's resignation in January 1781 and the promotion of John Cochran did quiet and competent leadership fall over the beleaguered organization.

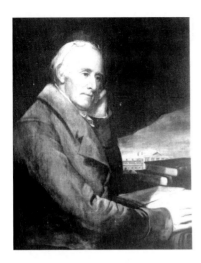

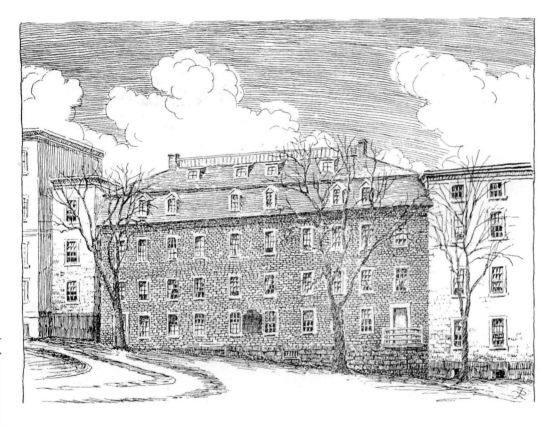

top left
Dr. Benjamin Rush, sign-
er of the Declaration
of Independence and
hospital commander of
the Continental Army in
the Revolutionary War.
National Archives.

center left
Bethlehem Hospital
in Bethlehem, Penn-
sylvania. More than
700 patients endured
filthy conditions here
during the winter of
1777–78. Poor diet and
unsanitary conditions
led to sickness afflicting
nearly 20 percent of the
Continental Army.
*Louis Duncan, Medical
Men of the American
Revolution, 1775–1783.*

One of the most important developments was
the Continental Congress's action in 1776
that gave the Director General the primary
responsibility for certifying the professional
credentials of all surgeons. This established his
authority to set and enforce professional standards for all medical officers in the Army.

Dr. Benjamin Rush created a useful guide in
March 1777. Published by the Board of War, it
was titled *Directions for Preserving the Health
of Soldiers, Addressed to the Officers of the Army
of the United States.* Dr. Rush was one of the

signers of the Declaration of Independence and
Physician General to the military hospitals.

The Hospital Department's system of general hospitals established in New Jersey and
Pennsylvania in 1777–78 had serious shortcomings. Many of their problems stemmed directly
from the undeveloped nature of medicine in
America, the absence of surgical skill, igno-
rance of the causes of diseases, and lack of
competent physicians with the experience
to run large hospitals. When the hospitals
mixed medical and surgical patients, diseases

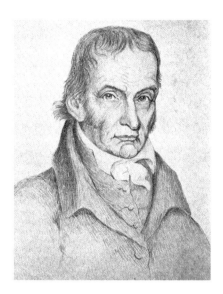

Dr. James Tilton, Physician General during the War of 1812. During the Revolutionary War he advocated small, scattered hospitals with good ventilation and plenty of fresh air. *Louis Duncan, Medical Men of the American Revolution, 1775–1783.*

often spread with great and deadly swiftness. Surgeons in the British Army had noticed this and considered general hospitals more perilous than the battlefield; American experience sadly confirmed this fact. Being a patient in some of these general hospitals was more dangerous than facing the Redcoats.

Soldiers considered duty in such hospitals as extremely hazardous and to be avoided at all costs. Line officers sent only their worst men to act as nurses and orderlies. No assigned and trained force of enlisted personnel existed to take care of the nursing, cooking, and routine functions of these military hospitals. Naturally, the quality of care was very poor and the patients suffered.

James Tilton, an able hospital director in the Princeton and Trenton areas of New Jersey and later the Physician General during the War of 1812, advocated small, scattered hospitals with good ventilation and plenty of fresh air. Tilton argued that the smaller, well-ventilated regimental and flying hospitals were better suited to a majority of the cases than the disease-ridden general hospitals which should take only the seriously wounded and chronically sick soldiers.

Although estimates vary and no reliable information on deaths from diseases was kept, it appears that during the Revolutionary War about 10 soldiers died from disease for every one who died in battle or from wounds. With an estimated 4,044 battle deaths, this meant the Continental Army lost at least 40,000 men to various illnesses.

A NEW NATION, 1783–1812

With the attainment of independence from Great Britain in 1783, the Continental Army and its entire medical organization disappeared. When the Constitution created a new form of government with a U.S. Army and Navy under a War Department, regular Army regiments were created which retained their surgeons and mates. However, no central military medical structure existed above the regiment until the Legion of the United States (1792–96) was established to defend the northwestern frontier.

In 1798, the possibility of a war with France led to significant changes in the American military and naval establishments. Washington was recalled to command an expanded army. Dr. James Craik, Washington's personal physician and a veteran of the Hospital Department, became Physician General in July. In March 1799, a Medical Department was established under him to oversee the Army's medical operations. The passing of George Washington in December 1799 preceded the end of the threat, and the new Army was disbanded. Craik and the nascent Medical Department were gone by June 1800—leaving only six surgeons and 12 mates. Once again the Army was without a formal medical establishment; the care of the soldiers fell entirely on the regimental surgeon, his mates, and whatever hospital facilities and medical supplies he could scrape together.

WAR OF 1812

Neither the Army nor its medical personnel were prepared for the second war with Great Britain which broke out in June 1812. It was not until nine months later, after the devastation wrought by disease along the Canadian front during the winter of 1812–13, that Congress took action. In March 1813, it resurrected the posts of Physician and Surgeon General and Apothecary General to provide some centralized control over medical operations. Dr. James Tilton, creator of the "Tilton hospitals" and now 68 years old and infirm, was selected to fill the new post of Physician and Surgeon General. His February 1813 book on hospitals and preventive medicine, *Economical Observations of Military Hospitals and the Prevention and Cure of Diseases Incident to the Army*, presented new concepts for dealing with these pressing issues and probably influenced his selection.

On the northwestern frontier, the Great Lakes, and in northern New York, military operations were at first inept and poorly organized adventures. The few regimental surgeons and mates in service marched off with their units, while hospital surgeons improvised hospitals with no assigned enlisted medical personnel.

Disease once again took the upper hand. Preventive medicine techniques were no less known than in the Revolutionary War, but again line commanders ignored the advice of even the most respected surgeons. Further complicating matters, the responsibilities of the surgeons were not spelled out in Army directives. This exacerbated the already contentious relations between medical and line officers. It was not until December 1814 that the War Department finally issued a general order establishing regulations for the Army and for the first time clearly defined the duties and responsibilities of medical officers and their place within the Army.

Tilton's Hospital, near Morristown, New Jersey, 1780. Drawing by Dr. James Tilton, the designer. The center section measured 31.5 feet by 19 feet. The external wings were 16 feet by 31.5 feet. *Louis Duncan, Medical Men of the American Revolution, 1775–1783.*

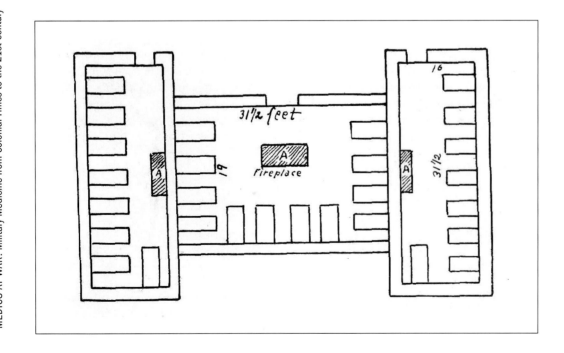

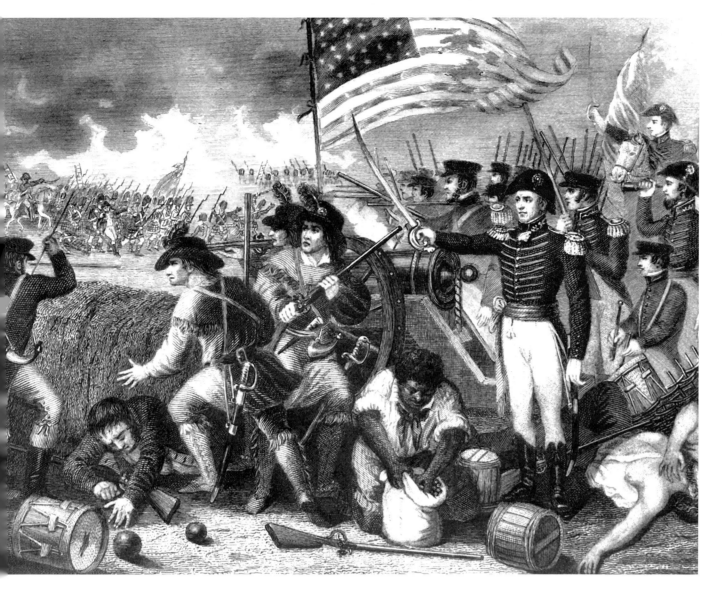

The Battle of New Orleans, January 1815. General Andrew Jackson's force of 3,500 men fought from entrenched positions, including cotton bales. They inflicted more than 2,000 casualties among the 5,300 British attackers. The U.S. Army's 7th Infantry Regiment earned the nickname "Cotton Balers" from their service in the battle. *Copy of engraving by H. B. Hall after W. Momberger. National Archives.*

Although American medicine had improved in the years since 1783, surgeons still knew little about the causes and spread of diseases. An important improvement in controlling smallpox was introduced in May 1812. Army surgeons were directed to vaccinate all soldiers using Dr. Edward Jenner's proven cowpox virus rather than inoculating with smallpox virus.

Surgical techniques were still relatively primitive. Amputation remained the only surgical option to treat serious wounds to the limbs and infected and gangrenous extremities. Thoracic and abdominal wounds were nearly always fatal, for surgical intervention could do little to save such cases.

Individual surgeons often overcame even the most daunting challenges to care for and save the sick and wounded. James Mann, Joseph Lovell, William Beaumont, and others worked diligently at general hospitals in Greenbush, Plattsburgh, Malone, and Williamsville, New York, and Burlington, Vermont, and other locations in 1812-13. Gradually, the deficiencies were corrected, and medical supplies were produced and distributed. Although aged and disabled, Tilton visited the fronts along Lakes Ontario and Erie and built a medical department to support the soldiers. By 1814–15, care in the general hospitals, especially in the North, had improved significantly.

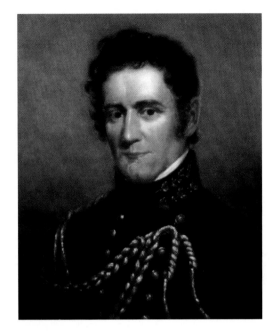

BUILDING A MEDICAL DEPARTMENT, 1815-60

The return of peace in 1815 resulted in a dismantling of the wartime Medical Department. The fundamental lesson of the War of 1812 for military medicine was clear: A permanent central staff organization was required to remedy its many problems. Such a structure and leadership were needed to build a strong professional corps of Army physicians who could care for the troops and undertake the systematic study of diseases and health conditions in all areas of the country where troops were stationed. Realizing the need to prevent the repetition of the disasters of 1812–15, Secretary of War John C. Calhoun in 1818 proposed a sweeping reorganization of the Army and created new staff departments to lead the revitalization.

On April 14, 1818, the Congress authorized the creation of a Medical Department under a Surgeon General within Army headquarters. As the staff officer for military medicine, the Surgeon General was responsible to the Secretary and commanding general for the health and well-being of the soldiers. Selected to fill this new post was the 29-year-old Joseph Lovell, whose work as a regimental surgeon with the 9th Infantry and a hospital director at Burlington, Vermont, early in the War of 1812 had been outstanding.

Lovell set about building a centralized Medical Department. He ended the division between regimental and hospital surgeons by creating a single Medical Corps that he and his office would eventually control in selection and assignment. In September 1818 he issued the *Regulations of the Medical Department*, which set out his responsibilities as Surgeon General as well as those of all medical officers in the Army, along with a clear command structure for the new department.

Lovell had a strong scientific bent and immediately set about the systematic collection of information from each post and regimental surgeon on the health of their soldiers. These reports permitted the first serious examination of the health of the Army and of the diseases that afflicted it. His directive to garrison medical officers to record and report weather and climatic conditions that he thought affected the soldiers' health laid the origins for the Army's Signal Corps and even the U.S. Weather Service.

Army surgeons on frontier duty sometimes had singular chances to conduct medical and scientific research. In 1822, William Beaumont, an Army surgeon at Fort Mackinac on Michigan's Upper Peninsula, used his physician skills to save the life of Alexis St. Martin. St. Martin suffered a shotgun wound to the midsection that resulted in a permanent abdominal fistula. The anomaly provided Beaumont a unique opportunity to study the digestive system by viewing it through the window of St. Martin's fistula. His investigations into the process of digestion won critical praise from the civilian medical world in the United States and Germany. His research emphasized how an Army surgeon without proper equipment or training could make significant contributions to emerging American medical science.

top
Dr. Joseph Lovell, first Surgeon General of the U.S. Army. His exemplary service with the 9th Infantry Regiment in the War of 1812 prepared him for invigorating the new department. *National Library of Medicine.*

bottom
Dr. William Beaumont, surgeon at Fort Mackinac, studied the digestive system via the fistula of a wounded trapper. His 1833 book, *Experiments and Observations on the Gastric Juice and the Physiology of Digestion*, advanced the practice of gastroenterology. *National Library of Medicine.*

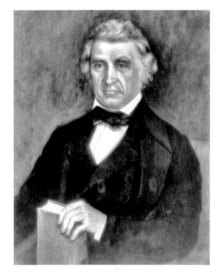

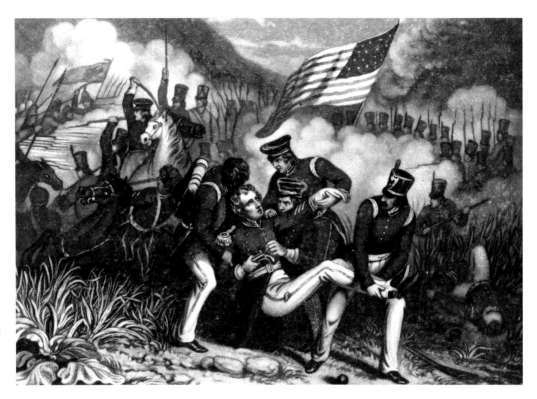

Fall of Lieutenant Colonel Henry Clay, Jr., killed leading his Second Kentucky Regiment in attack at Buena Vista, Mexico, on February 23, 1847. In two days of fighting, General Zachary Taylor's force of 4,594 soldiers defeated Mexican General Antonio Lopez Santa Ana's nearly 15,000 troops. The Mexican force sustained 591 killed, 1,048 wounded, and 1,894 missing. American casualties included 272 killed, 387 wounded, and six missing. *Library of Congress.*

When Lovell died suddenly in 1836, Thomas Lawson succeeded him and would guide the Medical Department through the next 24 years and into the first year of the Civil War. Lawson served with distinction as surgeon of the 6th Infantry in the War of 1812. After a number of frontier assignments, he was the medical director of forces assembling for the Seminole War when he succeeded Lovell in November 1836. Lawson's major challenge was maintaining medical support for an Army widely scattered in small forts and garrisons over the entire nation. Westward expansion stretched the Medical Corps's assets, and officers were often assigned to the exploratory expeditions that traversed the largely uncharted areas west of the Mississippi and Missouri rivers, especially in the years after the Mexican War.

MEXICAN WAR

The outbreak of the war with Mexico in May 1846 presented enormous challenges for Lawson. With only 71 regular Army medical officers including himself, he had to support Zachary Taylor's Army in Texas for operations into northern Mexico, Winfield Scott's subsequent expeditionary force headed for Vera Cruz and Mexico City, additional expeditions to California and New Mexico, and all existing garrisons. A volunteer force of 50,000 was called up, with one surgeon and one assistant surgeon per regiment.

Medical organization of the field armies was small and mostly in the regiments. Without a formal hospital structure and trained enlisted staff, medical directors of the armies and divisions sought medical personnel from regiments to staff any hospitals. But regiments could rarely spare enlisted personnel. Hospital directors often had to draft their patients to perform duties as stewards, nurses, and cooks. This utter lack of trained medical personnel degraded care in both the regiments and hospitals, with deadly consequences.

The Army's record in the fight against disease and sickness was pathetic. Medical science had made significant progress since the War of 1812. Contagious diseases were better understood. The recent introduction of ether for anesthesia promised easier surgery. However, some Army surgeons believed ether produced poor results and ceased using it.

On February 11, 1847, in an act to raise more regiments for the war, the Congress gave the officers of the Medical Corps an important victory: military rank, pay, and an equal footing with officers of the line and other staff departments. After 72 years, Medical Corps officers had finally gained the unquestioned right to command within their department and full status and privileges of officers of the U.S. Army.

Disease once again won virtually every skirmish. In the Vera Cruz and Mexico City campaigns, General Scott suffered the loss of nearly one-third of his command to disease. The same old litany was repeated—soldiers in poor health, poor provisions, poor field sanitation, and operating in areas in which deadly diseases such as yellow fever and malaria were endemic. As in previous wars, line officers often paid little attention to sound medical advice.

After the Mexican War, the expansion of the country to the Pacific with the acquisition of California and the areas of the Southwest strained the Medical Department. Organizing medical support for widely scattered units operating against hostile Indians on the western frontier was difficult given the limited number of medical officers. Removing casualties suffered in remote areas and treating arrow wounds challenged the field surgeons. In 1855, Lawson sought to remedy some of the department's most pressing problems, including the fact that he had only 94 medical officers to man 89 military posts and arsenals across the country. In 1856, Congress granted additional medical officers, the enlistment of hospital stewards, and extra-duty pay for hospital nurses and attendants detailed from the line. The first enlisted hospital stewards entered the Medical Department that year, marking a significant milestone in the history of the Army Medical Department.

Three years later, a board of officers evaluated models of wheeled ambulances as part of a larger plan for a field ambulance system.

NAVY MEDICINE: FROM 1775 TO THE EVE OF THE CIVIL WAR

EARLY DAYS, 1775-1842

The shots fired at Lexington and Concord on April 19, 1775, signaled the birth of a nation and the Continental Army. However, the British blockade of the Colonial American coast and the American desire to break the blockade and go on the offensive ultimately spawned the Continental Navy and Navy Medical Department.

In October 1775, the Continental Congress approved the creation of a navy to complement a polyglot force of privateers and state vessels. The ships in this tiny fleet—*Alfred, Andrew Doria, Cabot, Providence, Columbus,* and *Hornet*—contained the first sick bays where doctors of the Continental Navy practiced their healing art. Surgeons and surgeon's mates provided by the Continental Congress represented the early Navy Medical Department.

Among these medical pioneers were Drs. Joseph Harrison, Thomas Kerr, and Henry Tillinghast. Assisting in the daily care of the sick and wounded were the curiously named loblolly boys, enlisted medical personnel named after the thick porridge or "loblolly" they rationed out to the sick. Loblollies also had the dubious honor of providing containers for amputated limbs, hot tar for cauterizing stumps, and sand for spreading on decks to absorb blood shed during combat and surgical procedures.

The Continental Navy was a short-lived enterprise that did not long survive the Treaty of Paris. The new nation lived without a naval fleet until 1794 when Congress authorized six new ships to be built to defend its ever growing commercial interests. These vessels were to form the nucleus of the new United States Navy. Each warship was to have a surgeon, and, for the larger vessels of 36 guns, two additional surgeon's mates.

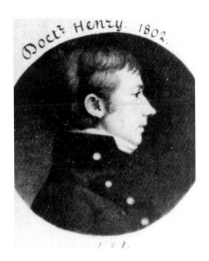

Dr. Isaac Henry. He entered U.S. Navy service as Surgeon's Mate in 1798 aboard the frigate USS *Constellation*, the first ship commissioned in the United States Navy. Promoted to surgeon in 1799, he saw action in the West Indies during the Quasi-War with France. *U.S. Navy Bureau of Medicine and Surgery.*

The Department of the Navy was born on April 30, 1798, during the so-called Quasi-War with France. A significant development during this period was in the shore hospitalization of sick and disabled seamen. By an act of 1798, Navy sailors could now be admitted to civilian hospitals designated by directors appointed in ports of entry. These directors paid the incurred expenses from a Marine Hospital Fund maintained by monthly deductions of 20 cents from every merchant and Navy seaman, naval officer, and marine. In subsequent years, Marine (later to be known as Navy) hospitals were established in Syracuse, Sicily (1804) and New Orleans, Louisiana (1810), but these were short-lived ventures.

On February 26, 1811, Congress approved "An Act establishing Navy Hospitals." The act directed that money collected from naval personnel and the unexpended balance from the Marine Hospital Fund should be paid to the Secretaries of the Navy, Treasury, and Army. These were to act as the so-called "commissioners" of Navy hospitals. The commissioners were to choose suitable sites for the building of permanent hospitals and then were to erect buildings at these locations.

Ten years elapsed before the selection of the first site at Washington, D.C., in 1821. This was followed by the purchase of other sites—Chelsea, Massachusetts (1823); Brooklyn, New York (1824); Philadelphia, Pennsylvania (1826); and Norfolk, Virginia (1827). In 1830, the Naval Hospital at Norfolk was the first of these facilities to open its doors to patients, followed soon thereafter by the Philadelphia Naval Hospital situated in the famed Naval Asylum, a multitasked institution that also served as the U.S. Naval Academy's first home.

What was health care like in the early days of the U.S. Navy? Fortunately, the writings of early Navy health practitioners provide some answers. While serving aboard the USS *United States*, Surgeon Edward Cutbush reported that venereal diseases and diarrhea were very common among the crew. He also noted their state of mental health. There were days, he said, in which sailors seemed "very low" and labored "under Nostalgia or a constant desire to return [home]." Scurvy also posed a problem for Navy surgeons until 1812 when citrus fruits were issued to naval ships regularly at the urging of Navy surgeon, and future chief of the Bureau of Medicine and Surgery, William P.C. Barton.

Following the Revolutionary War, the United States Navy fought sea battles with France, the Barbary Pirates, and with Britain in the War of 1812. Throughout these conflicts, the duties of the Navy surgeon were quite defined. He visited men under his care at least twice a day, supervised surgeon's mates, consulted with other surgeons in the squadron about difficult cases, informed the captain daily of the condition of his patients, and was expected to be prepared with his mates and assistants for battle. He kept a daybook, which contained the names of his patients, their prescriptions and methods of treatment, when and how they became ill or injured, when they recovered or died, and when they were discharged to duty.

From this daybook he made two journals, one a record of his "physical" practice, and the other a record of his "chirurgical" practice. At the end of each voyage he sent the two journals to the Navy Department. When ordering patients to hospitals, he was required to send with them a record of their cases. The Navy surgeon was permitted to send men to hospitals and sick quarters only when they could not be adequately cared for aboard ship. He had charge of the requisition, inspection, storage, accounting, and dispensation of all medical supplies used aboard his ship. Whenever the surgeon received faulty supplies, he was to notify the

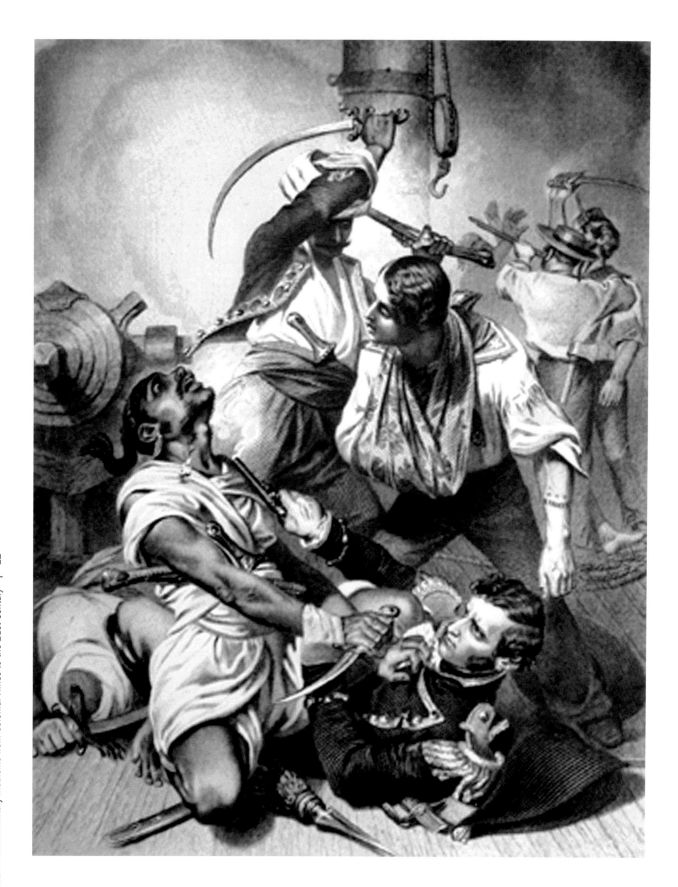

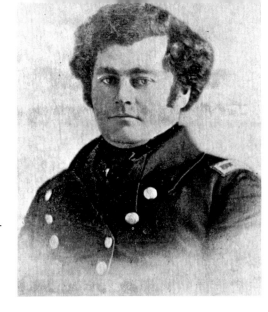

left
Captain Stephen Decatur, Jr., on deck with pistol, led a force of volunteers, including Boatswain's Mate Reuben James, arm in sling, center, into Tripoli harbor on the night of February 16, 1804, on a successful raid to burn the captured USS *Philadelphia*, to deny her to the Barbary Pirates. Reuben James took a sword blow from a pirate, saving his commander's life. He recovered from his wounds and continued in service with Decatur. *Engraving after Alonzo Chappel from the National Archives.*

top right
Dr. William Maxwell Wood, Fleet Surgeon of the Pacific Squadron under Commodore John D. Sloat. Wood's daring 1846 reconnaissance into Mexico City alerted Sloat that Mexico and the United States were at war. Sloat immediately claimed California for the United States of America. Wood's distinguished career, including the Civil War, culminated in appointment as the Navy's first Surgeon General in 1871. *U.S. Navy Bureau of Medicine and Surgery.*

captain. He forwarded accounts of medical supplies received and consumed to the accountant of the Navy at the end of each cruise.

Although the early Navy medical community was small, there were many giants who cleared a path to the organization we know today. Surgeon Edward Cutbush, a former doctor in the Pennsylvania militia, authored *Observations on the Means of Preserving the Health of Soldiers and Sailors*. Dr. Cutbush proposed methods of cleaning, disinfecting, ventilating, and drying ships. He advocated strict physical examinations of all men coming aboard in order to eliminate disease. He also urged all men to wear their hair short, to shave regularly, and to wash their clothing and bodies.

Surgeon William Paul Crillon Barton, the son of the designer of the Great Seal of the United States and nephew of a prominent American botanist, advocated that Navy ships be better equipped for the care of the sick and wounded. He also proposed a system of organizing Marine hospitals and adopting better physical standards in recruiting. Dr. Barton traced sick days compiled by the Navy to the practice of accepting mentally and physically unfit sailors for duty. He experimented with lime juice and lemonade aboard ships years before the Navy accepted the importance of antiscorbutic treatment for the dreaded vitamin C deficiency. Dr. Barton was also one of the first to propose that female nurses "be included among Navy personnel."

Surgeon Lewis Heermann, who served under Lieutenant Stephen Decatur in the war with Tripoli, would later establish a naval hospital in the bustling port of New Orleans at his own expense. Andrew Jackson's troops would use this hospital when they repelled a British invasion of New Orleans in 1815. A well-traveled and educated man, Heermann's organization of the short-lived hospital would serve as a model for future naval hospitals.

Surgeon Thomas Harris established what can be considered the first Navy medical school in 1822. This school instructed newly commissioned Navy medical officers on naval hygiene, military surgery, and naval customs.

It could be argued that the Navy Medical Department, or, more accurately, the doctors who made up the Navy medical community, was on an unequal footing with the rest of the Navy. For one, the Navy physician's salary was a great source of dissatisfaction. Drs. Barton, Cutbush, and Heermann protested against the paltry remunerations, stating that their pay should be at least equal to their counterparts in the U.S. Army, let alone the physicians in the British Navy.

Rank proved to be another concern. Navy medical men were simply surgeons, or surgeon's mates, and did not have relative rank with naval officers. The Act of May 24, 1828, for the "Better Organization of the Medical Department of the Navy" marked the first time that the status of personnel in the Navy Medical Department received serious attention. In this act, the designation for surgeon's mates was superseded by "assistant surgeon."

The same act created the title of "Surgeon of the Fleet," which authorized the president to designate and appoint to every fleet or squadron an "experienced and intelligent surgeon, then in the naval service." The Fleet Surgeon was to serve in the flagship and be generally responsible for all medical matters within the fleet or squadron in which he served.

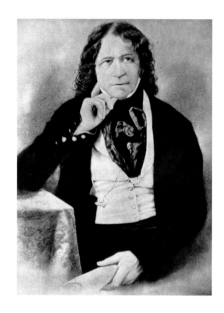

Dr. William Paul Crillon Barton entered U.S. Navy service in 1809 as surgeon aboard the frigate USS *United States*. His studies on diseases during cruises in tropical waters led to his 1830 book, *Hints for Medical Officers Cruising in the West Indies*. He became the first chief of the Navy Bureau of Medicine and Surgery when it was established in 1842. *U.S. Navy Bureau of Medicine and Surgery.*

In the Act of March 3, 1835, Congress first began to consider surgeons and assistant surgeons as officers when these positions were finally subject to the same pay scale as Navy line officers. The General Order of August 1846 finally conferred relative rank to doctors serving in the Navy. The order provided "Commanding and executive officers, of whatever grade, when on duty, will take precedence over all medical officers. This order confers no authority to exercise military command, and no additional right to quarters." By this general order, surgeons of the fleet and surgeons with more than 12 years' service were to have equivalent rank of commanders.

BUMED'S BEGINNINGS, 1842-60
Rank and pay aside, Navy medicine was not without its problems of organization. On August 31, 1842, Congress passed a Navy appropriations bill that was a blueprint for efficiency. The legislation provided for five bureaus to replace the outdated Board of Navy Commissioners—Yards and Docks; Construction, Equipment, and Repair; Provisions and Clothing; Ordnance and Hydrography; and Medicine and Surgery. A chief, appointed by the president, headed each bureau. William P.C. Barton became the first chief of the Bureau of Medicine and Surgery (BUMED).

BUMED became the central administrative headquarters for the Navy Medical Department, and those names became interchangeable. The General Order of November 26, 1842, which defined the duties of the new bureaus, charged BUMED with:

- All medicines and medical stores of every description, used in the treatment of the sick, the diseased, and the wounded;
- All boxes, vials, and other vessels containing the same;
- All clothing, beds, and bedding for the sick;
- All surgical instruments of every kind;
- The management of hospitals, so far as the patients therein are concerned;
- All appliances of every sort, used in surgical and medical practice;
- All contracts, accounts, and returns, relating to these and such other subjects as shall hereafter be assigned to this bureau.

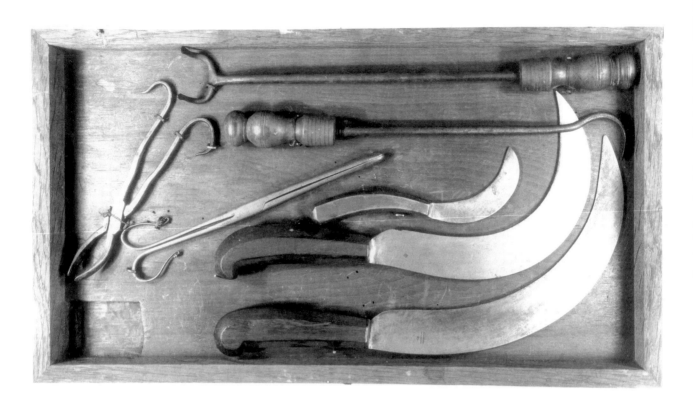

Surgeon's field case, American Revolution. Kits for both Army and Navy surgeons were similar and simple. Amputation was the treatment of choice for wounds to the extremities. *National Museum of Health and Medicine.*

BUMED's establishment contributed much to the development and efficiency of the Medical Department. Quantities and qualities of medical supplies and equipment improved. The year 1853 saw the construction of the naval hospital at Annapolis, Maryland, and the establishment of the Naval Laboratory in Brooklyn, New York. The lab, headed by Surgeon B.F. Bache and Passed Assistant Surgeon E.R. Squibb, experimented with chloroform and ether anesthesia. Squibb's major contribution was providing the Navy Medical Department with a reliable source of pure pharmaceuticals. In 1857, Dr. Squibb resigned from the Navy and founded the pharmaceutical house that bears his name.

What kind of medicine did Navy surgeons practice in the mid-19th century and how was it different from the practice of their Army colleagues? The instruments of civilian manufacture were similar. The surgical kit of an Army physician was almost identical to that of a Navy physician. A surgical scalpel was a surgical scalpel, a tourniquet a tourniquet, the treatment of choice for a shattered limb—amputation. After all, many Army and Navy surgeons attended the same medical schools.

The difference lay in the venue in which the naval surgeon practiced. The marine environment was decidedly different from the battlefield. Hazards unique to the marine theater ranged from dangers incident to storms or heavy weather at sea, falls from mast tops, spills down hatchways and ladders, and being caught between boats and gangways on ships and docks, among many others. The term "loose cannon" had an original and more deadly meaning. Sailors fell overboard and either drowned or died of hypothermia. Fire caused by spilled kerosene lamps below decks was a constant and sometimes fatal hazard. Contagious respiratory diseases ran through close-packed living spaces, leaving entire crews incapacitated.

By the eve of the Civil War, Navy medicine already had one foot firmly placed in the new age of steam. The technologies of ironclad ships and rifled guns would soon add a very new dimension to treating the sick and wounded.

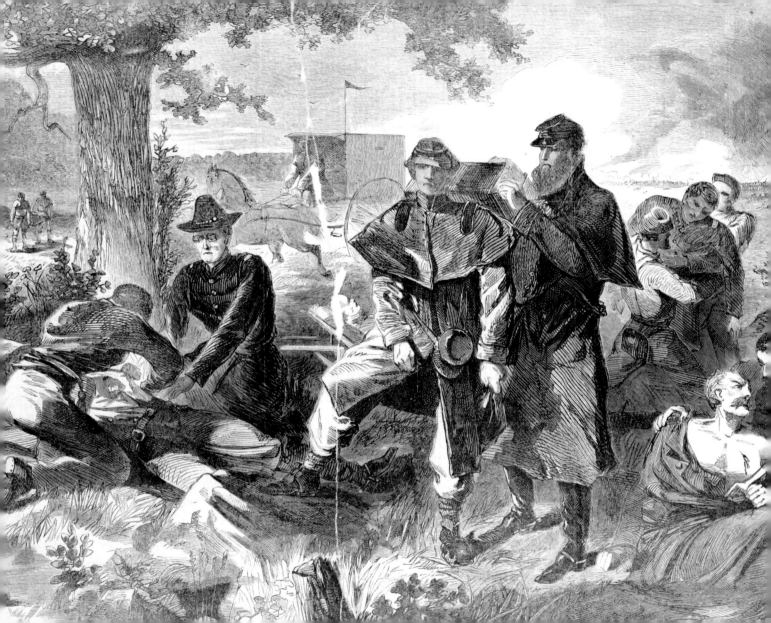

Chapter 2
Civil War, 1861-65

left
Surgeon of Army of the Potomac at work treating wounded soldiers during an engagement. The regimental surgeon of 1862 was responsible for care and evacuation of casualties, assisted only by a hospital steward and perhaps 20 to 30 untrained men. Drawing by Winslow Homer. *Library of Congress.*

ARMY MEDICINE UNREADY FOR WAR

MEDICAL DEPARTMENT LEADERSHIP AND COMPOSITION

The U.S. Army Medical Department entered the Civil War ill-prepared, disorganized, poorly supplied, and ineptly led by senior medical officers marked by their dogmatism, penny-pinching, and resistance to change. The appointment of 64-year-old Colonel Clement A. Finley, a man described as "utterly ossified and useless," as Surgeon General in May 1861 only confirmed that assessment.

Compounding the problem, the U.S. Congress provided insufficient funds for expanding and equipping the Medical Department. Concerned citizens established the U.S. Sanitary Commission in June 1861 to counteract what they saw as a disinterested Medical Department and to bring pressure for change on an uncaring Congress.

The Regular Army Medical Department began the war with 87 medical officers after 27 left to join the Confederacy. Another 92 regulars were added during the war, bringing the total to 179. These regulars formed the backbone of the Union Army's Medical Department and became its future leaders. Around them 547 surgeons and assistant surgeons from the new state and U.S. Volunteer units formed to share leadership and administrative duties. They became the medical directors of the armies, corps, divisions, and geographic departments for a Union Army that grew to 657,000 men by 1865; the medical inspectors who scrutinized the quality of care in the camps and hospitals; and the medical purveyors who provided the medicines and medical supplies.

Regimental surgeons and assistant surgeons were the first line of medical support in the Regular Army and the volunteer units. Working in regimental hospitals with enlisted hospital stewards, they were responsible for the health and medical care of the regiment's 1,000 men. During the war, a total of 2,109 surgeons and 3,882 assistant surgeons of volunteer units served at the regimental level.

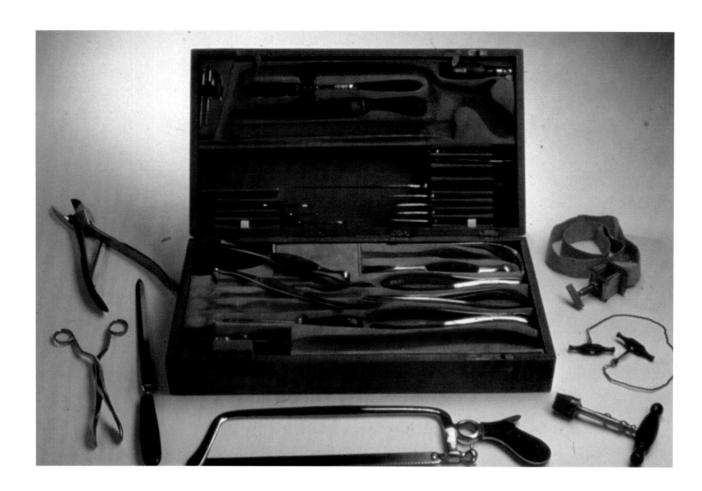

THE INITIAL CLASH: BULL RUN

The first major combat for the Union Army and its Medical Department came against Confederate forces in the Battle of Bull Run near Manassas, Virginia, on July 21, 1861. Surgeon William S. King had arrived from New Mexico to be General Irwin McDowell's medical director only days before the battle and had no time to correct the shortcomings he found: nonexistent evacuation and hospitalization plans, too few ambulances, no trained ambulance attendants, and no medical control over the volunteer unit surgeons or the ambulances.

The Union Army's medical support at Bull Run was a disaster. Evacuation was chaotic at best. Bandsmen assigned to stretcher duty deserted, and infantrymen fled battle under the guise of transporting the injured to the rear. Many wounded were left on the battlefield for days and weeks afterward.

The pathetic medical support witnessed at Bull Run hardly improved in subsequent operations. The continuing poor medical care and Finley's lack of leadership drove the Sanitary Commission to push even harder for reform. Using its political influence with the Congress and President Abraham Lincoln, in April 1862 the commission finally convinced the president and Secretary of War to reorganize the Medical Department and select a new Surgeon General.

top left
Surgical kit, circa 1864, made by Tieman and Co. The instruments are more numerous than those found in the Revolutionary War kit, but still serve mainly for amputations. *Photograph by Norman Watkins. National Museum of Health and Medicine.*

bottom right
Field hospital located in a clearing within the trees in Savage Station, Virginia, after the fighting of June 27, 1862, during the Seven Days Battle. When Union General George B. McClellan withdrew his army from the area, Confederate forces took custody of 2,500 Union casualties. *Library of Congress.*

TWO WHO REVOLUTIONIZED AMERICAN MILITARY MEDICINE

In April 1862, William A. Hammond was a first lieutenant serving as medical inspector of camps and hospitals in the Department of Western Virginia. The previous year Hammond's excellent work at hospitals in Hagerstown, Frederick, and Baltimore, Maryland, had established him as a dominating figure in an Army largely consisting of medical midgets and had drawn the positive attention of the Sanitary Commission's leaders. Finley had transferred the young officer to the remote assignment to reduce his visibility with the commission.

On April 25, 1862, Hammond was plucked from exile, promoted to brigadier general, and became the Army's Surgeon General. His meteoric promotion gained him many opponents and few supporters within the senior leadership of the Medical Department.

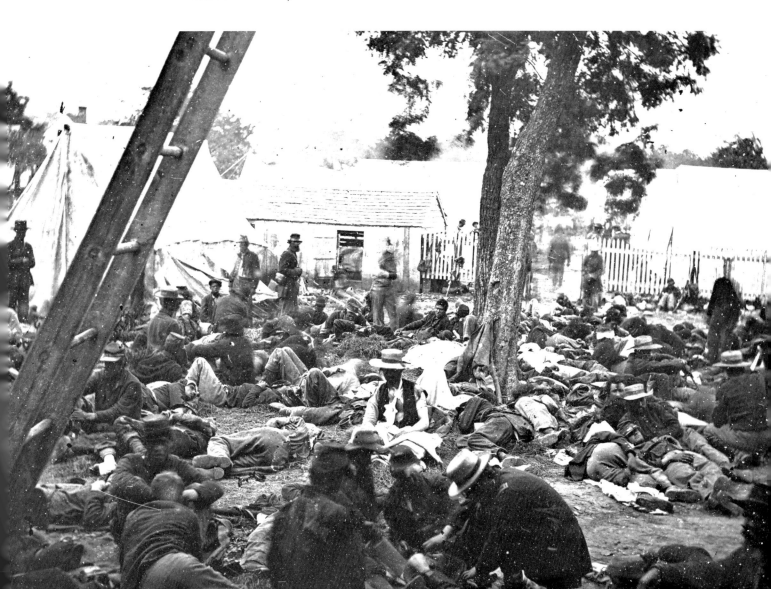

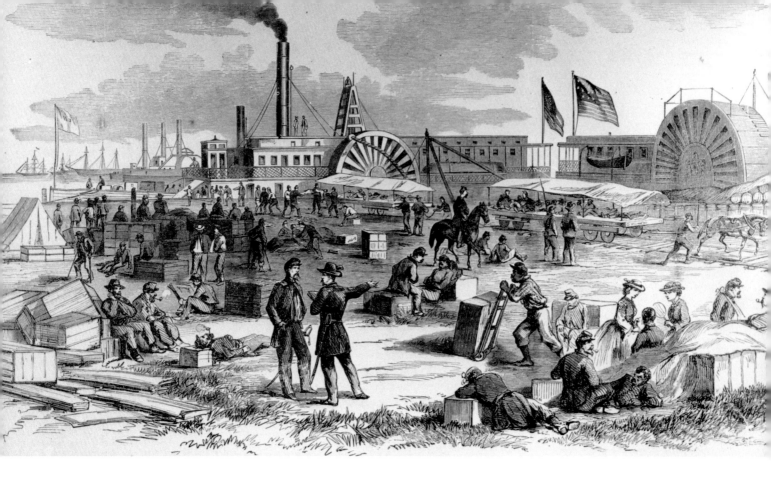

The 33-year-old Hammond set about reforming and revolutionizing the Medical Department. He remade the existing systems of field medicine, medical supply, military hospitals, selection and assignment of medical personnel, and the command and control of medical services. Dumping existing practices, Hammond selected medical directors for the field armies based on their competence rather than via the old boy network that stressed rank and connections.

To execute his programs, Hammond brought in medical officers who shared his reforming zeal. While in Western Virginia, he had worked with Jonathan A. Letterman, the department's medical director. Knowledgeable of Letterman's competence and capabilities, Hammond ordered him to Washington in May 1862 to serve as a medical inspector.

Hammond soon found a new task for Letterman. Medical support was inadequate for the Peninsula Campaign, where the Army of the Potomac, led by Major General George B. McClellan, was attempting to force its way to Richmond. Charles S. Tripler, McClellan's medical director, requested reassignment in June. Hammond selected the 37-year-old Letterman for this most crucial field medical post in the entire Union Army, choosing competence over seniority.

Letterman arrived at Harrison's Landing on the James River on June 23, 1862. Within a week, he had surveyed the generally deplorable medical conditions in the Army of the Potomac, met with McClellan, and asked Hammond for enough ambulances and hospital tents to move and care for the sick and wounded. Letterman also changed the rations to add fresh vegetables and bread. He knew that serious vitamin deficiencies in the Army rations harmed the soldiers' health, causing scurvy and other debilitating diseases. He then issued sanitary instructions to locate camps in the open and to observe basic field sanitation.

Hospital, Fortress Monroe, during the Seven Days Battle of June 26 through July 2, 1862. *Engraving from Harpers Weekly via the National Archives.*

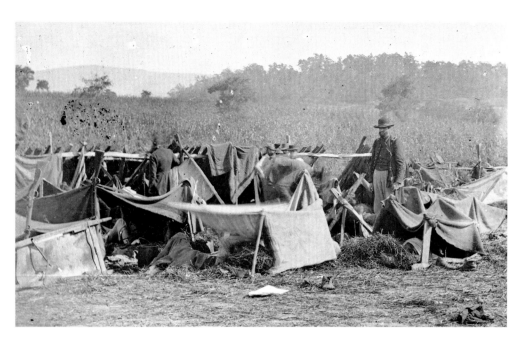

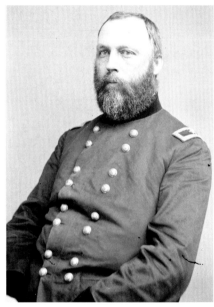

top
Dr. Anson Hurd, 14th Indiana Volunteers, treats Confederate wounded at Smith's Barn near Keedysville, Maryland, after Battle of Antietam, September 18, 1862. *Library of Congress.*

bottom
Brigadier General William A. Hammond, Surgeon General, Union Army. He led reform and innovation in the Medical Department during the Civil War. He faced stiff opposition and clashed with Secretary of War Edwin Stanton. *Library of Congress.*

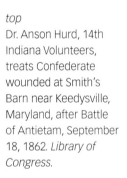

While still on the peninsula, Letterman prepared and McClellan approved the Army of the Potomac's Special Order No. 147 of August 2, 1862, that laid the foundations for the organization and operation of ambulances in the Union Army. Letterman placed the ambulances, horses, and equipment under the control of medical officers but commanded by "other officers, appointed for that especial purpose" who could respond quickly to the demands of the surgeons.

Letterman's new system was barely in place when it confronted a major test at the Battle of Antietam, near Sharpsburg, Maryland, on September 17, 1862. Despite some problems, the horrific casualties of that day were cleared within days, not weeks. With 13,000 of the 70,000 Union troops killed, wounded, or missing, field hospitals functioned as well as could be expected.

In four short months, Letterman had begun rebuilding the organization and management of the Union Army's entire field medical system. He established a field hospital structure that would properly care for the sick and wounded and revamped the medical supply system. After the war he wrote: "It will be perceived that the ambulance system, with that of supplies and of field hospitals, were ordered as essential parts of that new organization from which, I earnestly hoped, the wounded and sick would receive more careful attendance and more skilful [sic] treatment." His hope became a reality.

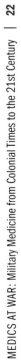
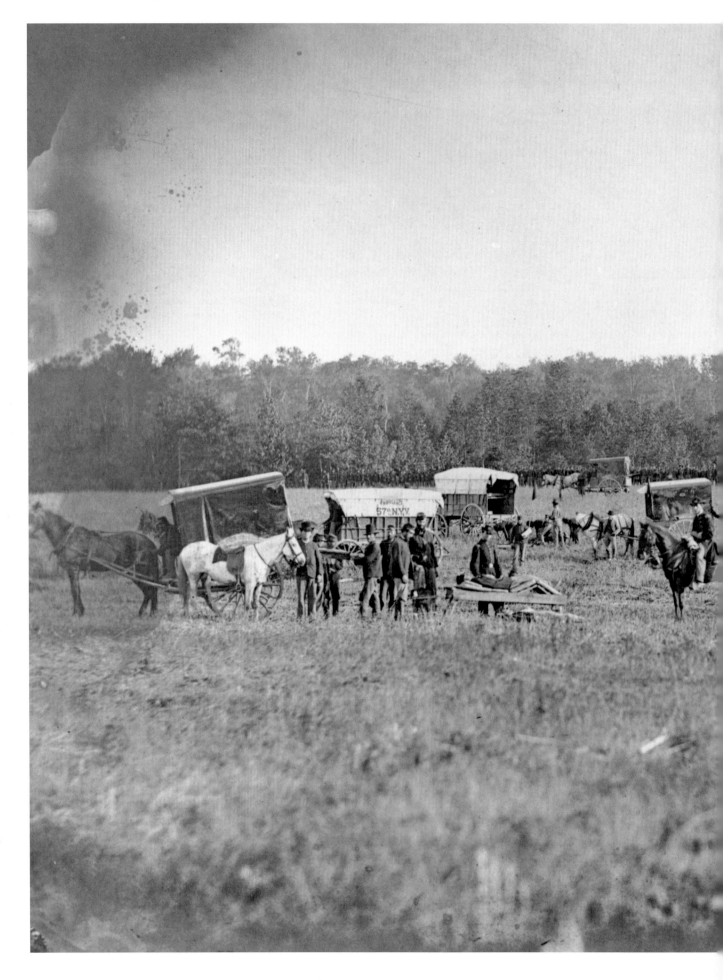

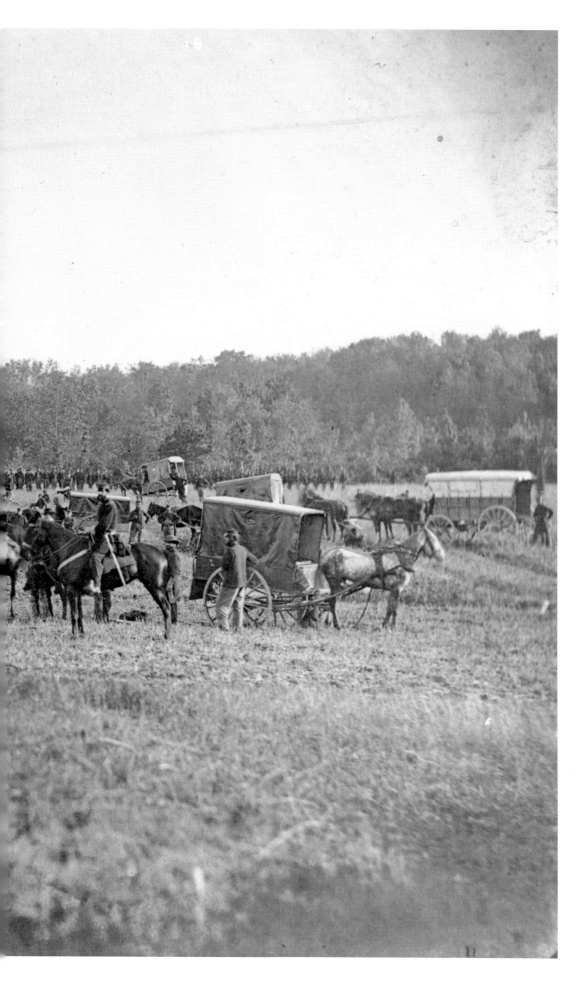

Horse-drawn ambulances at 57th New York Volunteer regimental aid station. Fragile two-wheeled Finley ambulances appear in foreground. The sturdier Tripler ambulance is in the left background. *National Archives.*

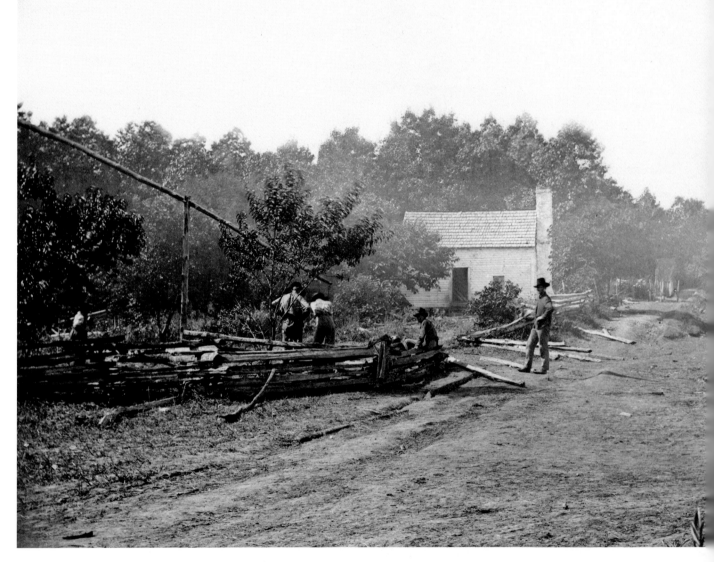

At Fredericksburg, Virginia, on December 13, 1862, each regiment's three ambulances and trained stretcher bearers cleared the awful casualties (12,600 suffered by the Army of the Potomac) of that battlefield by evening. Despite problems arising from restrictions imposed by the Army commanders at Chancellorsville in May 1863 and Gettysburg in July 1863, Letterman's system of ambulance corps and field hospitals showed its growing maturity. Letterman codified his system in the Army of the Potomac's General Order No. 85, "Ambulance Corps and Ambulance Trains," of August 24, 1863. After months of Army inaction, Congress took this general order and modified it into the Act of March 11, 1864, that mandated Letterman's system for the entire Union Army.

A Confederate field hospital near Cedar Mountain, Virginia, August 1862. *Library of Congress.*

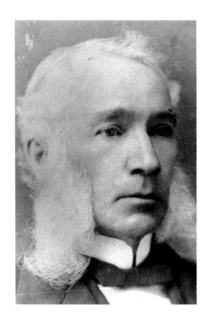

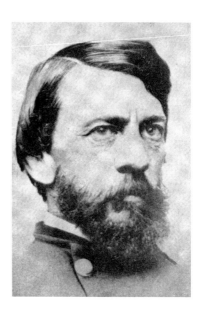

top

Samuel Preston Moore, M.D. A native of South Carolina, he resigned his commission in the U.S. Army to become Surgeon General of the Confederate States Army. He transformed the budding medical corps into an effective department. *Museum of the Confederacy.*

bottom

Dr. Jonathan Letterman, medical director, Army of the Potomac. His pioneering approach to immediate medical care and casualty evacuation revolutionized combat medicine. *Library of Congress.*

BATTLEFIELD CARE AND EVACUATION

Under Letterman's system, each ambulance carried a driver, two men, and two stretchers. Ambulances were organized by regiments, divisions, and corps—under sergeants at the regiment and officers at the corps and division. Personnel were screened, trained, and assigned to the Ambulance Corps, rather than merely detailed. This change relieved surgeons of personally supervising evacuation and allowed them to focus entirely on caring for the soldiers.

Field hospitals played a pivotal role in Letterman's system. These division hospitals were usually set up in field tents within one or two miles of the battlefield and grouped by corps. The three most competent surgeons in the division performed most of the surgery, while other less skilled surgeons tended the wounded and handled administrative duties.

The Ambulance Corps retrieved the wounded from the battlefield and transported them behind the lines to the nearest regimental aid station. Surgeons there controlled bleeding, applied tourniquets, cleaned and bandaged wounds, treated shock, and prepared the injured for transport. The Ambulance Corps then evacuated the wounded to a field hospital. Upon arrival, seriously injured soldiers were quickly evaluated, probed for bullets and bone fragments, and their wounds cleaned. The field hospital surgeons then decided upon their next course of action. Any major operations, mainly amputations or excisions, had to be performed within the first 24 hours to lessen the risk of infection.

By the time that General U.S. Grant launched his 1864–65 Virginia campaign against General Robert E. Lee, the Medical Department was soundly organized to handle large numbers of battle casualties and the sick. From May 5 to June 19, 1864, in an unrelenting campaign of bloody battles, Grant's army suffered the loss of 43,043 wounded. In most cases they were effectively evacuated and hospitalized.

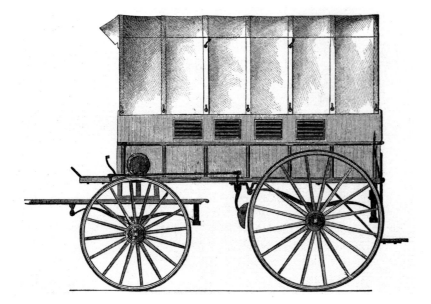

THE GENERAL HOSPITALS

Grant's campaign in Virginia showed how much the Union Army Medical Department had improved since the First Bull Run. Although Grant's forces suffered 52,156 gunshot wounds from March 1864 through April 1865, only 2,011 died of their wounds (3.6 percent). Such a rate was exceptional when compared with overall rates of 10 percent–25 percent for the three years from July 1861 to June 1864.

From 1861 to 1865, the Medical Department made its greatest progress in the organization and management of battlefield care and evacuation. The swift movement of the wounded to a large network of general hospitals in the rear for more complete treatment and recovery was to complete the system of echeloned care.

Before hostilities even began, medical officers questioned the ability of existing post and regimental hospitals to handle the anticipated number of sick and wounded soldiers. Surgeons preferred regimental hospitals so they could keep their men nearby, but many of the wounded were unable to make the journey when these hospitals packed up to follow their units. In response to this need, the old concept of general hospitals was revived early in 1861 in Washington, D.C.

The general hospitals were set up in barracks or unused buildings. Lacking surgeons, the Medical Department turned to "acting staff and assistant surgeons," usually local physicians who agreed to work part-time while maintaining their civilian practices. During the war, 5,607 contract surgeons staffed the Army's general hospitals and, on occasion, augmented field hospitals.

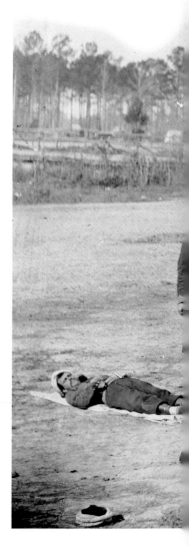

top left
The Rucker Ambulance, designed by Brigadier General Daniel H. Rucker, a Quartermaster officer, became the U.S. Army standard toward the end of the Civil War and for decades thereafter. *Medical and Surgical History of the War of the Rebellion.*

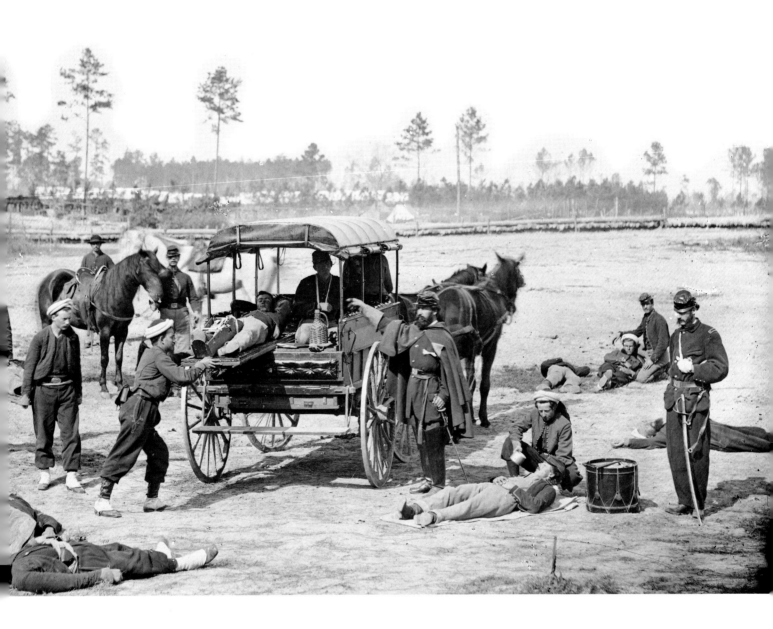

Ambulance drill at headquarters, Army of the Potomac, near Brandy Station, Virginia, March 1864. *Library of Congress.*

Other civilians complemented the hospitals' staffing needs—nurses, sisters of Catholic nursing orders, veterans, cooks, volunteers, attendants. Clara Barton organized the nursing aid and care for the hospitalized soldiers. Despite the Army's initial hesitation, more than 3,000 female nurses worked in the hospitals. Under the direction of Dorothea Dix, head of the Union Army's Women's Nursing Bureau, they made a crucial contribution to the soldiers' care. Without these thousands of dedicated civilians, the general hospitals simply could not have functioned.

The ever-increasing numbers of sick and wounded forced the expansion of the general hospitals far beyond anything ever imagined. With each successive campaign came a new wave of casualties that moved up the chain from the field hospitals to the general hospitals. That flow mandated additional general hospitals farther in the rear areas for those patients displaced to make way for the new arrivals.

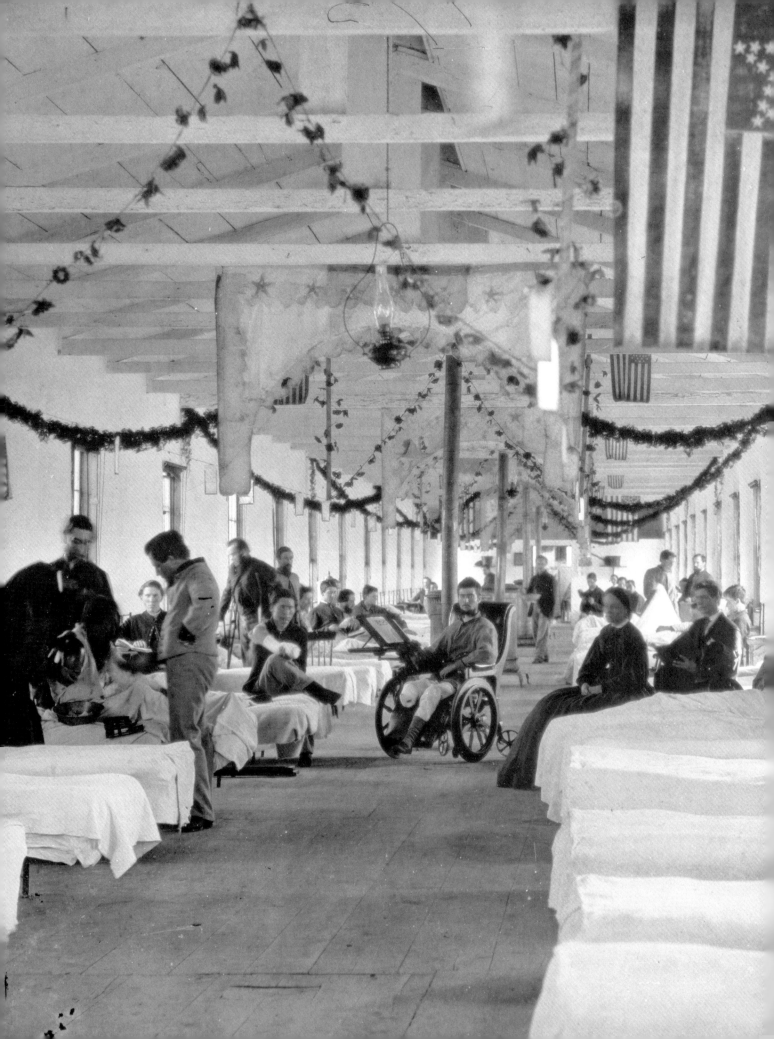

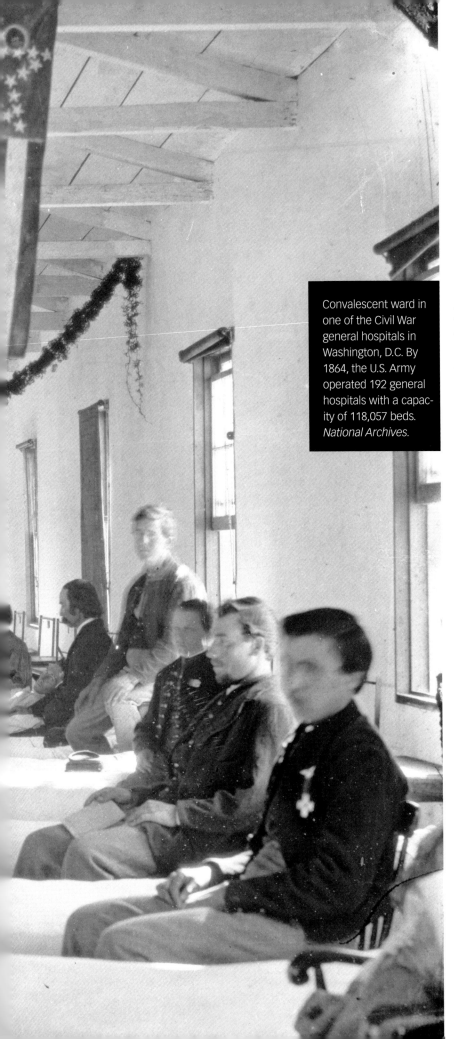

Convalescent ward in one of the Civil War general hospitals in Washington, D.C. By 1864, the U.S. Army operated 192 general hospitals with a capacity of 118,057 beds. *National Archives.*

Another one of Hammond's contributions was a new hospital construction program that replaced older facilities with innovatively designed structures. These new hospitals featured separate, small, well-ventilated, wooden pavilion-style 60-bed wards that were clustered to form a large general hospital. In the Washington, D.C., area, the 2,000-bed Harewood and the 2,575-bed Lincoln typified the breed. The success of these pavilion hospitals during the war influenced civilian hospital design until well after the First World War.

Special hospital trains and ships were soon introduced to move large numbers of patients under medical care from the front to rear area hospitals. River steamers converted to hospital ships plied the Mississippi, Ohio, Tennessee, James, Potomac, Susquehanna, and other rivers while ocean-going hospital ships served along the Gulf and Atlantic coasts. A major issue arose early when local line commanders asserted their control over the general hospitals and hospital ships against the will of the Medical Department and Surgeon General. This very contentious issue was not resolved until December 1864 when the Secretary of War placed the hospitals directly under the Surgeon General—a major change that finally clarified the Medical Department's command of medical facilities.

The administrative requirements for handling the hundreds of thousands of patients flowing into and out of the hospitals were enormous and essential. To account for patients and their treatment, the Medical Department created of an extensive patient administration and records system. These finishing touches linked the entire system of echeloned care from battlefield to general hospital.

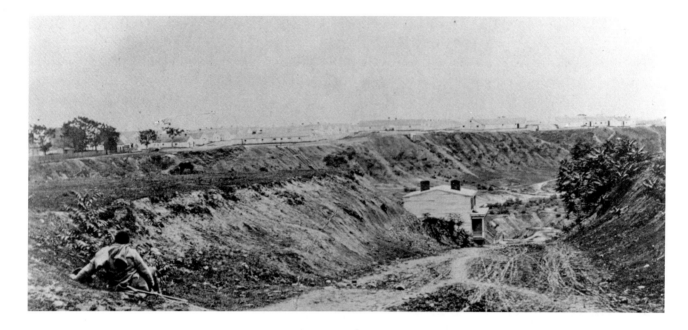

In its totality, the Medical Department's system of battlefield care and evacuation, hospital ships and trains to move the sick and wounded to the rear, and professional medical care in the general hospitals formed the basic chain of evacuation and hospitalization that, with some major modernization, is still in use today. It is this achievement, heavily based on the work of Hammond and Letterman, which underlies most concepts of battlefield care and evacuation that have existed since the Civil War.

WOUNDS AND SURGERY

Civil War surgery was primitive compared with today's standards. Neither aseptic nor antiseptic surgery was known or practiced. Antiseptic agents were used, but not to clean the surgeon's hands and instruments, wounds, or bandages. Surgeons would not learn of the importance of sterilization until 1867 when Lord Joseph Lister published his initial observations on antisepsis.

Gunshot wounds and trauma were extremely dangerous and difficult to treat. The large .58-caliber conoidal, soft lead rifled Minié ball that both sides employed produced nasty wounds and accounted for 76 percent of the wounds in which a causative agent was known. The round or musket ball of former conflicts produced much less damage and accounted for only 12 percent of wounds.

Minié balls flattened on impact, smashing tissue, organs, and bones. Even the most skilled surgeons lacked the knowledge and tools to save shattered limbs or repair massive internal trauma. Conservation, amputation, or excision of portions of limbs were the only techniques available with death rates of 18 percent, 26 percent, and 27 percent, respectively. Union surgeons performed 29,980 such procedures during the war; 6,147 of the upper extremities with a fatality rate of 12 percent and 13,833 of the lower extremities with a fatality rate of 40 percent. Minié ball wounds to the chest and abdomen were usually fatal, with 62 percent of chest wound and 87 percent of abdominal wound recipients dying. Surgeons simply did not know how to treat penetrating gunshot wounds.

Rifle balls and artillery fragments carried particles of dirt, clothing, and skin into the wound, breeding infection. At that time, surgeons knew little of what caused infections, how they spread, or how to cure them. Most of the infections—such as pyemia, a systemic septicemia with a death rate of 97 percent, and streptococcal hospital gangrene, with a death rate of 46 percent—occurred in the general hospitals. Surgeons did what little they could to treat the infections. Carbolic acid, tincture of iodine, and bromide were used with some success, but more on an experimental basis than as proven remedies.

Union surgeons examined and recorded 253,142 wounds during the Civil War. When they performed surgery, they used anesthesia 99 percent of the time. Depending on the circumstances, the anesthesia was chloroform, ether, or a combination of the two with a death rate of less than one percent.

Chimborazo Hospital in Richmond, Virginia, spans the horizon in the photo taken at war's end, April 1865. The hospital's 80 wards (in wooden huts) covered 40 acres and had a capacity of 3,000 beds. *Museum of the Confederacy.*

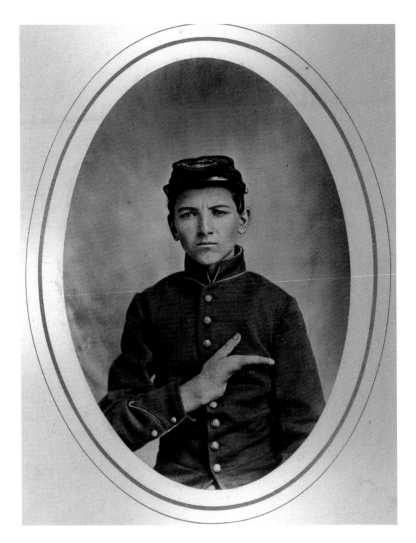

Private Robert Fryer, Company G, 52d New York Volunteers, was wounded at Hatcher's Run, Virginia, February 5–7, 1865. Surgeons amputated the third, fourth, and fifth fingers of his right hand. *National Museum of Health and Medicine.*

DISEASES AND NUTRITION

The rush to fill the volunteer units in 1861–62 often resulted in enlisting men who were physically and mentally unfit for strenuous military duty. Disregarding the tradition of pre-induction physicals, the states rejected few men because of poor health, which caused many problems later. Moreover, many of the men from rural areas had never been exposed to the common childhood and other communicable diseases that urban dwellers often brought. The lack of discipline of new and young soldiers, poor hygiene, and inadequate sanitation in overcrowded camps soon produced epidemics of typhoid fever, diarrhea, dysentery, measles, chicken pox, and mumps.

Diseases disabled large numbers of soldiers for lengthy periods at critical times, which certainly affected the conduct of operations. For example, 208,539 soldiers under the command of Grant during the Virginia campaign of 1864–65 fell ill to disease with 2,235 (1.1 percent) dying. This death rate was astonishingly low when compared to earlier years or even to more modern wars, and indicated the general success of the Medical Department's efforts.

The two most prominent causes of death from disease during the war were typhoid fever, which killed more than 28,000 Union soldiers, and chronic diarrhea, which accounted for more than 29,000 deaths. Medical officers recognized the symptoms of typhoid fever, malaria, dysentery, and diarrhea but they lacked the ability to determine what caused the diseases and were therefore unable to treat them. However, they knew from experience that good field sanitation and hygiene were the best measures for curing dysentery and many other diseases, and that foul drinking water was a possible cause of typhoid.

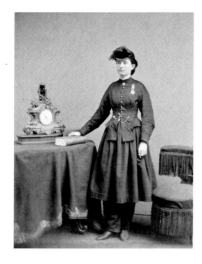

Malaria posed an ever-present threat throughout most areas of the South where the Union Army operated. To reduce the incidence and severity of malaria, Union surgeons gave the soldiers daily prophylactic rations of whiskey laced with quinine. This kept the troops happy and malaria largely under control. Quinine or not, 1,121,919 cases of malaria were reported. Malaria was then a disabler rather than a killer; only 5,217 deaths were reported for a fatality rate of 0.5 percent. The real cost of malaria was in the large number of troops that it rendered ineffective and the size of the medical contingent required to care for them.

Smallpox, the former killer disease, was mostly under control. The vaccination method introduced by Dr. Edward Jenner had been used in the Army since 1812, and once again proved effective in preventing the disease. While only 16,609 cases of smallpox were recorded, smallpox was still a potent killer of the unvaccinated and 6,181 died (37 percent).

Typical Army rations had very poor nutritional value. Fresh fruits and vegetables—rich sources of Vitamins A and C—were critically lacking from the soldiers' diets. The resultant vitamin deficiencies compromised the health of the soldiers and made them vulnerable to more serious diseases such as scurvy, which made its appearance in 1861. Many medical officers, including Letterman, tried to improve the rations to counteract the debilitating effects of vitamin deficiency. This problem, which was never really solved during the Civil War, remained a challenge for years to come.

SUMMARY

The Civil War formed an important chapter in the history of medicine, both in America and the American military. More than 12,000 physicians served in the Union Army as regular and volunteer surgeons or as contract surgeons. The individual and collective experience gained in treating more than 250,000 wounds and 6 million disease cases was significant in the subsequent development of American medicine. Physicians learned by experience and were taught new concepts of medical care and treatment as well as new surgical techniques and principles. They often packed a lifetime of surgical and medical learning into a few short years of wartime service. With the experiences thus gained, many returned to civilian life and eventually reshaped postwar American medical and surgical practice and education.

The list of major medical advances from the Civil War is neither extensive nor revolutionary. While few new surgical advances emerged, extensive experience was gained in use of quinine to control malaria; bromides, carbolic acid, and iodine to combat infections; and anesthetics. Neurological studies undertaken with the war-wounded and amputees produced a wealth of information. Female nurses played a prominent role in the general hospitals. That experience motivated Clara Barton to establish the American Red Cross in 1880, and the Catholic nursing orders to set up hospitals throughout the country. Hygiene and sanitation were once again confirmed as important in preventing diseases and saving lives, even if the reasons remained unknown.

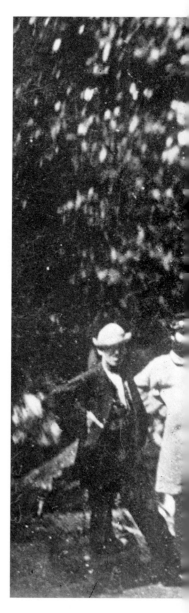

top left
Dr. Mary E. Walker, civilian contract surgeon during the Civil War. She served at the battles of First Bull Run, Chickamauga, and Atlanta, and at hospitals in Washington, D.C. She also was a prisoner of war for four months. For her service, Dr. Walker received the Medal of Honor. *National Archives.*

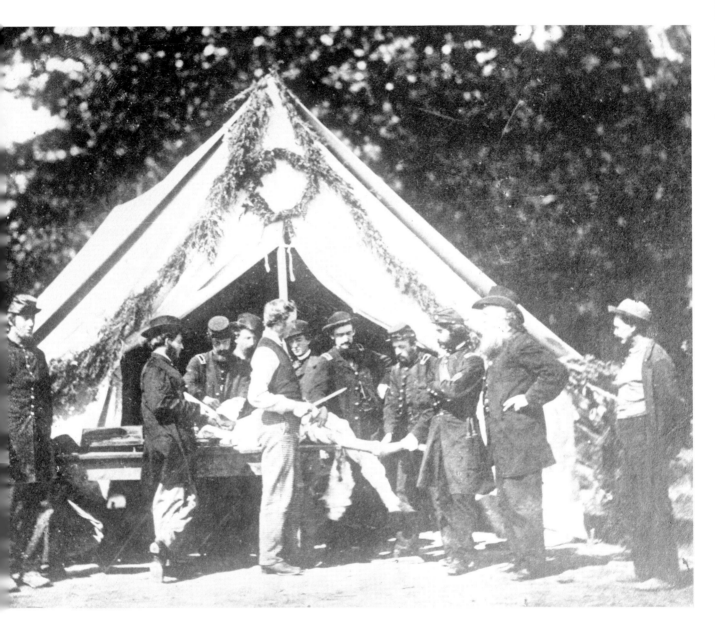

Amputation being performed in a hospital tent, Gettysburg, Pennsylvania, July 1863. Sterile conditions were unknown. Anesthetics were usually ether or chloroform, or a combination of the two. *National Archives.*

The Civil War claimed almost as many American lives on both sides as all other wars combined, but the precise figures remain in dispute. Union losses totaled 364,511, of which 140,414 were battle deaths (including those who died as prisoners of war) and 224,097 were non-battle deaths from disease, injury, and other causes. The number of those who actually died from disease is difficult to determine. The statistical volume of the Surgeon General's monumental six-volume *Medical and Surgical History of the War of the Rebellion* (1875) concluded that the Union Army suffered 186,216 deaths from disease and an additional 24,184 deaths from unknown causes. The Union Army probably lost more than 190,000 men to disease and the Confederates lost about another 165,000, so American losses to disease alone easily topped 355,000.

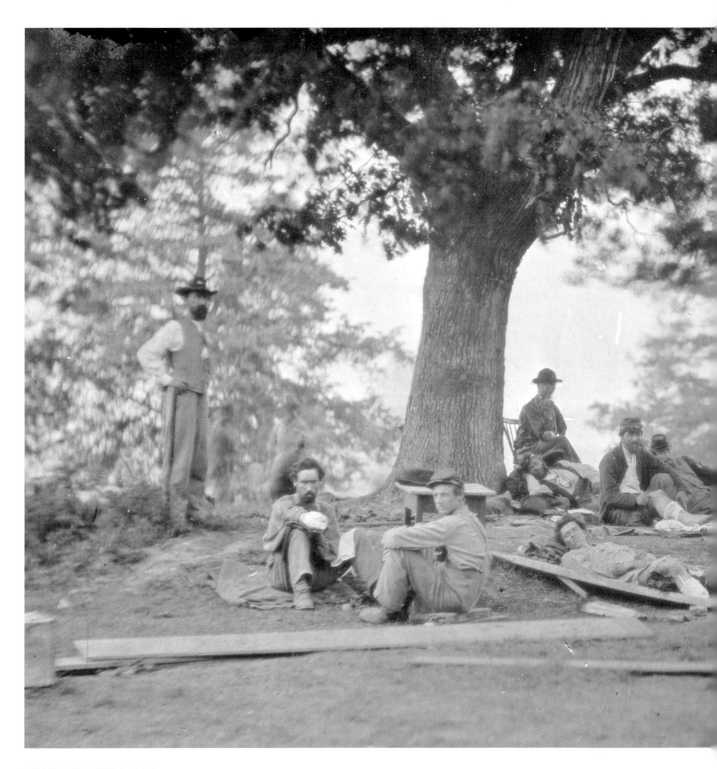

ENDURING LEGACIES

William Hammond and Jonathan Letterman transformed the Army Medical Department during the Civil War into the world's finest military medical organization. They saw what was wrong. They fought against stubborn opposition to carry out the reforms that they thought were required to protect the soldiers' health and to care for the sick and wounded. Their reforms lived on and have saved the lives of countless American soldiers. Many of the concepts which they strove so hard to put into practice continue to guide the Army Medical Department and to serve American soldiers today.

MEDAL OF HONOR RECIPIENTS IN THE CIVIL WAR

Twenty-nine medical officers were killed in action, 10 died of wounds, 35 were wounded

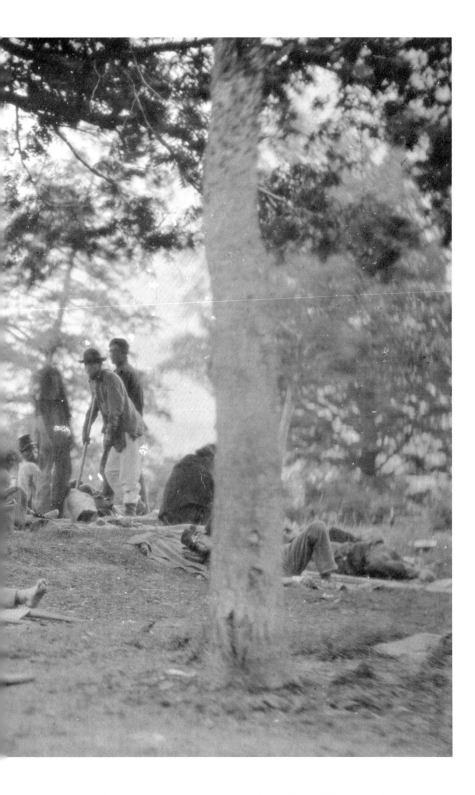

ARMY MEDICAL DEPARTMENT MEDAL OF HONOR RECIPIENTS IN THE CIVIL WAR

WILLIAM R.D. BLACKWOOD

JOSEPH K. CORSON

RICHARD CURRAN

ANDREW DAVIDSON

GABRIEL GRANT

GEORGE E. RANNEY

JACOB F. RAUB

J. (JAMES) HARRY THOMPSON

DR. MARY E. WALKER

Wounded soldiers from the Battle of Spotsylvania, May 8, 1864, under trees at Marye's Heights, Fredericksburg. Regimental surgeons provided immediate medical care in the field. *National Archives.*

in action, and 297 died of disease and other causes, bringing the total to 371 medical officer casualties during the war. In recognition of their heroism and contributions on the battlefield, nine medical officers were subsequently awarded the newly created Medal of Honor. Among them was Dr. Mary E. Walker, a contract surgeon, one of only seven women physicians to serve in some capacity in the Union Army.

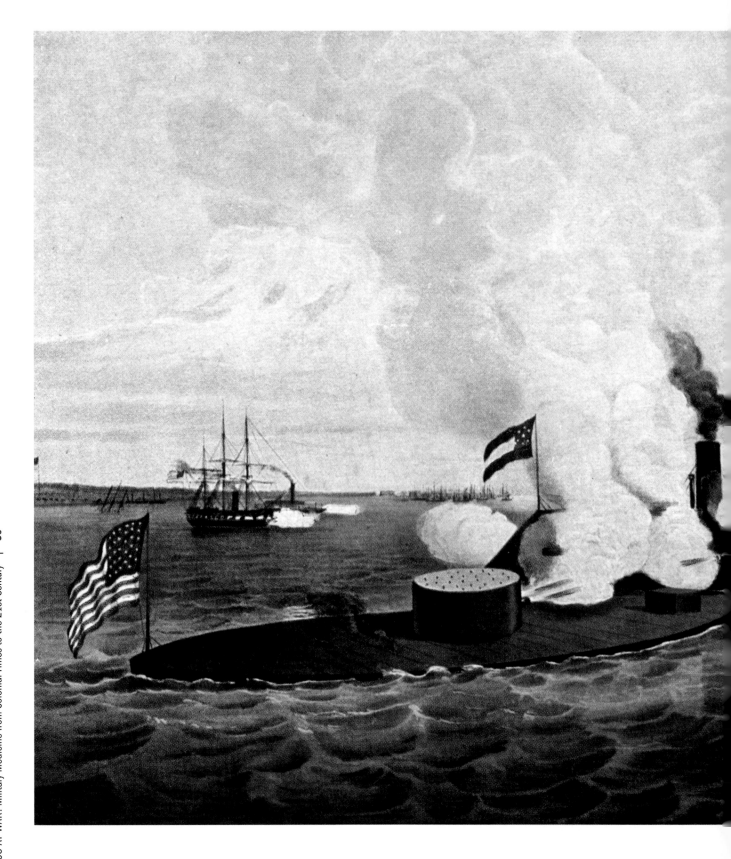

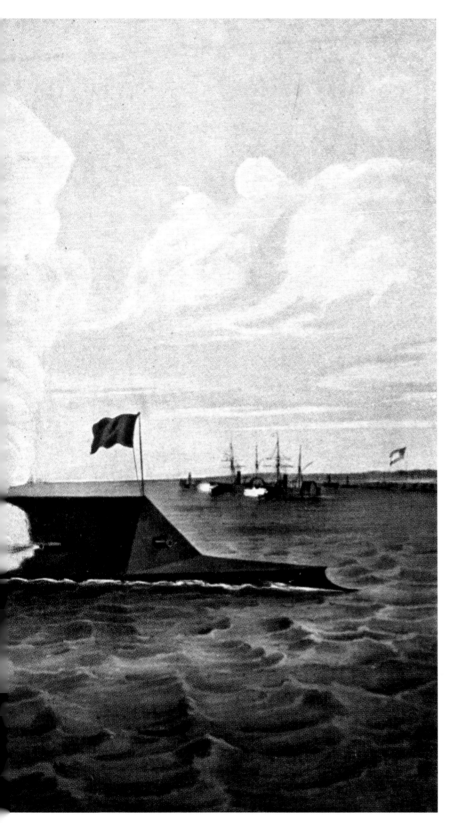

NAVY MEDICINE DURING THE CIVIL WAR, 1861–65

FIRST BATTLE OF IRONCLAD SHIPS

The legendary fight between the ironclads USS *Monitor* and CSS *Virginia* off Hampton Roads, Virginia, on March 9, 1862, transformed naval warfare and naval medicine. U.S. Navy physician Charles Martin described the battle this way:

> David goes out to meet Goliath and every man who can walk to the beach sits down there, spectators of the first ironclad battle in the world. . ... The day is calm, the smoke hangs thick on the water. The low vessels are hidden by the smoke. They are so sure of their invulnerability they fight at arm's length. They fight so near the shore, the flash of their guns is seen and the noise is heard of the heavy shot pounding the armor.

That image of the Yankee cheese box on a raft versus the slope-sided, ungainly ex-*Merrimack* depicted the naval transition from wood and sail to iron and steam. After all, the once U.S. Navy sloop of war, now in Confederate service as CSS *Virginia*, had prevailed over three Union warships the day before. She set the USS *Congress* afire, rammed and sank the USS *Cumberland*, and ran the USS *Minnesota* aground. On March 9 she headed out to finish off the grounded *Minnesota*. But the *Monitor*, her low-freeboard decks nearly awash, popped into view and saved the day, fighting the *Virginia* to a draw.

"The First Fight between Iron Ships of War." The battle between USS *Monitor* and CSS *Virginia* (ex-USS *Merrimack*) on March 9, 1862, off Hampton Roads, Virginia. Newport News, Virginia, is depicted in the far left distance. *Currier and Ives lithograph courtesy Naval Historical Center.*

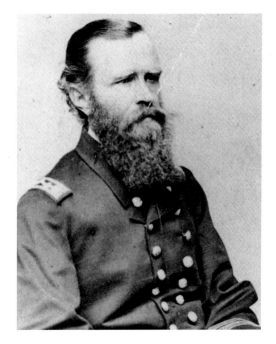

What was the medical aftermath of that now legendary combat? No fatalities. On the Union side, three men injured on the *Monitor*; the *Virginia* suffered a few wounded. Toward the close of the action, the Confederate ironclad inflicted its last and most significant casualty. A shell from the *Virginia* fired at 10 yards' range smashed into the *Monitor's* pilothouse and exploded. Lieutenant S. Dana Green, the *Monitor's* executive officer, reported that Lieutenant Commander John L. Worden, the *Monitor's* skipper, received the force of the blow, stunning him, filling his eyes with powder, and blinding him. Worden directed Green to take command. Green led Worden to his cabin. Dr. Logue examined Worden's eyes, removing tiny scales of iron and a small quantity of paint, and then made cold applications to them.

Worden left the ship for hospitalization in Washington after the battle. The other two patients returned to duty the following day. Worden was the only serious casualty of the battle, losing the sight in one eye and incurring a disfiguring facial scar.

NEW TECHNOLOGIES, NEW HAZARDS

Although this first great combat between the ironclads ended in a draw, war at sea had changed forever and with it the practice of naval medicine. The advent of the ironclad ship made the naval environment different from the Civil War battlefield. Designer John Ericsson's *Monitor* incorporated numerous technical advances, including forced ventilation of living spaces, a protected anchor which could be raised and lowered without it or the crew being exposed to enemy fire, and a protected pilothouse.

The new technologies of iron and steam introduced brand-new hazards—exploding boilers, scalding steam, burn injuries, and primary and secondary wounds resulting from large caliber, rifled naval guns. Ironclad vessels also introduced environmental and occupational concerns for sailors aggravated by badly ventilated and hell-hot engine rooms. It is estimated that a typical low ranking coal heaver aboard a poorly ventilated ironclad routinely endured temperatures approaching 130 degrees Fahrenheit. Aboard the *Monitor* in summer, temperatures of 125 degrees were recorded on the berth deck and 150 degrees in the galley.

Ironclad crews endured other new hazards. With negligible freeboard, many ironclads of both navies were literally only inches from disaster. One day out of New York en route to Hampton Roads where she would fight the USS *Virginia*, the *Monitor* encountered a storm. Heavy seas cascaded over her deck, washing out turret caulking, flooding her berth deck, disabling her blowers, and nearly extinguishing her boiler fires. Her crew fought for survival against steam, gas, and smoke that engulfed the between decks area. That nightmare played out again at the end of 1862 off Cape Hatteras. *Monitor's* pumps failed to stem the incoming seas, and the ironclad pioneer plunged to the sea bottom, with the loss of several crewmen.

John L. Worden, USN, commanding officer of USS *Monitor* during the battle of March 9, 1862. He was one of three *Monitor* crew members wounded in the battle. Photograph probably taken soon after his July 16, 1862, promotion to the rank of commander. *Naval Historical Center.*

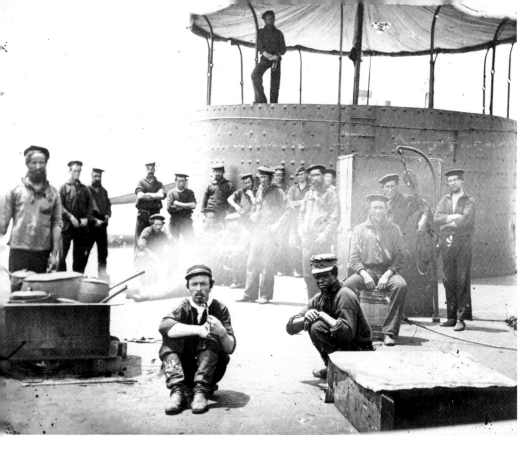

Aboard USS *Monitor*, on the James River, Virginia, crew members cook on deck, July 9, 1862. The view is forward from the port quarter. Note cook stove supported on bricks at left and awning above the turret. *Naval Historical Center.*

Coal, the fuel that fired an ironclad's boilers, was also a threat. Coal had the potential of becoming a silent killer. Civil War engineers did not yet understand that fossil fuels require proper ventilation. Wet, unventilated coal produces high levels of the dangerous gas carbon monoxide. Casualties occurred when crewmen either loaded wet bituminous coal in below-deck bunkers or bilge water contaminated the coal. Sailors were discovered either dead or unconscious below deck. The more fortunate revived when exposed to the fresh air.

DIFFERENT WOUNDS TO TREAT

Many differences existed between wounds sustained in battle on the old wooden ships and those encountered aboard ironclads. Shots striking wooden vessels tended to throw splinters which, as secondary projectiles, caused many of the wounds. Burns were uncommon.

In yardarm engagements and during the hand-to-hand fighting resulting from boarding an enemy's vessel, many wounds were caused by small arms, cutlasses, bayonets, and pikes. In ironclad fighting, splinters might be fewer, but burns and fragment wounds became commonplace. The so-called protected environment an ironclad warship provided was illusory. If anything, it presented fatal hazards the crew of a wooden ship rarely experienced. Take the example of the monitor USS *Nahant*. Engaged in Samuel DuPont's attack on the Charleston forts in April 1863, shellfire from the forts slammed against her pilothouse and turret with such velocity that broken bolts ricocheted about like bullets, killing one man and injuring two others, including her captain.

Iron cannons now shot rounds weighing more than 150 pounds, making the 24- and 32-pound size thrown by earlier guns seem quite puny in comparison. Moreover, a newer generation of rifled guns that could pulverize masonry forts inflicted worse damage to those enclosed within an iron-sheathed hull. The "the garbage can effect" was the result. With blood dripping from nose and ears, crewmen were sometimes driven mad under the barrage of both rifled and unrifled artillery impacting against iron armor. And if not driven mad, many sailors had their eardrums ruptured or, at the very least, suffered temporary or permanent deafness. Civil War sailors frequently described ringing in the ears or tinnitus. Noise levels aboard Civil War ironclads routinely exceeded 130 decibels, surely causing hearing damage among these warriors.

As similar as the practice of medicine may have been for both Army and Navy physicians—certainly in the treatment of battle injuries—the marine environment offered some very unique circumstances. Sailors on blockade duty experienced little battle and much boredom. Under these conditions, the psychological health of sailors was often in question. "Give me a discharge and let me go home," a distraught coal heaver begged his skipper after months of duty outside of Charleston. "I am a poor, weak, miserable, nervous, half crazy boy. Everything jarred upon my delicate nerves."

NUTRITION AND SANITATION

Adding to the misery of this dull routine was an unbroken diet of moldy beans, stale biscuits, and sour pork. Commanding officers and medical officers assigned to the James River Flotilla complained of the lack of fresh provisions and vegetables. Following a July 1862 inspection, Fleet Surgeon of the North Atlantic Squadron, Dr. James Wood, recommended that vessels be furnished with fresh provisions twice a week. His inspection report also contained a recommendation for improving the water supply for the vessels. He said that the "turbid and objectionable" river water in use tended to produce diarrhea. He saw no reason for continuing to use impure river water, since steam vessels could condense more pure water than their crews needed.

Sanitary conditions aboard ship were often superior to those ashore, and both navies probably fared better than the armies when it came to the frequency of disease. However, rheumatism and scurvy kept the Navy doctors busy; so did typhoid, dysentery, break bone fever, hemorrhoids, and damage done by knuckles. In the southern climes, insect-borne malaria and yellow fever laid low many a crew. And, regardless of what they had to work with, surgeons aboard the ironclads, and indeed every vessel, had no medicine for the ills of the spirit brought on by the strain of monotony, poor

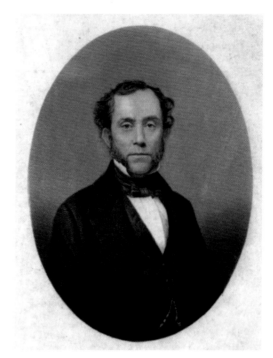

Fleet Surgeon Ninian Pinkney. Dr. Pinkney was responsible for establishing the USS *Red Rover* as the "first naval hospital ship." *U.S. Navy Bureau of Medicine and Surgery.*

food, and unhealthy living conditions which produced much longer casualty lists than did Confederate shells or mines.

HOSPITALS ASHORE AND AFLOAT

Whether victims of disease or hostile action, sailors required treatment and convalescence. Much Navy medicine took place in the three existing hospitals at Chelsea, Massachusetts; Brooklyn, New York; and Philadelphia, Pennsylvania. By the fall of 1862, all three were "filled to their utmost capacity."

Following their recapture by Union forces, two naval hospitals in the South at Portsmouth, Virginia, and Pensacola, Florida, were put back into operation. At least four other new hospitals came on line between 1862 and 1865 at Mound City, Illinois (1862); Memphis, Tennessee (1863); New Orleans, Louisiana (1863); and Port Royal, South Carolina (1864). Located within the theater of operations of the blockading river squadrons, they acted as receiving hospitals, taking patients on a short-term basis.

One of the medical stations capable of long-term care was not stationary at all. In 1862, Union forces captured a Confederate side-wheeler, *Red Rover*. Under the order of Naval Fleet Surgeon Ninian Pinkney, the ship was converted into the Navy's first hospital ship (however, there is evidence that Navy ships used during the Tripolitan Wars were used as floating hospitals). According to a Navy General Order of June 1862, "only those patients

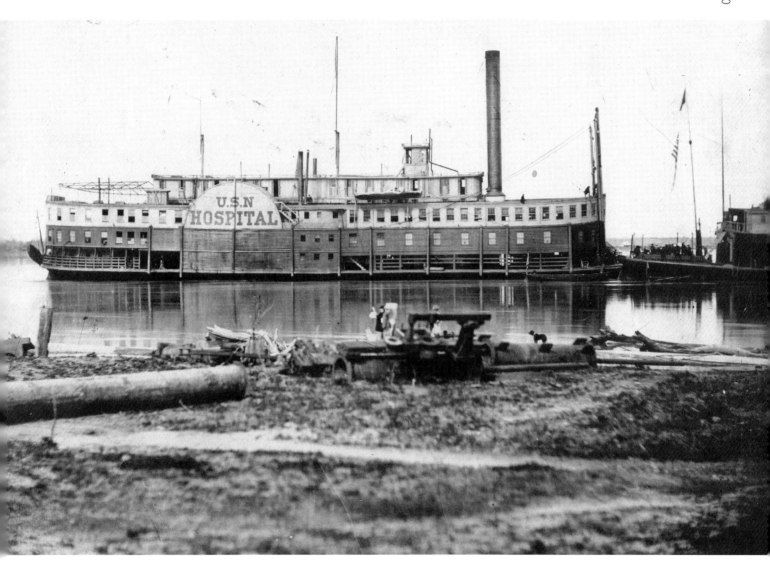

USS *Red Rover,* Navy hospital ship on the western rivers during Civil War. From 1862 until 1865, the medical staff on board the *Red Rover* cared for 2,450 casualties, including 300 wounded Confederates. *Naval Historical Center.*

are to be sent to the hospital boat who it is to be expected to be sick for some time, and whose cases may require more quiet and better attention and accommodation than on board the vessels to which they belong."

It was also the first ship to have a staff of female nurses trained in the medical arts. On Christmas Eve 1862, Sisters of the Order of the Holy Cross of St. Mary's of Notre Dame in South Bend, Indiana, reported aboard the *Red Rover* to care for sick and wounded seamen. One hundred years later the Navy helped to honor these women at a ceremony on the Notre Dame campus as true "pioneers of the Navy Nurse Corps."

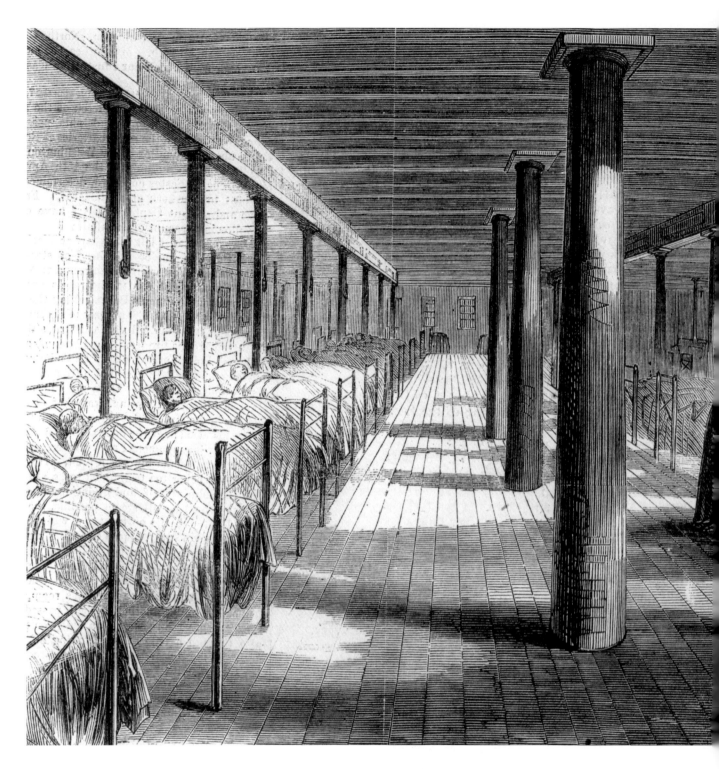

The war took a heavy toll on the Navy Medical Corps, killing 33 surgeons. Assistant Surgeon William Longshaw, Jr., was one of them. Secretary of the Navy Gideon Welles and Rear Admiral John Dahlgren acknowledged Dr. Longshaw's "gallant behavior" for his action on November 15, 1863. Under heavy fire, he volunteered to retrieve the monitor USS *Lehigh*, which had run aground. In January 1865, Dr. Longshaw was killed in an assault on Fort Fisher, North Carolina, while binding the wounds of a dying man. His heroism under fire encapsulates Navy medicine's true Civil War legacy.

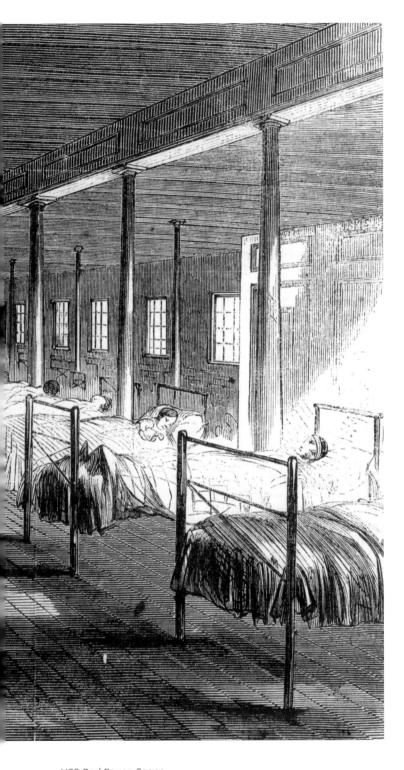

USS *Red Rover*. Scene in the ward. The vessel boasted a laundry; an elevator that could transport the sick from lower to upper decks; and gauze blinds to keep flies, mosquitoes, cinders, and smoke from annoying the patients. *Naval Historical Center.*

NAVY MEDICINE COPES WITH POSTWAR CHANGE

A new United States Navy emerged at war's end in 1865, even though hard-bitten conservatives in Washington had been loath to trade traditional wooden hulls and canvas for an all-iron fleet. By the late 1870s and certainly by the turn of the 20th century that fact was a reality. Medical planners and health care providers would now have to face squarely the realities that Civil War surgeons encountered during their war. The new steel ships now carried rifled, breech-loading artillery. What their muzzle-loading predecessors had inflicted upon human flesh and bone had already been demonstrated.

Traumatic amputations, penetrating fragment wounds, and horrific burns had become commonplace during the Civil War. In the postwar environment, these wounds would increase exponentially as would new kinds of injuries merely hinted at during the Civil War—primary and secondary blast injuries, scalded skin and flesh caused by ruptured steam pipes and boilers, toxic smoke inhalation—the products of fire below decks. The problems first encountered during the war of the ironclads would now have to be dealt with aboard ships of the all-steel, all-steam Navy.

CIVIL WAR SERVICE AND CASUALTIES 1861-65

Total U.S. Service Members (Union)	2,213,363
Battle Deaths (Union)	140,414
Other Deaths in Service (Union)	224,097
Non-Mortal Woundings (Union)	281,881
Total Service Members (Confederate)	1,050,000
Battle Deaths (Confederate)	74,524
Other Deaths in Service (Confederate)	59,297*
Non-Mortal Woundings (Confederate)	Unknown

* Does not include 26,000 to 31,000 who died in Union prisons.

Source: Department of Veterans Affairs from Department of Defense.

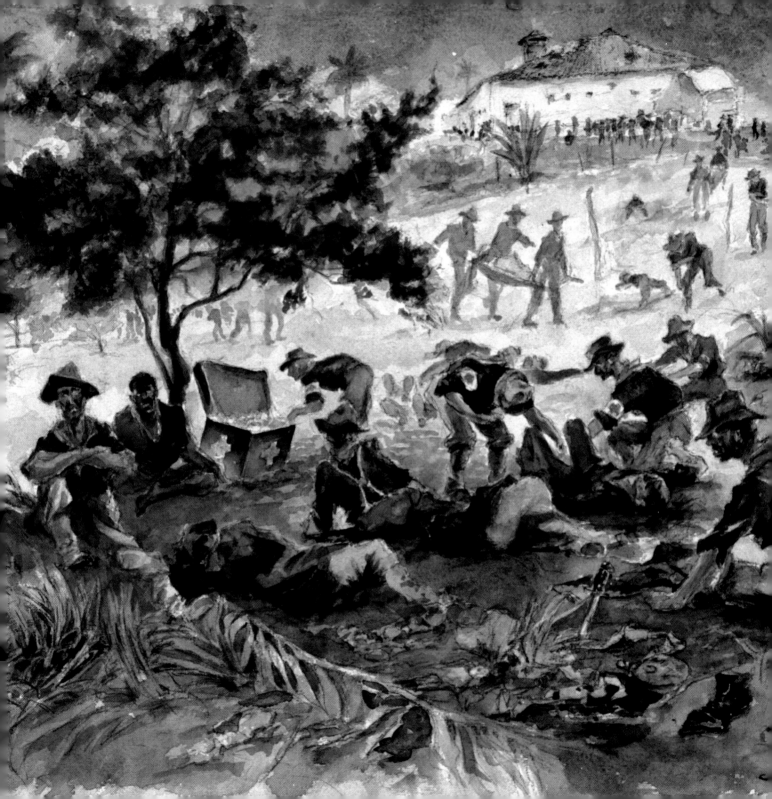

Chapter 3
From Civil War to World War, 1865–1917

left
Field hospital back of the lines, July 1, 1898. A makeshift first aid post set up on the slopes of San Juan Hill below the Block House. *U.S. Army Art Collection.*

right
Bernard J. D. Irwin received the Medal of Honor in 1894 for conspicuous gallantry in action at Apache Pass, Arizona Territory, on February 13–14, 1861. *National Library of Medicine.*

LESSONS FORGOTTEN AND RELEARNED

THE DAY OF SMALL THINGS IN THE U.S. ARMY, 1865-98

Soldiers serving in the tiny postwar Army of the late 19th century described the period as "The Day of Small Things." The Army's medical failings in the war against Spain in 1898 provoked and stimulated dynamic transformations that prepared the Medical Department for bigger things: the enormous challenges of a world war in Europe.

The Union Army shrank swiftly from more than 600,000 soldiers at the end of the Civil War to 54,000 a year later. The superb medical organization perfected during the war disappeared by the end of 1866. The postwar Army did not need the excellent system. However, the Prussian military grasped its importance and employed it successfully in the 1870–71 Franco-Prussian War.

In July 1866, the Army's 216 medical officers and 264 contract surgeons served at posts where they and the hospital stewards formed the soldiers' first and only line of medical support. By 1874, the Army had only 145 medical officers on duty and 187 contract surgeons, less than half the requirements.

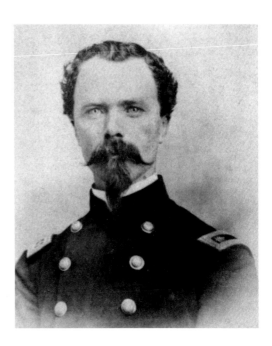

Medical personnel assigned to units campaigning against the Indians cared for soldiers under harsh field conditions, and often shared their fate. Among the six Army medical personnel who received Medals of Honor during the Indian Wars, two stand out. Assistant Surgeon Bernard J.D. Irwin was honored for bravery against Cochise's Apaches on February 13–14, 1861, the first action for which a Medal of Honor was awarded and the earliest in the Indian Wars. He retired in 1894 as a colonel. Assistant Surgeon Leonard Wood earned recognition for gallantry against Geronimo's Apaches in the summer of 1886. Dr. Wood later transferred to the cavalry, commanded the 1st U.S. Volunteer Cavalry ("Rough Riders") in the war with Spain, and became the only Medical Corps officer ever to serve as Chief of Staff of the Army (1910–14).

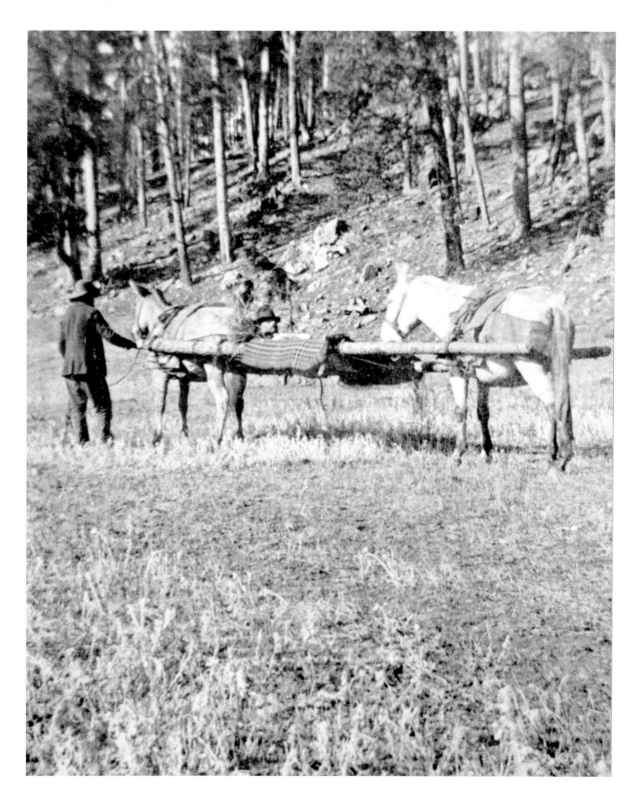

Major milestones marked the latter part of 19th century Army medicine. By the mid-1880s, antiseptic surgical techniques were being practiced throughout the Army. In November 1886, the Army introduced first aid instruction, a significant step in safeguarding soldiers' lives on the battlefield. On January 17, 1887, the Army opened its first permanent general hospital, the Army and Navy General Hospital located in Hot Springs, Arkansas. Another significant development was the establishment of the Hospital Corps and creation of the medical enlisted force on March 1, 1887. Enlisted men and hospital stewards (non-commissioned officers) were now available for a wide range of medical and hospital duties and for peacetime training with medical officers for wartime missions.

left
Two-horse litter carrying a wounded man from the Battle of Slim Buttes along French Creek, Black Hills, Dakota Territory, September 9, 1876. The soldier is covered with a plaid blanket. Tree boughs serve as a headrest. *National Archives.*

right
George Sternberg, Civil War veteran and Army Surgeon General during the Spanish-American War. Author of the first American bacteriology text, he pushed the Army into modern scientific medicine. *National Library of Medicine.*

The Army was concentrated on fewer and larger posts with the waning of the Indian Wars in the early 1890s. Medical officers found more opportunities for research, professional development, and interaction within the Medical Department and the larger American medical community. This professional awakening coincided with the major advances in modern scientific medicine emanating from Europe where Louis Pasteur, Lord Lister, Robert Koch, Rudolf Virchow, and others were discovering pathogenic microorganisms as the source of infection and disease.

George M. Sternberg's selection as Army Surgeon General in 1893 clearly exemplified this new scientific direction. Sternberg was a leader in the new field of bacteriology that was critical to advances in public health, sanitation, and preventive medicine.

Sternberg, in his nine years as Surgeon General (1893–1902), led the Army into modern scientific medicine. Under his guidance, first aid packets were developed to control bleeding and prevent infection on the battlefield. He encouraged research and built post laboratories and modern operating rooms. He started the Army Medical School, first proposed by Hammond in 1862. The school, which opened in Washington, D.C., in late 1893, gave all new Medical Corps officers an introductory course in the Army and military medicine. It also became the Army's research institute in public health and preventive medicine, a role it continues today as the Walter Reed Army Institute of Research.

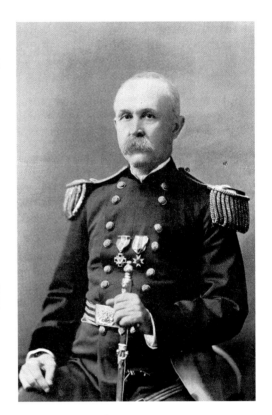

**ARMY MEDICAL DEPARTMENT
MEDAL OF HONOR RECIPIENTS
IN THE INDIAN WARS**

WILLIAM C. BRYAN

OSCAR BURKARD

BERNARD J.D. IRWIN

JOHN O. SKINNER

HENRY R. TILTON

LEONARD WOOD

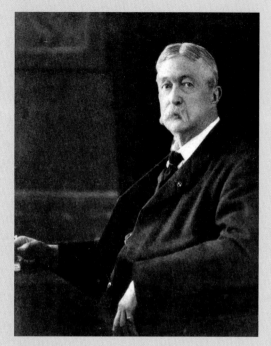

JOHN SHAW BILLINGS

Colonel James M. Phalen, writing for the *Army Medical Bulletin*, subtitled his biographical sketch of John Shaw Billings "A Many-Sided Genius." Billings was probably the most remarkable person ever to serve in the Army Medical Department.

Billings graduated from Miami of Ohio in 1857 and received his medical degree in 1860 from the Medical College of Ohio in Cincinnati. He became a contract surgeon at the outbreak of the Civil War and was commissioned in July 1862. In March 1863, he reported to Jonathan Letterman, Medical Director of the Army of the Potomac. He served as surgeon with the 11th Infantry and later 7th Infantry of Sykes' Division, V Corps (Regulars) and was a field surgeon at Chancellorsville and Gettysburg. From March 1864, he was Medical Inspector with the Army of the Potomac from the Wilderness through the siege of Petersburg. Invalided back to Washington and assigned to the Surgeon General's office, he assumed responsibility for the Library and Medical Museum, his life focus for the next 30 years.

With funds from disbanded Army hospitals, he accumulated medical literature wherever he could find it. Billings built the collection from 1,800 volumes to more than 116,000 volumes and 191,000 other reference works. He directed the cataloguing of every item in the collection, laying the foundation for the *Index Catalogue* of

medical books and the *Index Medicus*, a monthly listing of new library acquisitions. Today, both publications remain essential bibliographical guides to medical literature. The collection that Billings built became the Army Medical Library, the most comprehensive medical library in the world and the core collection of the National Library of Medicine since 1956.

Billings' reports on Army hospitals and hygiene in the 1870s earned him a reputation for hospital design and construction. His design proposals for Johns Hopkins Hospital and organization of its School of Medicine underpinned development of those institutions in the 1870s and 1880s. Billings was also instrumental in selecting the faculty for the School of Medicine, including William Welch, William Halsted, and Sir William Osler, medical and surgical giants who reoriented American medical education and practice.

In charge of vital statistics for the federal censuses in 1880, 1890, and 1900, Billings identified and corrected significant problems with the 1880 census figures and methodology. He recommended development of mechanical and electrical tabulating equipment for the 1890 census and convinced his associate, Dr. Herman Hollerith, to do so. Hollerith created a system based on punch cards and tabulating machines to tabulate and sort the data. Hollerith's Tabulating Machine Company of 1896 evolved into International Business Machines (IBM).

Billings retired from the Army in 1895, and in 1896 became director of the budding New York Public Library. He organized the city's library system and designed the main library building. He convinced his friend Andrew Carnegie to underwrite establishment of neighborhood branches.

This man of enormous talent and energy, truly "A Many-Sided Genius," left an enduring legacy to the Army Medical Department and American medicine.

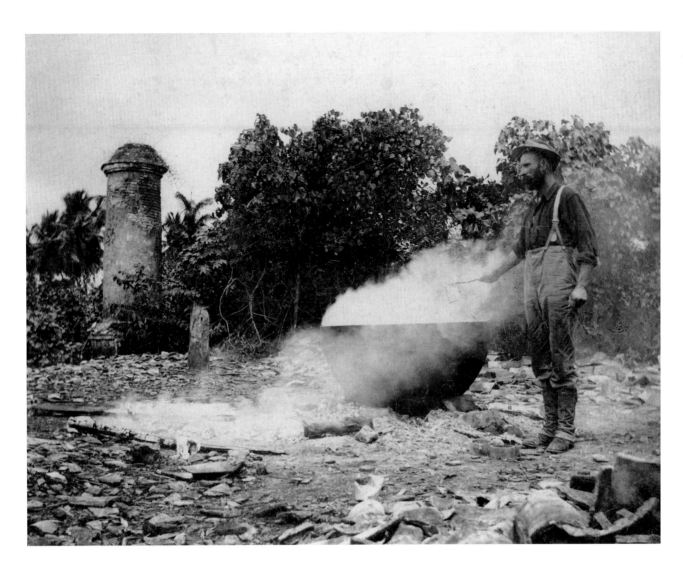

Boiling drinking water for 21st Infantry Regiment near Santiago, Cuba, 1898. Potable water was essential to soldier's health. *National Archives.*

SPANISH-AMERICAN WAR, 1898

The Army and its Medical Department, having failed to maintain the reforms instituted by Hammond and Letterman during the Civil War, was unprepared for the war against Spain in April 1898. It entered battle lacking personnel, medical equipment and supplies, funding, field medical units, and plans.

The Army once again had to rely on state and U.S. Volunteer surgeons to fill corps, division, and brigade posts. Sternberg wanted to put medical support closer to the soldiers by assigning medical troops from the regiment to corps, but the required personnel simply did not exist. In addition, he knew that tropical diseases endemic, and often epidemic, in Cuba, Puerto Rico, and the Philippines posed great threats.

Camp and unit commanders routinely ignored their medical officers' advice about sanitation. As mobilization surged, thousands of undisciplined volunteers crowded into the hastily organized, unsanitary camps at Chickamauga, Georgia; Tampa and Jacksonville, Florida; Falls Church, Virginia; and Middletown, Pennsylvania. Typhoid fever quickly became epidemic.

At the time, medical officers believed that typhoid fever was a water-borne disease. They did not know that it could spread by other means: poor camp sanitation and improper disposal of human wastes, preparation and handling of food by infected soldiers, person-to-person transmission by typhoid carriers, and flies.

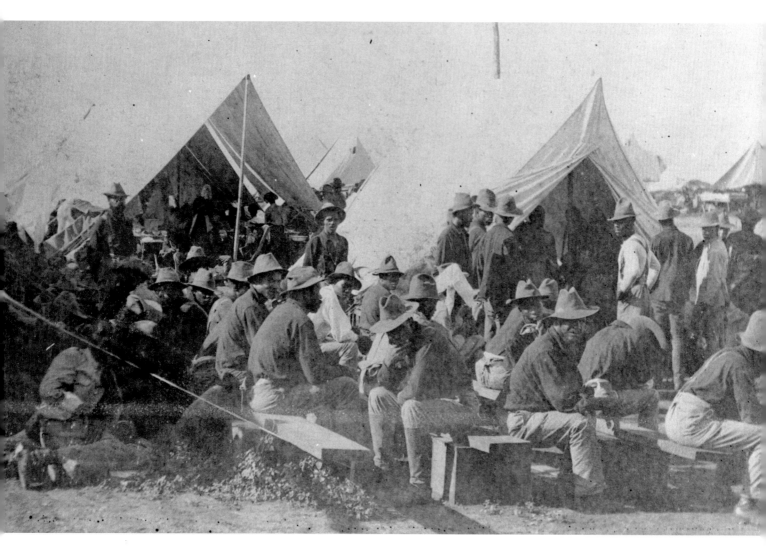

Typhoid stricken soldiers crammed and immobilized regimental and field hospitals. The general hospitals also soon filled. The five main mobilization camps alone accounted for 20,738 cases of typhoid fever and 1,590 deaths, or 86.8 percent of all deaths from disease within them. Of all the disease-related deaths in the Army from May–December 1898, 2,620 out of 4,430 (59.1 percent) were due to typhoid fever.

Under duress and lacking trained Hospital Corps personnel for his hospitals, Sternberg accepted the offer of trained female contract nurses from the Daughters of the American Revolution. Anita Newcomb McGee, M.D., who soon joined Sternberg's staff, directed the program. She changed the Medical Department and military medical care forever. Through July 1, 1899, more than 1,500 female nurses served—working first in the general hospitals and later in field hospitals in the U.S., Cuba, and the Philippines. They also staffed the Army hospital ship, *Relief*. They proved to be dedicated, skilled, efficient, and valuable.

top left
2d Infantry Regiment attending sick call at Siboney, Cuba, 1898. Regimental surgeons encountered more casualties from disease than wounds. *National Archives.*

top right
Army contract nurses aboard U.S. Army Hospital Ship *Relief* (AH-1) in Cuban waters, 1898. Esther Voorhees Hasson, back row, center, became first superintendent of the Navy Nurse Corps, 1908–11. She served in World War I as chief nurse of two Army base hospitals in France. *Naval Historical Center.*

bottom left
U.S. Army Hospital Ship *Relief* (AH-1), converted from a civilian passenger ship for hospital service off Cuba, 1898. The Army transferred her to the U.S. Navy in November 1902. Beginning in 1908, she saw active Navy service as USS *Relief* until 1919. *Naval Historical Center.*

bottom right
A patient ward aboard U.S. Army Hospital Ship *Relief* (AH-1) in Cuban waters, 1898. She also served in the 1899 Philippine campaign. The large skylight at upper right brightens the ward. *Naval Historical Center.*

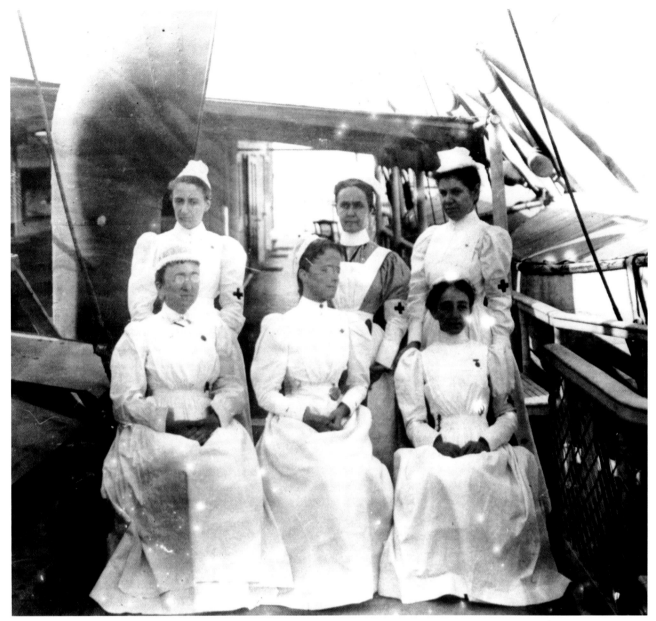

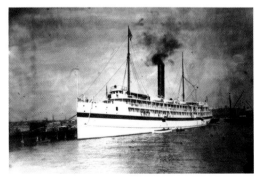

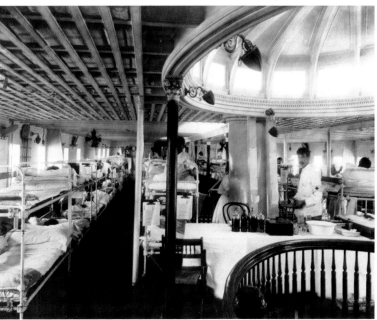

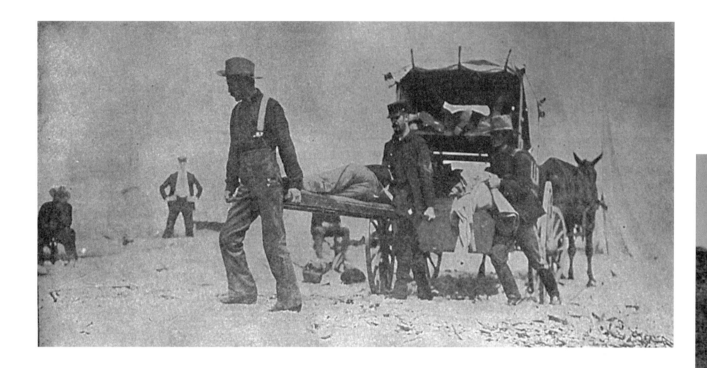

MEDICS IN COMBAT

Enormous medical problems confronted the expeditionary V Corps (Regulars) destined for Santiago, Cuba. Divisional field hospitals had been improvised from the regimental hospitals that arrived at Tampa, Florida, but much of their medical equipment and supplies had to be left. On arrival at Daiquiri, Cuba, on June 22, the landing of the hospitals lagged. Once ashore few wagons were available to move them. Major Louis A. LaGarde and then Lieutenant Merritte W. Ireland, later Chief Surgeon in France (1917–18) and Army Surgeon General (1918–31), set up their base hospital at Siboney.

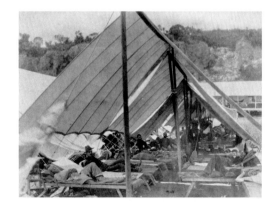

Meanwhile, the field hospitals with the 1st and Cavalry divisions pushed toward Santiago and the Spanish defenders. In a clash at Las Guasimas on June 24, 1898, Assistant Surgeon James Robb Church of Leonard Wood's 1st U.S. Volunteer Cavalry earned the only Medal of Honor awarded to a medical soldier during the war. Three more medical officers received Medals of Honor during the postwar Philippine Insurrection of 1899 to 1902. They would be the last Medical Corps officers to receive the nation's highest award for heroism.

In the short Cuban campaign, medical personnel were up front with troops. Assistant Surgeons Harris, Brewer, Fuller, and Church were active on San Juan and El Caney hills, treating and evacuating the wounded during the fighting on July 1. Without ambulance companies, dressing stations were few and evacuation was poorly organized. Acting Assistant Surgeon H.W. Danforth, 9th Cavalry, was killed on July 2, the only medical officer to be killed by hostile action in the war.

The use of smaller caliber metal-jacketed bullets produced less damaging wounds than the Civil War. The first aid packets proved to be remarkably effective in preventing bleeding and the septic infection of wounds. Surgeons found the new X-ray machines to be of great diagnostic value, but little else was learned surgically because so few men were wounded.

top left
Carrying the wounded: horse-drawn ambulance and litter bearers, Cuba. Evacuation was poorly organized in the campaign. *Wright's Official History of the Spanish-American War, courtesy St. Petersburg Museum of History.*

bottom left
Army field hospital tent at Siboney, Cuba, July 8, 1898. Field hospitals were improvised and primitive. *National Archives.*

right
A U.S. Army surgeon and his assistants attend wounded soldiers in an improvised hillside field hospital in Cuba, 1898. *Library of Congress.*

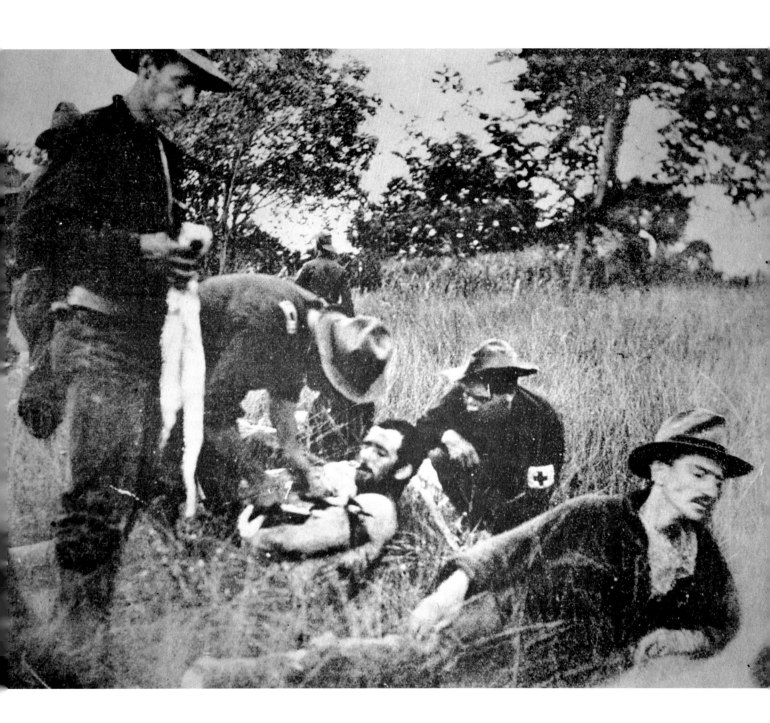

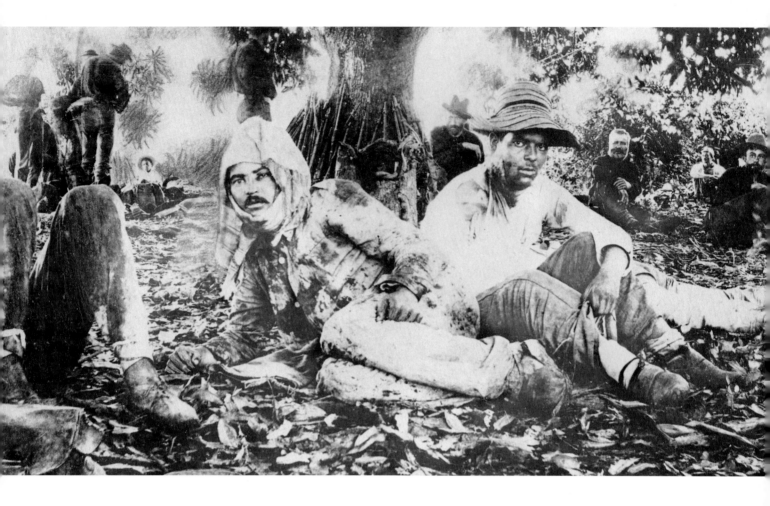

The endemic malaria and yellow fever were far more dangerous to American troops that summer than the Spanish soldiers. The first case of yellow fever was confirmed at Siboney on July 6 when LaGarde and many others already had malaria. On July 9, Major William C. Gorgas, a future Surgeon General (1914–18), took over care of contagious patients until he contracted yellow fever. How the diseases were transmitted remained a mystery, but both relentlessly attacked the American soldiers.

By early August, typhoid and dysentery had joined malaria and yellow fever on sick call. The situation was so serious that the entire V Corps was evacuated from Cuba to Camp Wikoff at Montauk, Long Island, before it was destroyed. Both at home and at the front, the Medical Department learned again that disease was a deadly enemy.

The war with Spain was for the Medical Department a costly lesson in what not to do. A staggering 2,565 soldiers died of disease, compared with 280 killed in action and 1,577 wounded. Unlike the Civil War, this war was over so quickly that there was no time to correct many of the problems resulting from the lack of readiness. However, the lessons were learned and soon would change the entire Army.

TRANSFORMING THE MEDICAL DEPARTMENT, 1898-1917

Change and modernization dominated the years following the Spanish-American War. A postwar commission led by retired Major General Grenville Dodge pointed out the Army's shortcomings during the war and recommended corrective actions.

The War Department's reorganization of February 1901 began a major transformation. The most critical change came in 1903 when Secretary of War Elihu Root created a General Staff under a Chief of Staff to coordinate centralized military planning and operations.

Army medics tend to Spanish casualties at brigade hospital, San Juan Hill, Cuba, on July 3, 1898. *National Archives.*

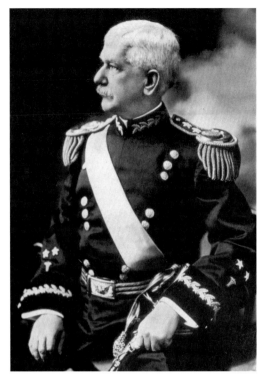

William C. Gorgas's programs of mosquito control enabled the building of the Panama Canal. Gorgas later became Army Surgeon General and received the first Distinguished Service Medal ever issued (1918). *National Library of Medicine.*

Beginning in 1904, new doctrine was developed and codified in Field Service Regulations (FSRs), and unit structure was spelled out in tables of organization. All Army schools were thoroughly revamped based on these changes. Majors Edward L. Munson and Paul F. Straub, who received a Medal of Honor in the Philippine Insurrection, introduced medical instruction for line officers in advanced Army schools. The Medical Department updated and periodically revised its *Manual for the Medical Department* to align its doctrine, organization, supply tables, and procedures.

In the first FSR of 1904, medical personnel were incorporated into regiments. Each infantry division was allocated ambulance companies and field hospitals. The 1914 FSR, the last before World War I, put four ambulance companies and four field hospitals in the sanitary train of each 18,000-man division. The 1914 tables of organization attached 28 medical personnel to each infantry regiment. The combination of the FSR, tables of organization, and *Medical Manuals* converted the chaos of 1898 into order and prepared the Medical Department for war.

By 1910, the framework of the Army's evacuation system from the battalion aid station to base hospital was complete. A permanent structure of medical units was laid out in a chain of evacuation that carried the wounded man from injury at the front until he occupied a bed in a permanent hospital.

Although authorized in the 1904 FSR, the Hospital Corps companies were not converted into the first four regular ambulance companies and field hospitals until 1911. The major work of restructuring Army medical assets began when the New York National Guard organized the first field hospital in March 1906 and then the first ambulance company in November 1911. By early 1917 the National Guard contained 59 ambulance units and 47 hospital units along with 267 sanitary detachments.

An early test of the Army's mobilization capability came at Fort Sam Houston, Texas, in 1911 when a field division mobilized for the first time since 1898. The ambulance companies and field hospitals made up the first complete sanitary train organized since the Civil War. A far better test came when many regular and National Guard units served on the Mexican border during the Punitive Expedition of 1916–17.

ARMY MEDICAL DEPARTMENT MEDAL OF HONOR RECIPIENTS IN THE SPANISH-AMERICAN WAR AND PHILIPPINE INSURRECTION

SPANISH-AMERICAN WAR

JAMES ROBB CHURCH

PHILIPPINE INSURRECTION

GEORGE W. MATHEWS

GEORGE F. SHIELS

PAUL F. STRAUB

THE MEDICAL DEPARTMENT

Following the Dodge Commission's lead, the War Department's February 1901 reorganization began reforming the Medical Department. First, it created an Army Nurse Corps of trained female nurses within the Medical Department to be responsible for the care of sick and wounded soldiers. This action freed the enlisted men in the Hospital Corps to fill positions in field medical units and hospitals as well as in infantry and cavalry regiments. The transition from Hospital Corps to field medical soldiers and today's combat medics was under way.

Second, the War Department authorized a Dental Corps of contract dentists to care for dental health, an increasingly important aspect in the overall physical well-being of the soldier. On March 3, 1911, the Dental Corps became a commissioned service and integral part of the Medical Department.

In 1908 another Army medical reorganization act corrected major deficiencies in the 1901 act. The most significant provision was the creation of the Medical Reserve Corps, the first integral voluntary reserve for war ever established in the American military. It was the model for the creation of the Navy's medical reserve and the Army's Organized Reserve Corps of 1916. By early 1917 more than 3,000 officers, trained and ready for duty, were members of the Army's medical reserve.

The Medical Reserve Corps also attracted some of the best-known and most influential American physicians and surgeons. By 1916, Harvey Cushing of Harvard Medical School, George Crile of the Lakeside Hospital in Cleveland, Charles and William Mayo of the Mayo Clinic, and many others belonged to the Medical Reserve Corps.

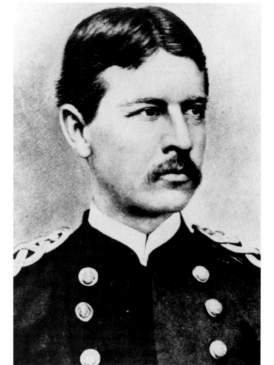

Major Walter Reed. He headed the 1900–01 yellow fever research commission in Cuba. The researchers' heroic sacrifices captured the world's imagination. Several died, but the team proved the disease was mosquito-borne. This medical triumph soon changed life in the tropics and the economic and trade structure of the world. *Library of Congress.*

GENERAL HOSPITALS

Advances in American medicine and surgery, the development of specialization, and the evolution of the American hospital after 1898 coincided with the establishment of a system of large, permanent Army general hospitals. The expansion of Army operations into Cuba, Puerto Rico, and the Philippine Islands required general hospitals on a permanent rather than temporary wartime basis. Moreover, larger hospitals and staffs were now needed to provide the sophisticated equipment and specialized care for soldiers and their families that small post hospitals could not give. Army general hospitals possessed the medical and surgical services that could restore the sick and wounded to being useful soldiers and citizens.

In addition to the Army and Navy General Hospital, three other permanent general hospitals existed before 1917: Walter Reed General Hospital, Washington, D.C., in the East; Letterman General Hospital at the Presidio of San Francisco in the West; and Fort Bayard, New Mexico, which received only tuberculosis cases.

PREVENTIVE MEDICINE

The Spanish-American War shocked the Army and the Medical Department into the realization that preventive medicine and field sanitation were critical to combating disease and maintaining the Army's fighting strength.

Major General (Dr.) Leonard Wood earned the Medal of Honor in 1886 during the Indian Wars, commanded the "Rough Riders" volunteer cavalry regiment in the Spanish-American War, and served as military governor of the Philippines and Cuba. Later he became Army Chief of Staff, 1910–14. *National Library of Medicine.*

Sternberg organized the Typhoid Board under Major Walter Reed of the Army Medical School to study the causes of the 1898 typhoid fever epidemic. The board's preliminary report in 1899 identified some, but not all, of the epidemic's causes and recommended corrective actions. It also highlighted the commander's responsibility for maintaining his unit's health. Typhoid fever remained a concern until Major Frederick F. Russell of the Army Medical School developed and produced a typhoid vaccine based on a British Army strain. The Army then began a voluntary vaccination program in 1909–10.

Sternberg also sent Reed to Cuba in 1900 to head the Yellow Fever Board to investigate that deadly disease. His board concluded that the *Aedes aegypti* mosquito spread yellow fever. This discovery led to the development of mosquito control programs in Cuba under Colonel William C. Gorgas to destroy the breeding places of the mosquitoes and mitigate the danger of the disease. Gorgas took his lessons and moved on to Panama. His efforts after 1903 not only made the completion of the Panama Canal possible, but also made him the Army Surgeon General in January 1914.

After 1898, the Medical Department devoted significant attention and effort to preventing disease in the field. Army medical officers studied tropical diseases, especially malaria, in the Philippines, Cuba, and Puerto Rico. Much research and development was devoted to field sanitation, the disposal of garbage and excreta, water purification, fly and mosquito control, and prevention of intestinal and insect-borne diseases.

Major Carl R. Darnall, who discovered water chlorination in 1910, solved the critical problem of purifying large quantities of water for drinking, bathing, and cooking. In 1913, Major William J.L. Lyster developed a technique using calcium hypochlorite in a large "Lyster Bag" for quickly purifying water in the field.

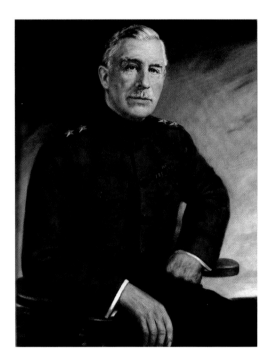

Division maneuvers at Fort Sam Houston, San Antonio, Texas, in the summer of 1911 demonstrated the Army's success with preventive medicine. Overall health was excellent and disease rates were low. The entire 15,000-man force underwent compulsory immunization using Russell's typhoid vaccine. Only two cases of typhoid fever were reported. The effectiveness of Russell's vaccine and compulsory vaccination were proven. To protect the entire Army from potential attacks, typhoid vaccination of all soldiers became mandatory in September 1911. As a result of Russell's work and mandatory vaccination, the Army in World War I suffered only 1,897 cases of typhoid fever and 227 deaths in stark contrast to 1898.

MEDICAL PREPAREDNESS

The Medical Department's lack of cooperation with the American Red Cross during the Spanish-American War was unnecessary and justly criticized. By 1912, the Medical Department rebuilt its relations with the Red Cross and established a strong cooperative relationship that provided substantial dividends even before the war.

In 1916, Dr. George Crile, a leading surgeon and Medical Reserve Corps officer just back from operating an American hospital in France, proposed that the Red Cross and Army Medical Department establish 500-bed Red Cross Base Hospitals affiliated with major hospitals and medical schools around the country. The affiliated hospital units provided a major enhancement in the Medical Department's overall readiness in 1916–17 and a vast increase in the quality of the Army's medical and surgical capabilities when called to duty. Thirty such hospitals existed by the time America entered the war.

The National Defense Act of June 3, 1916, was a major milestone for the Medical Department's preparation for World War I. This act for the first time authorized the Medical Corps and Enlisted Force, which now replaced the Hospital Corps, to be manned as a fixed percentage of the Army enlisted strength so they varied automatically with the total. The act also created the Veterinary Corps and assigned it to the Medical Department with responsibility for all veterinary medicine activities, including food inspection for the Army.

The failures of the war with Spain had driven Army and medical transformation and modernization after 1898 and were an ever-present reminder of why preparedness was necessary. Well before the conflict in Europe began in August 1914, the Medical Department and its leaders were preparing for the eventuality that the United States might be drawn into war.

NAVY MEDICINE BETWEEN THE WARS, 1866–1917

SHRINKING AND NEGLECTED

After the Civil War, the U.S. Navy lapsed into dramatic decline. Naval appropriations were cut and the number of ships and men on active duty shrank dramatically. The Navy and its Medical Department were truly landlocked.

Medical Department resources were deemed entirely inadequate. Few young physicians joined the Navy, deterred by poor pay, low entry rank, and scant opportunity for promotion. In his 1867 report to the Secretary of the Navy, Phineas Horwitz, Chief of the Bureau of Medicine and Surgery, complained bitterly about the discouraging outlook. He noted 48 vacancies in the Medical Corps, impossible to fill "properly." The postwar vacancies were in danger of increasing to such a degree that some feared the Navy Medical Department would simply fade away. Dr. Horwitz urged Congress to act promptly on legislation to increase the opportunities for promotion in respect to both

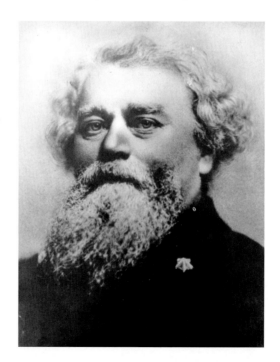

below

William Maxwell Wood, first Surgeon General of the U.S. Navy. Dr. Wood was Chief of the Bureau of Medicine and Surgery when the Naval Appropriations Act of March 3, 1871, grouped medical officers in a separate corps with grades established by law. *U.S. Navy Bureau of Medicine and Surgery.*

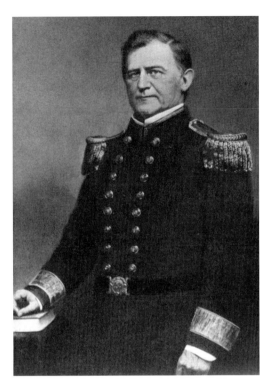

Dr. Jonathan M. Foltz, nicknamed "Surgeon of the Seas," served in the Navy Medical Department from 1831 to 1872. He was second Surgeon General of the Navy. *U.S. Navy Bureau of Medicine and Surgery.*

rank and pay. Congress acted on March 3, 1871, with the Naval Appropriations Act that granted medical and other staff officers of the Navy "relative rank" with grades "equal to but not identical with the grades of the line."

This act surpassed any previous congressional action in transforming and enhancing the Navy Medical Department. The Chief of the Bureau of Medicine and Surgery (BUMED) now had the additional title of Surgeon General, with relative rank of commodore. William Maxwell Wood, a surgeon entering his 42nd year of unusual and varied service, took the helm of this revitalized organization. Dr. Wood had served aboard the USS *Poinsett,* one of the first steam vessels of the Navy, during the Seminole War. Wood served ashore at Sackett's Harbor in New York and at Baltimore, as Fleet Surgeon of the Pacific Fleet, and under Commodore John D. Sloat during the Mexican War. He served less than two years as Surgeon General and Chief of BUMED, being succeeded by Jonathan M. Foltz.

SAILORS' HEALTH IMPROVEMENTS

The health of the Navy's personnel steadily improved following the war, partly due to the new emphasis on preventive medicine and hygiene. The transition from the age of wooden hulls and sail power to the all-steel, steam-powered Navy required better measures to vent the pollution caused by below-deck storage of coal and the exhaust gases generated by its combustion. The foul condition of many ships' bilges had become a regular theme of Navy Surgeons General's reports to the Secretary of the Navy. The conditions aboard many naval vessels were blamed for yellow fever outbreaks and led to the 1887 establishment of the short-lived, and underutilized, Navy quarantine hospital on Widow's Island, Penobscot Bay, Maine.

On March 20, 1878, the Navy Department created a board of officers to examine and ascertain the best system to ventilate Navy ships. The board advocated an aspirator ventilation plan consisting of a network of tubes reaching every part of the ship and terminating in a large main through which the air was drawn by a steam blower. Surgeon General Phillip Wales urged rapid introduction of the new ventilation system.

During the 1870s the naval hygiene movement was given new life by Medical Directors Joseph Wilson, Jr., author of *Naval Hygiene* (1870), and Albert L. Gihon, author of *Practical Suggestions in Naval Hygiene* (1871). As early as 1879 the Bureau of Medicine and Surgery established a laboratory for investigating hygiene-related matters and began collecting items which would comprise the collection of the Naval Museum of Hygiene, established in Washington, D.C., in 1882. Until it merged into the Navy Medical School in 1902, the museum exhibited ships' ventilation systems and housed displays of disinfection techniques. It also was a leader in promoting environmental and occupational medicine and went beyond its role as a museum by becoming an education center for the promotion and development of laboratory research, particularly with chemical, bacteriological, and microscopic investigations.

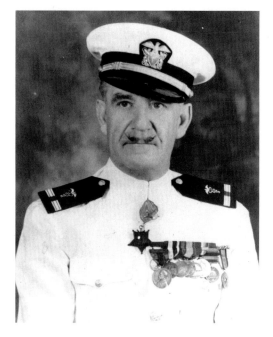

INTERNATIONAL PRESENCE CREATES NEW DEMANDS

The scope of the Navy Medical Department widened to the Pacific in the 1870s as American interest in the Far East increased. During the years 1867–69 the USS *Idaho*, converted into a hospital ship and kept anchored at Nagasaki, Japan, served as a floating hospital for the American Squadron in the Far East. To handle Pacific requirements, the Navy constructed a new hospital in 1870 at Mare Island, California, and at Yokohama, Japan, in 1872.

Throughout the 1880s and 1890s, U.S. Navy vessels became increasingly evident throughout the world. Besides routine cruises, Navy missions included protecting American citizens and American interests, providing assistance to disaster victims, and carrying out special explorations.

Medical officers went ashore at hundreds of international ports. Their reports detailed climate and medical conditions, the people, quality of medical facilities available, endemic diseases, and the methods being employed to combat them. Many of these observations were published in the *Annual Reports of the Navy Surgeon General* from 1871 through 1959.

ORGANIZATIONAL IMPROVEMENTS

With the outbreak of war with Spain in April 1898 the Navy unveiled its first floating hospital since USS *Red Rover*. The former liner *Creole*, renamed USS *Solace*, was the first vessel to fly the Geneva Red Cross flag. She rendered service treating casualties after the naval engagement off Santiago, Cuba, on July 3, 1898. She later served as a transport between San Francisco and the Philippines.

On June 17, 1898, a century after the first "loblolly boy" reported for duty aboard the USS *Constellation*, Congress established the Navy Hospital Corps. Navy Surgeons General had long advocated well-trained professional corps to provide medical care in the field, but Congress acted only after the war began. The first group of 25 hospital corpsmen were pharmacists (apothecaries) with rank, pay, and privileges of warrant officers.

The Hospital Corps came just in time. Following the Spanish-American War, the world's newest colonial power had to govern places such as Guam, the Philippines, Puerto Rico, Cuba, and Samoa. As a Pacific power, the United States participated in the China Relief Expedition of 1900. Naval medical officers had to confront tropical diseases few had ever seen: dengue, yaws, leishmaniasis, leprosy, yellow fever, intermittent fever, filariasis, dysentery, elephantoid fever, and the ubiquitous venereal maladies sailors acquired in exotic liberty ports.

The Navy Medical Department dealt with these issues through enhanced training. The Navy Medical School moved in 1902 from Brooklyn, New York, to the Naval Museum of Hygiene in Washington, D.C. Its mission was simple and straightforward: "the instruction and training of newly appointed medical officers in professional branches peculiar to naval requirements." Newly commissioned physicians learned medicine they would not have encountered in civilian medical schools. Examples

U.S. Navy Hospital Apprentice Robert Stanley earned the Medal of Honor for conspicuous gallantry in Peking during the China Relief Expedition, June 1900. In later Navy service, he became Chief Pharmacist. *U.S. Navy Bureau of Medicine and Surgery.*

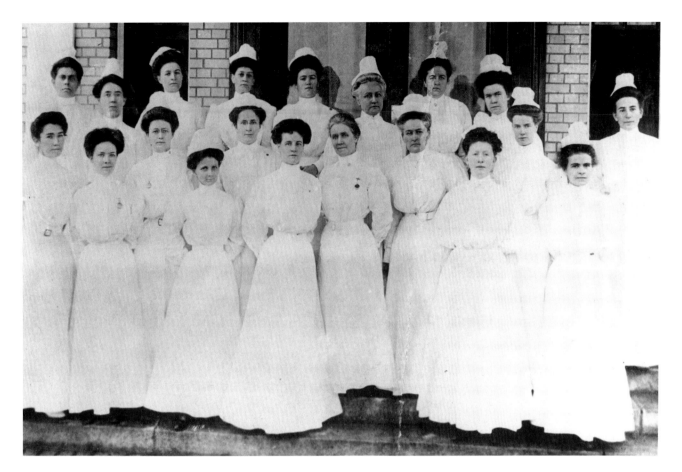

"The Sacred Twenty," the first U.S. Navy nurses, at the Naval Hospital, Washington, D.C., circa October 1908. Esther Voorhees Hasson, first superintendent of the Navy Nurse Corps 1908–11, appears fourth from right in the front row. *Naval Historical Center.*

included tropical medicine, the treatment of ballistic wounds, and burns—the grist of naval medicine. The curriculum of a five-month course covered microscopy, naval hygiene, and military law, plus a program of physical exercise and military drill akin to a military school or service academy.

Tropical disease was a chief focus of attention at the school since it caused many of the casualties suffered in the war with Spain. Edward Rhodes Stitt, a pioneer in tropical medicine, taught at the school and was one of its first commanding officers. He served as Surgeon General of the Navy for eight years, 1920–28.

NEW CORPS ESTABLISHED

Following the creation of the Army Nurse Corps in 1901, BUMED campaigned for its own nurse corps. The struggle finally paid off on May 13, 1908, when the U.S. Navy Nurse Corps was established. The first nurses in the Navy were known as the "The Sacred Twenty." They reported later in 1908 for orientation and duty at the U.S. Naval Hospital, Washington, D.C. Esther Voorhees Hasson, a former U.S. Army nurse, was appointed as the Nurse Corps' first superintendent on August 8, 1908.

The Medical Department continued to grow. President William Howard Taft signed a bill on August 22, 1912, authorizing "not more than 30 acting assistant dental surgeons to be part of the Medical Department of the United States Navy." On the eve of World War I, Surgeon General held the rank of Rear Admiral and the Navy Medical Department had grown in size to four separate corps, with added responsibilities for two hospital ships and 17 naval hospitals.

On April 9, 1914, General Victoriano Huerta's soldiers arrested U.S. Navy personnel seeking supplies in Tampico, Mexico. The Mexicans released the sailors, but without the apology that President Woodrow Wilson demanded. Wilson ordered naval forces under Rear Admiral Frank F. Fletcher to occupy the Mexican port of Vera Cruz. The U.S. intervention and occupation resulted in Mexican resistance and an outbreak of hostilities which generated casualties on both sides. Navy Surgeons Middleton Elliott, Cary Langhorne, and Hospital Apprentice 1st Class William Zuiderveld received the Medal of Honor for their heroic actions treating the wounded under fire. This was a prelude to larger actions. In less than four years, Navy medical personnel would brave U-boats in the North Atlantic and fight on the Western Front.

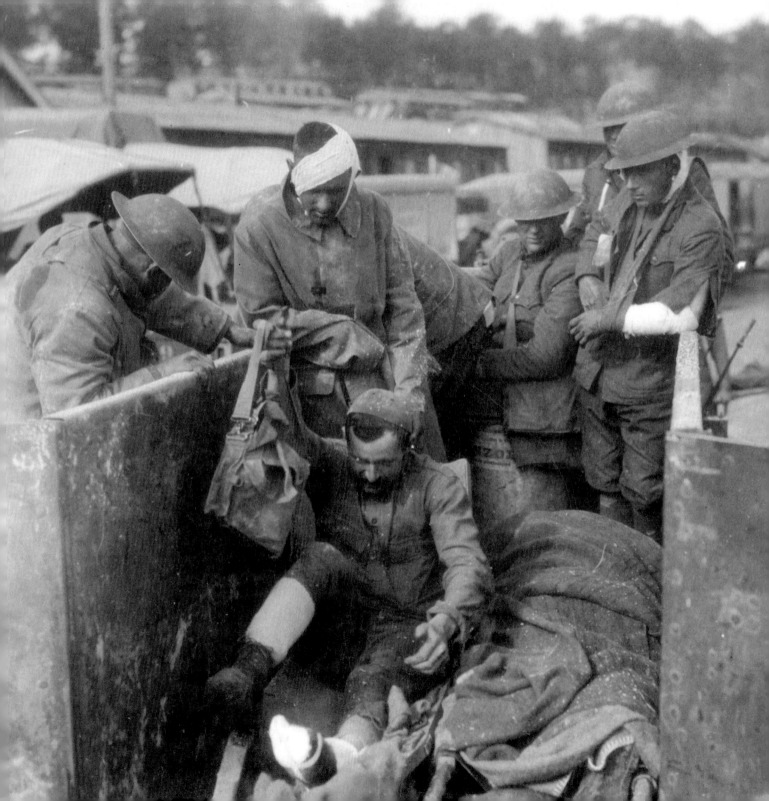

Chapter 4
World War I, 1917–18

left
Unloading wounded soldiers from truck that just arrived from the front. Souilly, France. September 28, 1918. *National Museum of Health and Medicine.*

right
British General Hospital No. 16 in the French fishing village of Le Treport had a capacity of 2,232 patients and was constructed entirely of huts. U.S. Base Hospital No. 10 from the University of Pennsylvania School of Medicine ran this hospital during the war. *National Archives.*

"SEND US DOCTORS"

The United States entered the war in Europe in April 1917, almost three years after it began. Although the Army Medical Department was better prepared for war than ever before, its preparation fell short of what lay ahead.

Late in April 1917, Sir Arthur Balfour and a British military mission arrived in Washington to discuss the Allies' most pressing needs. He pleaded, "Send us doctors," because Britain had too few physicians for its civilian and military requirements.

No regular Army hospital units could answer the plea, but a number of 500-bed Red Cross Base Hospital units were trained and ready for service. Six of these units (Base Hospital Nos. 2, 4, 5, 10, 12, and 21) were ordered to France in May 1917 to support the British Expeditionary Force (BEF). The first unit to go was George Crile's Base Hospital No. 4 from Western Reserve and Lakeside Hospital in Cleveland, Ohio. It left New York on May 8 and on May 25 assumed full responsibility for British General Hospital No. 9 at Rouen, France.

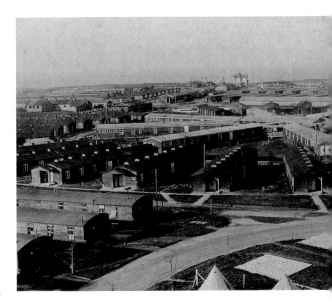

By war's end, more than 1,600 American medical officers served with the BEF down to the level of battalion surgeon. More than 3,000 American medical personnel per month were in service with the BEF through early 1919. They called themselves the "Lost Legion," because so few Americans or British knew of their contributions and sacrifices; 25 medical officers died in battle and 96 others died from non-battle related causes. Harvey Cushing's Base Hospital No. 5 (Harvard University) at BEF General Hospital No. 11 suffered the first U.S. military losses to hostile action. A German bombing raid on the night of September 4, 1917, killed 1st Lieutenant William T. Fitzsimons, MC, and several enlisted men.

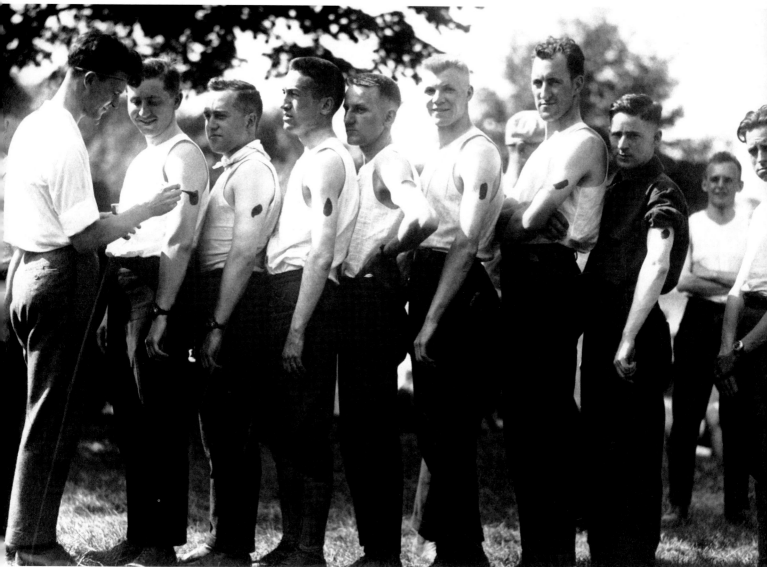

MOBILIZATION AND THE HOME FRONT

Prewar mobilization plans envisioned an Army of perhaps 300,000. By the summer of 1917, the planned force grew to 38 divisions and two million men for deployment to France. The Medical Department assumed enormous tasks:

- to complete physical and mental examinations of recruits and inductees,
- to maintain the health of the mobilized and deployed Army through its camp and general hospitals in the United States and its base and camp hospitals in France, and
- to recruit, train, deploy, and supply field medical units to support this large expeditionary force.

The burden of shaping the medical force fell to Major General William C. Gorgas, Surgeon General since January 1914, and his office. Gorgas estimated that an Army of two million soldiers required 20,000 medical officers based on a ratio of 10 medical officers per 1,000 men. Large numbers of dentists, veterinarians, nurses, and enlisted personnel were required. Against those estimated needs, Gorgas had a small but highly qualified cadre of personnel in the Medical, Dental, Veterinary, and Army Nurse Corps of the regular Army, Reserve, and National Guard around which to build. There were 491 medical officers, 86 dentists, 62 veterinarians, and 233 nurses in the regular Army in April 1917. They were augmented by 1,246 medical officers and 249 dentists from the National Guard, and about 3,000 personnel from the medical officers' reserve.

above
Men of the Ambulance Training Corps of Allentown, Pennsylvania, being iodined before receiving inoculation, January 1, 1917.
National Archives.

right
U.S. Army mobile dental service in France, 1918.
National Archives.

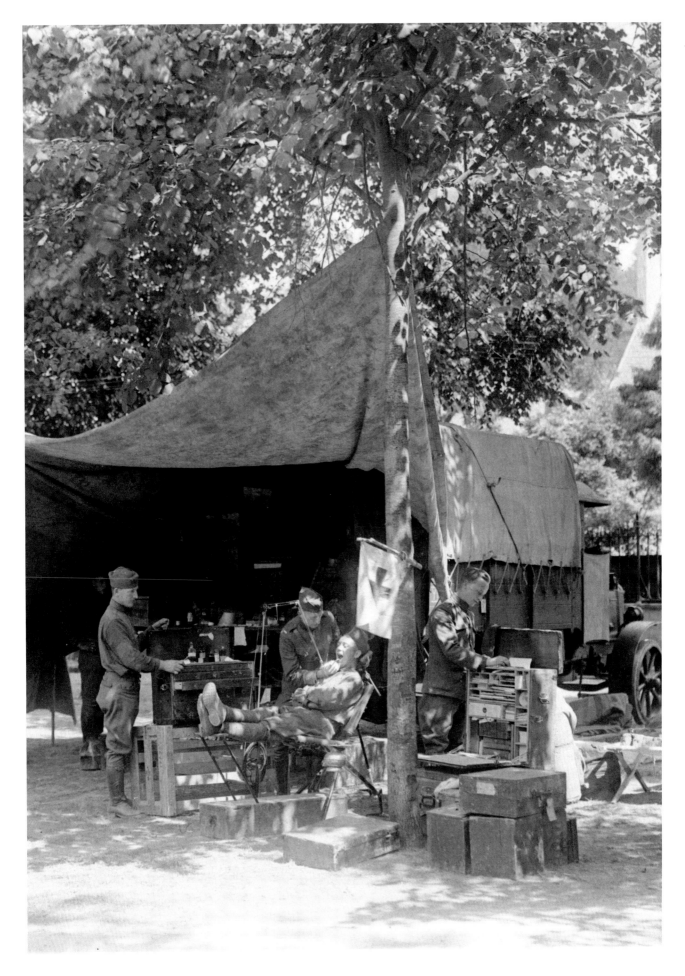

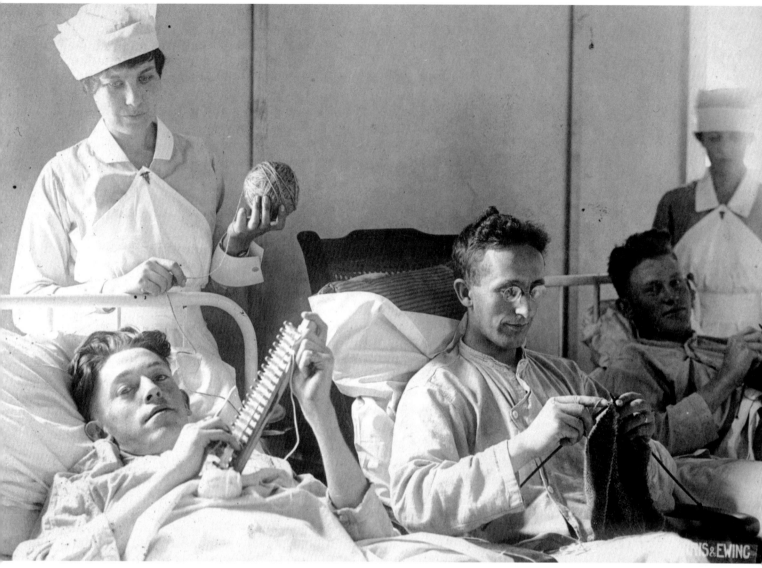

Soon the estimate of the force needed in Europe by the end of 1919 mushroomed to four million men and 98 divisions. Gorgas's estimates required serious revision.

By the time of the Armistice in November 1918, Gorgas had succeeded with the help of all elements of the American medical professions. The Medical Department expanded to more than 336,000 personnel in only 18 months.

The Medical Corps numbered 30,591 (roughly 27 percent of all American physicians), the Dental Corps 4,620, the Veterinary Corps 2,002, and the Army Nurse Corps 21,480. Enlisted strength grew from 6,619 in April 1917 to 264,181 in November 1918. The new Sanitary Corps, with 2,919 officers, was added in June 1917 as a wartime organization of allied health professionals and medical administra-

tors. The civilian work force grew from 450 to 10,695 and included physical and occupational therapists as well as dietitians. New technologies, typified by the Air Service, created unique medical needs. Thus the new field of aviation medicine was born.

Adding new personnel was one thing; training medical personnel and creating field medical units was quite another. The Medical Department opened Officers' Training Camps for whites and African-Americans to familiarize new medical, dental, and veterinary officers with the Army and military medicine.

The combat force came from the regular, National Guard, and National Army divisions. The August 1917 reorganization created the "square division" of two infantry brigades each with two infantry regiments and 27,120 men. The

Knitting was an important element of the occupational therapy for these wounded recuperating soldiers at Walter Reed General Hospital, Washington, D.C., circa 1918–19. *National Archives.*

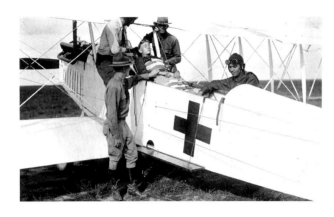

The field of aviation medicine originated in World War I. Physicians assigned to the U.S. Army Air Service quickly reconfigured various aircraft for patient evacuation. This Curtiss JN-4D "Jenny" modified by Major S.M. Strong, U.S. Army, was one of the first experimental aerial evacuation planes. Kelly Field, San Antonio, Texas, February 1918. *U.S. Air Force Medical Service.*

division had a medical structure of 104 officers and 1,455 enlisted men—54 officers and 543 men served in headquarters, infantry, artillery, engineer, and signal units. The other 50 officers and 912 staffed the Sanitary Train of four ambulance companies and four field hospitals (three motorized and one horse drawn). The medical detachment of each infantry regiment had only 55 officers and men to care for 3,775 soldiers, which proved far too few.

The hospital structure in the continental U.S. burgeoned enormously to support the vastly expanded Army. By November 1918 the Medical Department managed 92 large hospitals (89 of them new construction) with 120,916 beds. Instead of its four prewar general hospitals, 37 now existed that accepted all patients and were under the control of the Surgeon General.

Certain hospitals were also designated for patients requiring special treatment, such as for tuberculosis, psychiatric conditions, and orthopedic, oral, and plastic surgery. New amputation centers pooled orthopedic surgeons, physical and occupational therapists, reconstruction aides, and prosthesis manufacturing and fitting. More than 25,000 disabled soldiers received special reconstructive surgery and therapy plus rehabilitation and occupational training to enable them to reenter civilian life with job skills as productive members of society once again.

AMERICAN EXPEDITIONARY FORCES IN FRANCE

After the first six hospitals joined the BEF, another eight Red Cross Base Hospitals (Base Hospital Nos. 6, 8, 9, 15, 17, 18, 27, and 39) deployed to France to support the arrival of American troops. The first of these, Base Hospital No. 8 from Johns Hopkins in Baltimore, Maryland, sailed from New York on May 28, 1917, aboard the S.S. *Baltic* with Major General John J. Pershing and his staff of the American Expeditionary Forces (AEF) headquarters.

Pershing brought his medical team from the Southern Department at Fort Sam Houston, Texas. He wanted Colonel Merritte Ireland, MC, former commander of the post hospital at Fort Sam Houston, as his chief surgeon. However, he deferred to Gorgas's choice of Colonel Alfred Bradley. Ireland became Bradley's deputy but actually assumed chief surgeon responsibility due to Bradley's poor health. Ireland was promoted to chief surgeon in April 1918. His superb work in France and Pershing's recommendation led to Ireland's succeeding Gorgas as Army Surgeon General in October 1918. He served in the post until May 1931.

During the voyage to France, Reserve Major Hugh Young, a leading American urologist from Johns Hopkins, convinced Pershing and his staff of the need for a strong program to control venereal disease. They paid heed. From the outset, the AEF's venereal disease control was the strongest and most successful in the war, stressing unit discipline, prophylaxis, and prevention through condom use.

THE HOSPITAL SYSTEM

The early arriving base hospitals soon doubled to 1,000-bed units, but usually without additional personnel. All hospitals fit into the prewar concept of Advanced, Intermediate, and Base Sections of the Lines of Communications (Services of Supply) that supported the Zone of the Armies. The AEF aligned the entire chain of evacuation and the hospital system along the rail lines to support its sector in Lorraine.

The urgent need for more combat troops in France revised shipping priorities and meant that medical units, equipment, and personnel did not arrive as originally planned. Instead of receiving the 14.5 percent of AEF strength it required, the Medical Department was limited to an arbitrary 7.65 percent. It never recovered from this constriction, and operated with serious shortages throughout the war.

By July 1918, only eight of the required 52 evacuation hospitals were in France to support the 26 combat divisions. Prewar medical doctrine made these units the critical link in the chain of evacuation that stretched from frontline field hospitals to rear area base hospitals. Evacuation hospitals took the wounded from the field hospitals for initial treatment, stabilization, resuscitation, and life-saving surgery and passed them by hospital train to the rear for more definitive care. Lacking evacuation hospitals, Ireland, the chief surgeon, had to improvise from the existing base hospitals, often with negative consequences. In the summer of 1918, Ireland took personnel from the 46 base hospitals and organized shock and surgical teams to augment the stressed evacuation hospitals. This solved one problem but created another by removing surgical personnel when they were most needed to care for wounded arriving from the front.

Ireland also realized that the U.S. Army needed mobile surgical units similar to those that the French were already using to augment their hospitals. In February 1918, 20 mobile hospitals and 20 mobile surgical units were organized to move surgical aid forward to the seriously wounded soldier rather than moving the soldier to the surgeon. The surgical units provided critical reinforcements during combat operations.

Luckily, the medical and surgical personnel in the Red Cross Base Hospitals that were tapped for the new units came from some of the finest medical schools and hospitals in the United States. They formed the cadres for virtually every new hospital unit from camp hospitals to mobile hospitals to surgical teams, and whatever else the AEF chief surgeon needed anywhere in France.

AEF hospital bed requirements were based on a percentage of its total strength (10 percent for normal admissions and 10 percent for combat admissions—20 percent total) and grew as the AEF expanded. A massive construction and renovation program was undertaken to support American hospital requirements because few suitable hospitals were available. By November 1918, 221,000 beds (338,000 in emergency) were available for a force of 1.9 million and plans called for 541,000 beds for a projected force of 3.2 million men.

During 1918, the chief surgeon began grouping several base hospitals and convalescent camps into 17 hospital centers to reduce administrative overhead and free the hospitals of recuperating soldiers. Some centers had as many as 20,000 beds and their total capacity increased from 30,890 in July to 163,368 in December 1918.

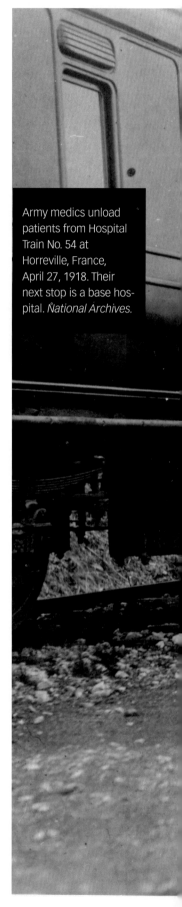

Army medics unload patients from Hospital Train No. 54 at Horreville, France, April 27, 1918. Their next stop is a base hospital. *National Archives.*

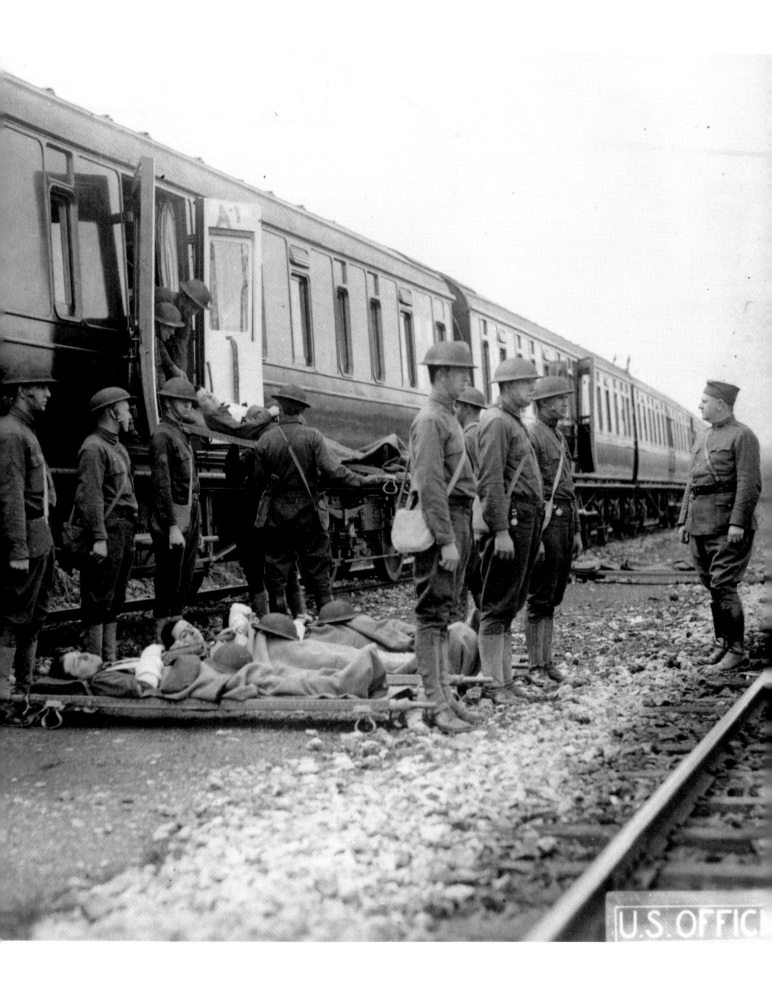

U.S. OFFICI

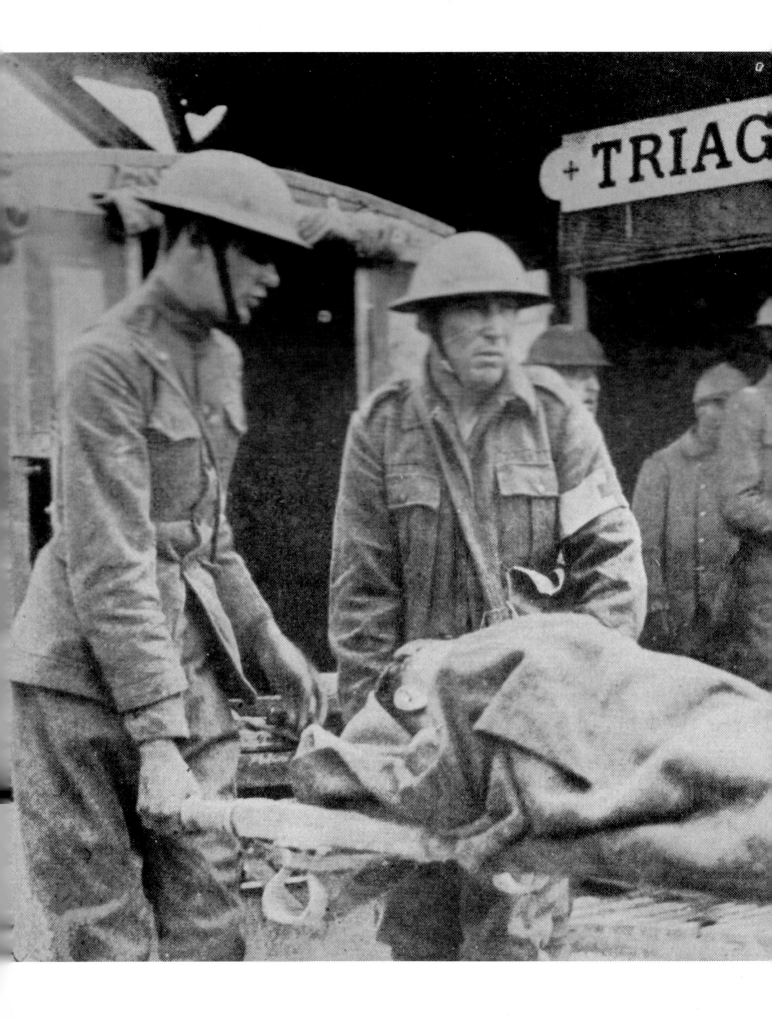

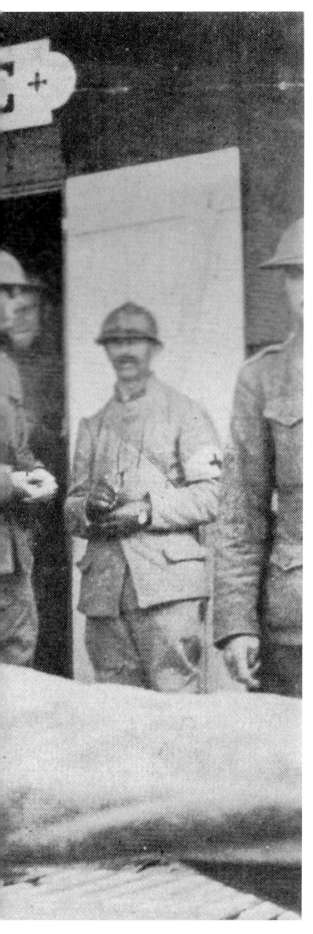

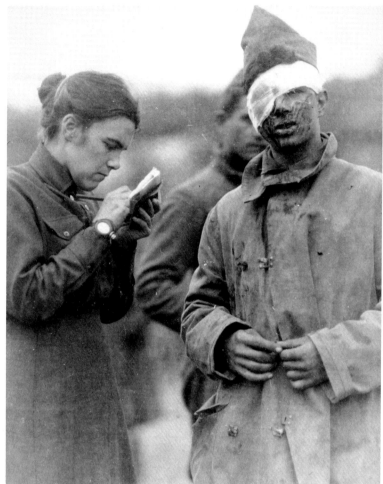

left
Triage point, 42d Division, near Suippes, France, July 17, 1918. At a triage point, medical officers sorted patients into three groups: those who could return to duty, the minor walking wounded, and the severely wounded litter patients. *National Archives.*

top right
Salvation Army worker writes a letter to the home folks for a wounded soldier, circa 1917–18. The Salvation Army dispatched about 500 men and women to assist the American Expeditionary Force. *National Archives.*

The AEF's Medical Department grew slowly and never reached its programmed strength. From seven officers and two enlisted men in June 1917, the AEF Medical Department grew to 5,198 officers, 2,539 nurses, and 30,674 enlisted men on June 1, 1918. By early October and the opening phase of the Meuse-Argonne Offensive, it had 14,483 officers, 7,522 nurses, and 104,557 enlisted men—126,562. It peaked at 174,083 in January 1919, or more than 50 percent of the entire Army Medical Department.

MEDICAL AND SURGICAL ADVANCES
The chief surgeon set up an AEF field medical school at Langres, France, to train arriving Medical Department officers and receive updates from British and French medical officers on wartime developments. After three years of war, the French had developed new practices and surgical procedures. The AEF adopted the French system of *triage,* or sorting of casualties by the severity of the wounds and need for immediate surgical care. Triage has since become standard practice in all emergency medicine.

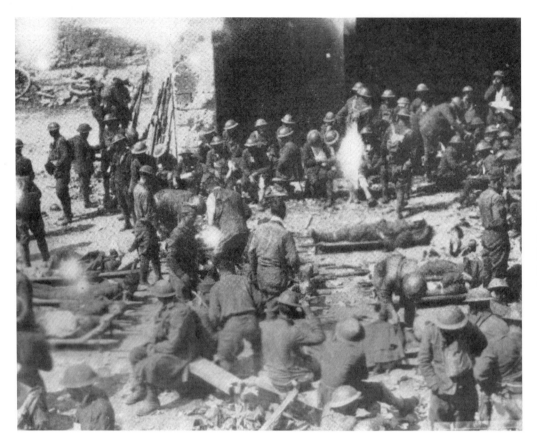

First aid station of the 1st Division set up immediately behind the frontline trenches near Missy-aux-Bois, July 17, 1918. *National Archives.*

A second technique adopted from the French was *débridement*, the surgical removal of all foreign objects and dead or damaged tissue from a wound that would prevent proper healing or cause infection. Wounds resulting from artillery fire were normally infected with soil and other foreign objects and demanded immediate attention because these infections developed quickly and were often fatal.

Surgical units were moved as close as possible to the front line to reduce the time before surgery. To prevent further infection, medics followed the Carrel-Dakin method of cleansing and irrigating wounds with an antiseptic solution. Fixation of extremity wounds with bandaging and splints prior to movement from the battlefield was seen as critical to prevent further injury.

Major advances during the war included these, among others:

- blood transfusions,
- the understanding and treatment of shock,
- shell shock and other psychiatric issues,
- reconstructive and plastic surgery,
- primary suture and delayed primary suture,
- diagnostic use of X-ray machines,
- maxillofacial and oral surgery,
- treatment of gas casualties,
- the increased importance of orthopedic surgery, and
- physical therapy and rehabilitation.

American medical officers would soon have enormous experience in all of these areas.

The increased specialization in American medicine and surgery was clearly seen when the AEF chief surgeon followed the lead of the Surgeon General and created a consultants' advisory group. AEF consultants arranged for selected base hospitals to specialize. Thus, Base Hospital No. 20 received all tuberculosis cases and No. 9 all orthopedic cases. Such specialization produced improvements in care and significant advancements in procedures and techniques from the experience gained by treating thousands of cases. This experience improved and benefited American medicine and surgery in the postwar years.

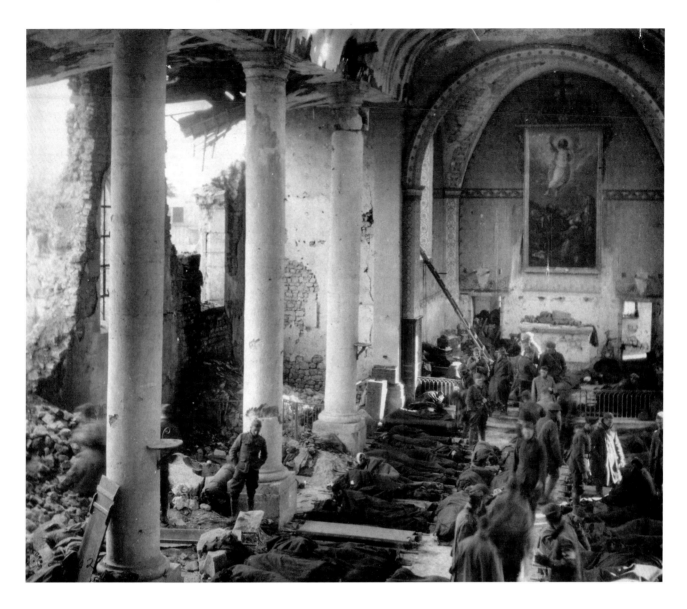

This shattered church in the ruins of Neuilly, close to the Argonne Forest, furnished temporary shelter for American wounded on the first day of the Meuse-Argonne offensive on September 26, 1918. *National Archives.*

BATTLEFIELD EVACUATION

Ironically, the refined Letterman system of echeloned care, which the Medical Department took to France in 1917, required the most seriously wounded soldiers to travel the farthest to receive potentially life-saving surgery. The greatest challenge remained to reduce the time between injury and treatment.

The regimental surgeon oversaw all medical care for the combat soldier. Care began at the company level, where bandaging and first aid were the responsibility of two enlisted litter bearers. Regiments had too few medical personnel and stretcher bearers for the battalion and companies effectively to recover the wounded on the battlefield and care for them. Battalion aid stations performed basic first aid, checked bandages and tourniquets, and often functioned within 250 yards of the front line.

Casualties then moved to ambulance company dressing stations, the forward element of the divisional sanitary train.

At these stops, medical officers checked the patients and triaged them into three groups: those who could return to duty, the minor walking wounded, and the severely wounded litter patients. From dressing stations the wounded moved three to four miles to the field hospitals which provided more complete treatment. The roads to and from the front lines were often impassable, heavily traveled by troop and supply convoys, and always subject to enemy shelling and even air attack. Evacuation presented a dangerous and time-consuming route to safety and the next echelon of medical care.

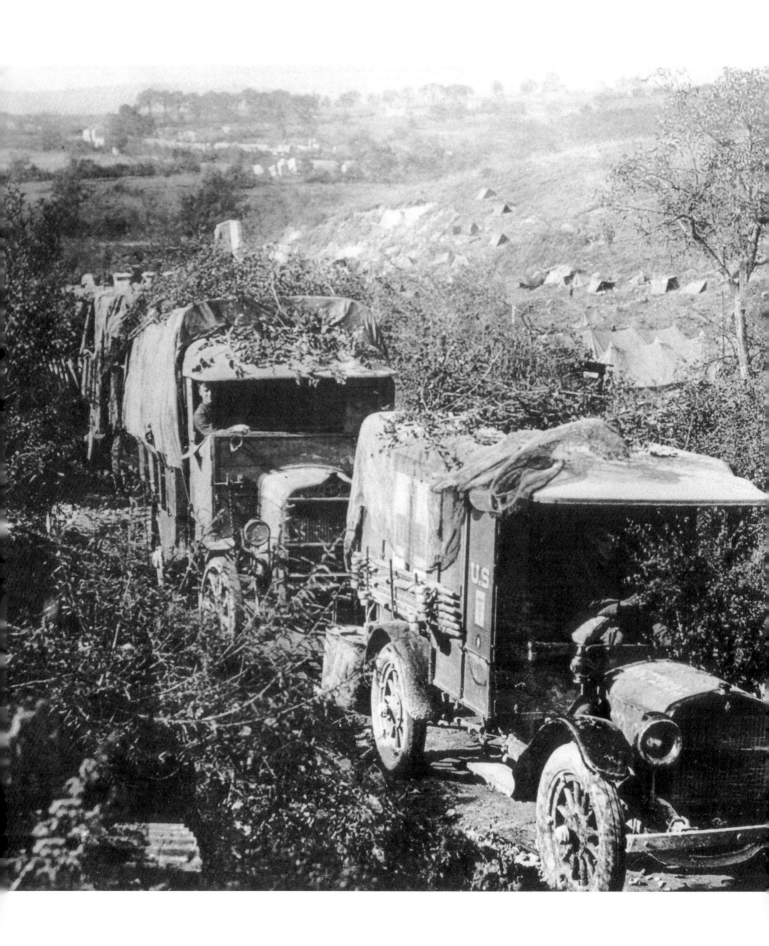

left
Trucks of Field Hospital No. 13 on the move near Véry, Meuse Sector, France, on October 3, 1918. *National Archives.*

right
Latex tent for convalescents at an Army hospital in France, 1918. *National Archives.*

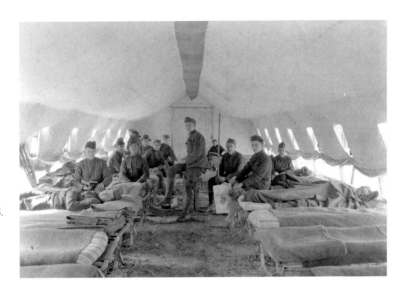

Field hospitals had to be mobile to move with their division, but they were modified to hold patients for longer periods depending on the type and severity of the wounds. Learning from British and French experience, one of the four field hospitals in each division specialized in gas casualties. Another field hospital added a mobile surgical unit so that it could hold and treat patients. The other two field hospitals were unchanged and could move with the division. Mobile hospitals, mobile surgical units, and special surgical and shock teams provided important additional surgical support to field and evacuation hospitals during major offensive operations.

Field hospitals relied on horse-drawn and motorized evacuation ambulances to move their patients to the evacuation hospitals on the rail lines. However, too few ambulances reached France during 1918. Significant French assistance averted serious problems during major operations. There were never enough evacuation hospitals to provide two for each division, so field and base hospitals were augmented and frequently called upon to act as evacuation hospitals.

From the evacuation hospitals, hospital trains transported the wounded back to the base hospitals for definitive treatment. The smooth operation of the entire hospital system depended on having sufficient hospital trains to move patients from evacuation hospitals to base hospitals and to keep the forward hospitals clear of patients in order to receive new casualties. The Medical Department often borrowed hospital trains from French forces when casualties from major offensives overloaded its train capacity.

The Meuse-Argonne Offensive of September to November 1918 was the AEF's largest of the war. The offensive reflected the magnitude of the Medical Department's challenges, but it also stretched an already badly overextended medical force to the breaking point. In the course of the operation, 69,832 American and 2,635 German wounded were treated along with 18,664 gas victims and 2,029 shell shock cases (1,204 returned to duty in three days), for a total of 93,160 casualties.

WORLD WAR I SERVICE AND CASUALTIES 1917–18

Total U.S. Service Members	4,734,991
Battle Deaths	53,402
Other Deaths In Service	63,114
Non-Mortal Woundings	204,002

Source: Department of Veterans Affairs from Department of Defense.

Another 68,760 medical cases were admitted to hospitals, many of them with influenza. Deaths in hospitals numbered 3,528, and 143,051 patients were evacuated. Ambulances made 24,521 trips carrying 126,883 patients to evacuation hospitals, and hospital trains made 408 trips and evacuated 151,045 to rear area hospitals, including 93,437 American casualties and 55,698 medical patients.

DISEASE

The Medical Department had learned its lesson about disease from the Spanish-American War. Its prewar preventive medicine program was strong with a proven vaccination program against smallpox and typhoid fever. However, neither it nor any other medical organization in the world could do much to cope with the influenza pandemic of 1918–19. Modern medicine had no answers to this virulent virus that swept across the globe, killing millions.

With millions of soldiers in close quarters in the U.S. and France, the Army suffered heavily from the flu and its associated respiratory consequences, especially pneumonia. The Army had 762,000 flu victims: 534,000 admissions with 16,571 deaths in the U.S. and 228,000 admissions with 7,366 deaths in Europe. Most of the victims in Europe came during the St. Mihiel and Meuse-Argonne operations from September through November 1918. Pneumonia and other diseases brought the respiratory deaths to 26,540 in the U.S. and 16,241 in Europe out of an Army total of 44,270.

Deaths from the flu and respiratory disease accounted for 80 percent of the 55,868 disease deaths during war. Disease once again claimed more American lives than the enemy.

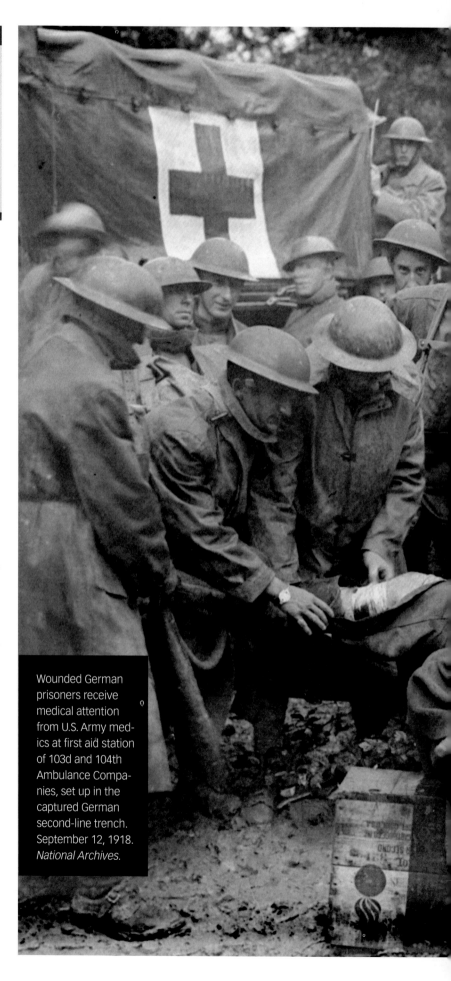

Wounded German prisoners receive medical attention from U.S. Army medics at first aid station of 103d and 104th Ambulance Companies, set up in the captured German second-line trench. September 12, 1918. *National Archives.*

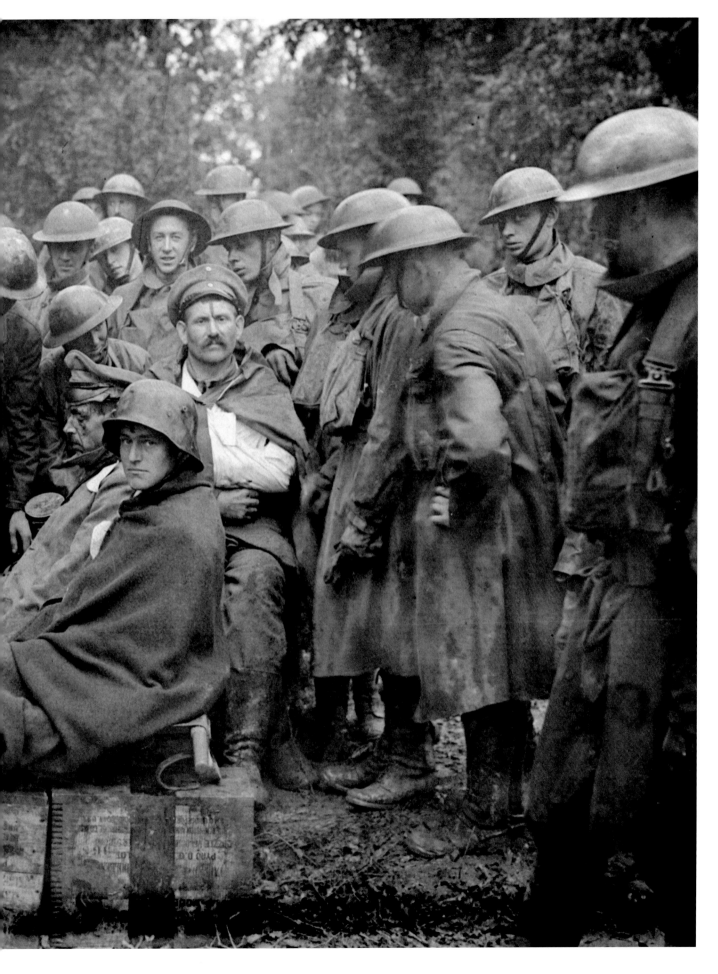

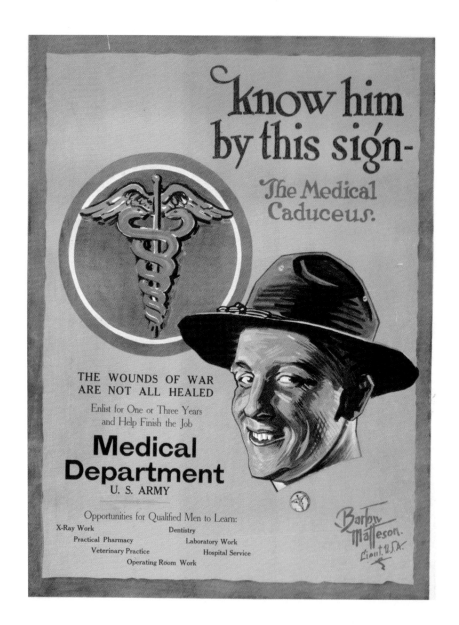

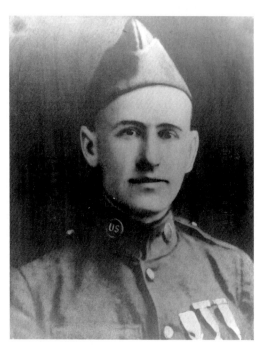

top
"Know him by this sign." This Medical Department recruiting poster appeared late in the World War I era. *Library of Congress.*

bottom two portraits Private First Class Charles D. Barger, left, and Private First Class Jesse N. Funk, of Company L, 354th Infantry Regiment of the 89th Division, on October 31, 1918, learned that two daylight patrols had been caught out in no-man's-land and were unable to return. Upon their own initiative, Barger and Funk made two trips 500 yards beyond friendly lines under constant machine gun fire, and rescued two wounded officers. They received the Medal of Honor for their gallantry above and beyond the call of duty. *National Archives.*

NAVY MEDICINE IN WORLD WAR I

SACRIFICE AND HEROISM

In World War I, the Medical Department suffered 5,506 battle and non-battle deaths in the U.S. and Europe and 3,772 wounded in action. The Medical Corps loss included 47 killed in action, 450 wounded, and 27 wound-related deaths. The heaviest losses were among enlisted personnel who were closest to the fighting. Their losses numbered 120 killed in action, 3,265 wounded, and 209 wound-related deaths, plus another 4,382 disease and non-battle deaths. Many of the deaths occurred during the influenza pandemic which claimed a large number of caregivers both at home and abroad.

In recognition of their heroism, medical personnel received 265 Distinguished Service Crosses—174 enlisted personnel, 88 Medical Corps officers, and three Army Nurse Corps. Two stretcher bearers, Private First Class Charles D. Barger and Private First Class Jesse N. Funk, Company L, 354th Infantry Regiment of the 89th Division, had the unusual distinction of receiving their Medals of Honor during the same action. These were the only Medals of Honor awarded to medical personnel.

In many ways, World War I opened the curtain for a century of conflict. From the outset in France, the Medical Department was forced to make due without its planned medical units, personnel, supplies, and equipment and to operate with constant shortages. By November 1918 this situation had reached a major crisis point that only the Armistice ended. Ireland and the Medical Department improvised an evacuation and hospital system that supported massive casualty bills from combat operations and the everyday health care needs of nearly two million American soldiers. The Army Medical Department learned many hard lessons about manning, building, and operating a functional medical system for an enormously expanded Army and for an expeditionary force fighting far from its homeland and base of support.

MOBILIZING FOR WAR

In April 1917, after President Woodrow Wilson called for a declaration of war against Germany, and American isolationism headed for temporary retirement, the Navy Medical Department had to recruit and train hundreds of physicians, dentists, and nurses, as well as thousands of hospital corpsmen.

Although the U.S. Navy never engaged an enemy fleet during its participation in the conflict, its medical personnel performed admirably. They served with Marine Corps units on the Western Front; aboard every man-of-war, troop transport, and supply ship; with submarine divisions and aviation groups; and with the United States Railway Battery in France. In 1917, the Navy deployed 38 physicians, five dentists, and 348 hospital corpsmen to France; nurses also went. They encountered the frightful realities of warfare: trench foot, disease, rats, vermin, complete lack of the most rudimentary hygiene, and the terrifying results of mustard, phosgene, and chlorine gases.

Navy medical personnel who supported the Marine Brigade on the Western Front also had to deal with other war trauma. They handled shrapnel wounds, blast injuries, high-velocity projectile wounds, and psychiatric disorders, then collectively known as shell shock. From that terrible conflict in Europe, medical personnel became skilled in trauma resuscitation, the treatment of wounds and infectious disease, and the psychological wounds of war.

Preventive medicine was a major component of a Navy doctor's day-to-day job, especially with the prevalence of communicable diseases. Indeed, illness could be acquired in places other than the battlefield. According to one Navy physician, venereal disease in wartime France increased because control of licensed prostitution had become less rigid. By his account, 50 percent of French prostitutes were infected with syphilis in its primary or secondary stages.

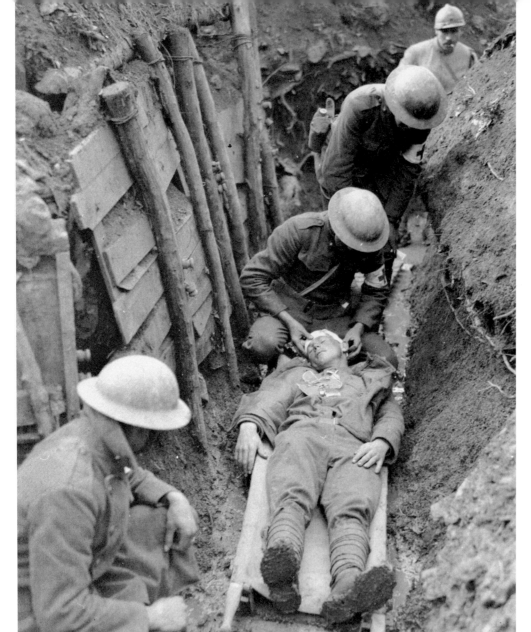

U.S. Marine receiving first aid before being sent to hospital in rear of trenches, Troyon Toulon Sector, Verdun, France. March 22, 1918. Navy medical personnel served with the Marine Brigade as part of the Army's 2d Infantry Division. *National Archives.*

World War I saw the birth of two specialties—aviation and submarine medicine. Both fields were logical consequences of the first extensive use of airplanes and submarines by the combatants. These new technologies would later keep many Navy personnel busy between the wars learning how to protect the human body in both hypobaric and hyperbaric environments.

HOSPITALS AND HOSPITAL SHIPS
To support the American Expeditionary Force, the Navy established five hospitals in Europe. They included Navy Base Hospital Nos. 1 and 5 at Brest, France; Navy Base Hospital No. 2 at Strathpeffer, Scotland; Navy Base Hospital No. 3 at Leith, Scotland; and Navy Base Hospital No. 4 at Queenstown, Ireland.

NAVY MEDICAL DEPARTMENT MEDAL OF HONOR RECIPIENTS IN WORLD WAR I

JOHN H. BALCH

JOEL T. BOONE, MC

DAVID E. HAYDEN

ALEXANDER G. LYLE, DC

WEEDON E. OSBORNE, DC

ORLANDO H. PETTY, MC

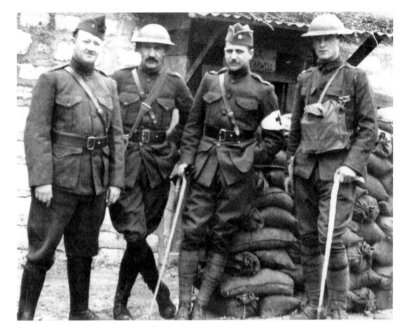

top
Navy Lieutenant Joel T. Boone, MC, second from right, 1918. Lieutenant Boone earned the Medal of Honor for conspicuous gallantry in action with the 6th Marine Regiment at Vierzy, France, on July 19, 1918. In later years, Boone served as White House physician for three presidents and in combat during World War II and the Korean War. *Naval Historical Foundation.*

bottom
World War I Navy nurse Hazel Herringshaw, wearing the indoor duty uniform with cape, flanked by two convalescing U.S. Marines. *Naval Historical Center.*

The base hospitals in Brest were especially notable. That city served as a major port where American troops disembarked and thousands of wounded were sent home. Navy Base Hospital No. 5 had a minimum capacity of 500 beds and, throughout the war, it averaged 400 patients. During the influenza epidemic, that number reached 800. The hospital had all the facilities necessary for providing advanced medical and surgical care, and received patients from other naval stations in France, from the Merchant Marine, and from U.S. naval facilities of all classes. The hospital remained in operation until March 1919.

The Navy added to its fleet of hospital ships in 1918 with the acquisition of two former steamships, the *Havana* and the *Saratoga*. They became the USNS *Comfort* (AH-3) and the USNS *Mercy* (AH-4), respectively. Although hospital ships were protected under the Geneva Conventions, Navy officials noted that the German government did not abide by these agreements. As a result, both vessels remained in American waters until the final month of the war when they were used as troop transports.

Navy medical personnel exhibited great valor during World War I. A total of 684 citations and awards were presented to the 331 Navy medical personnel who served in France. One such honoree was Navy Cross recipient Lena H. Sutcliffe Higbee, Superintendent of the Nurse Corps. When trained nurses were in short supply, she helped to pioneer a new training program to augment the supply of nurses being deployed to France. The Vassar Training Camp served as a finishing school for many of these nurses. During Higbee's tenure, the Navy Nurse Corps grew from 160 in April 1917 to 1,386 by November 1918.

A total of 60 Medical Corps officers, 12 Dental Corps officers, and 500 hospital corpsmen were assigned to field service with the Marine Corps. By the time the war ended in 1918, two physicians, two dentists, and two hospital corpsmen had earned the Medal of Honor.

Fighting in Europe ended with the signing of the Armistice in November 1918. The experience gained by Navy medical personnel in the Great War prepared them and their successors for multiple and varied challenges in the decades ahead.

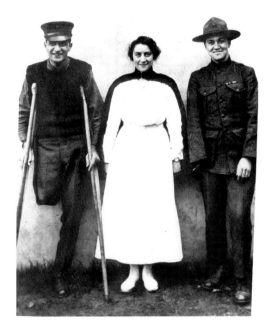

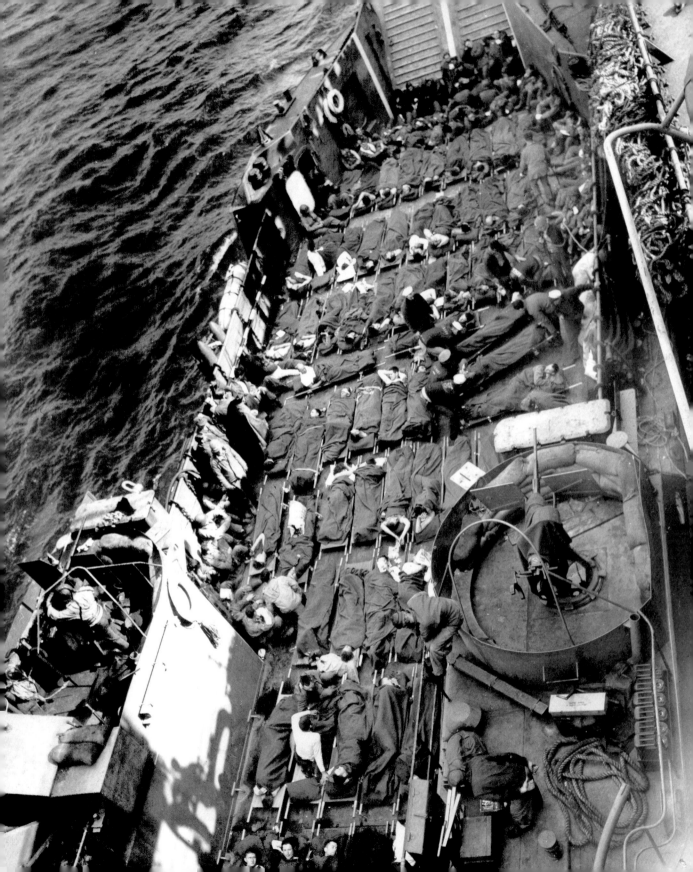

Chapter 5
Prewar Buildup and World War II in Europe, 1919–45

Rows and rows of wounded in stretchers cover the deck of a Coast Guard LCT (landing craft, tank) bringing out American and British troops from the beachheads of France. D-Day, June 6, 1944. *U.S. Coast Guard.*

SHRINK AND PREPARE

ACTIVITIES BETWEEN THE WARS

The medical departments of the armed forces dwindled in size in the two decades after World War I. However, the medics who remained in service applied the lessons learned in the war, supported U.S. military activities worldwide, contributed to medical advances, and prepared for the conflict that would soon engulf the entire nation.

Army and Navy medical personnel supported U.S. participation in postwar foreign interventions, including the Russian expeditions of 1918–20, and occupations in Haiti and Nicaragua. During the Haitian occupation (1915–34), Navy medical officers and hospital corpsmen served in the public health arm of the newly created Haitian gendarmerie, supervising drainage of low-lying areas, cleanup of streets, and control of disease-carrying mosquitoes.

During the interwar period, the United States was the only nation to maintain hospital ships. The aging and obsolete *Solace* was decommissioned in 1921 and replaced by the *Relief* (AH-1), the first U.S. vessel to be built as a hospital ship from the keel up and the second to carry the name. She was commissioned on December 28, 1920, with a bed capacity for 500 patients. The new *Relief* was also the first Navy hospital ship to allow Navy nurses aboard as regular staff.

In the 1920s and 1930s, the specialized field of aviation medicine developed in the United States and Europe. The U.S. Naval Medical School instituted a course in aviation medicine that addressed issues such as human endurance and adverse effects of accelerative forces, anoxia, fatigue, and psychological stress.

Meanwhile, Japanese aggression in the Far East and German armed expansion in Europe in the 1930s were harbingers of larger conflicts to come.

PREPARING FOR WAR

As war clouds darkened, President Franklin D. Roosevelt and military planners launched a preparedness program in early 1939. Germany's attack on Poland on September 1, 1939, ignited war in Europe and hastened American mobilization.

From June 1939 to June 1941, the number of active duty Navy physicians went from 841 to 1,957; its Dental Corps increased from 255 to 511; the Nurse Corps increased its rolls from 439 to 524; and the Hospital Corps grew from 4,467 to 10,547. By the summer of 1941, the Navy had 23 hospitals and two hospital ships in commission.

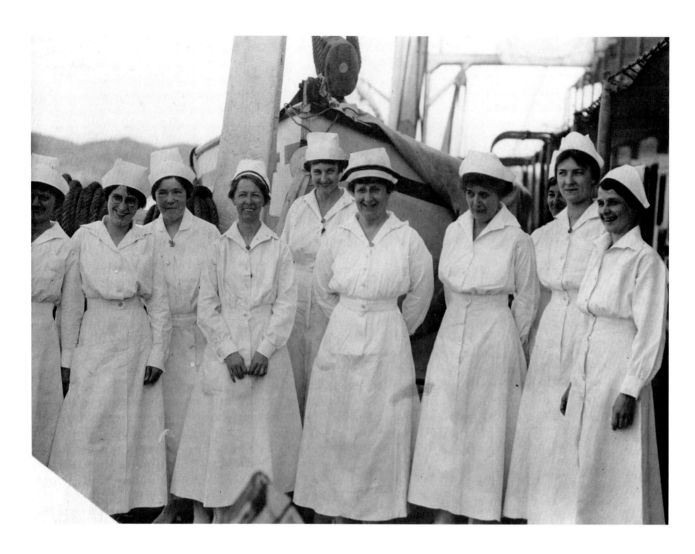

President Roosevelt approved the Victory Program in September 1941 that called for an army of 8,765,658 men and 215 divisions (only 90 divisions were actually fielded). When the Japanese attacked Pearl Harbor on December 7, 1941, the Army Medical Department counted 11,342 physicians, 7,043 nurses, and 107,867 enlisted men on active duty.

WARTIME EXPANSION

Following the Victory Program guidance, Army Surgeon General Major General James C. Magee (1939–43) shaped the wartime Medical Department. Throughout the war, Magee and his successor, Major General Norman T. Kirk (1943–47), constantly adjusted medical unit and personnel numbers in response to fluctuating troop numbers. The Medical Department reached its largest magnitude at 688,537 in August 1944 when enlisted strength peaked at 567,268. The officer strength peaked in July 1945 at 145,342. Among the number were 47,990 Medical Corps, 14,325 Dental Corps, 19,848 Medical Administrative Corps (MAC), and 55,702 Army Nurse Corps.

Combat forces, service forces, and the training base required hundreds of medical units. Station hospitals and named general hospitals operated in the continental United States, where, by 1945, 66 general hospitals provided more than 150,000 beds. Overseas, there were station and numbered general hospitals and divisional and non-divisional field medical units.

Reserves again reinforced the Army's mobilization efforts. By mid-1941, 8,025 reserve medical officers served on extended active duty when the regular Army had only 1,210 medical officers. The prewar mobilization would have been impossible without these dedicated reservists, many of them World War I veterans. In 1922, the War Department reinstituted the "affiliated" reserve hospital program. However, it faded away before revitalization in 1939. By June 1941, 41 general, 11 evacuation, and four surgical hospitals were formed in this program, and 52 general and 20 evacuation hospitals served in all theaters during the war.

Nursing staff aboard USS *Relief* (AH-1), circa 1920. Principal Chief Nurse J. Beatrice Bowman stands in center, fourth from right. Bowman served as Superintendent of the Navy Nurse Corps from 1922–35. She was the last of "The Sacred Twenty" Navy Nurses on active duty. *Naval Historical Center.*

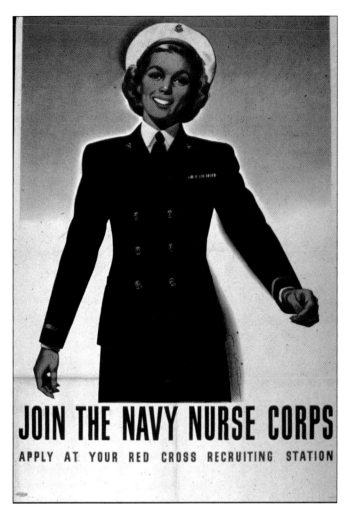

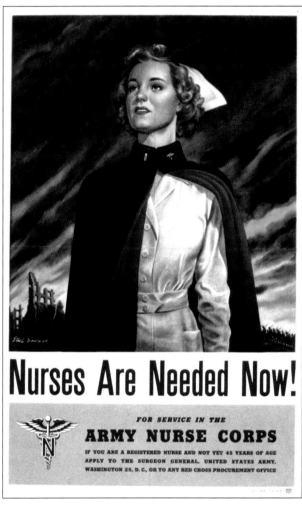

top
"Join the Navy Nurse Corps." Navy nurse recruiting poster of World War II. Five hundred and twenty-four women staffed the Navy Nurse Corps in June 1941. *National Archives.*

right
"Nurses are needed now." World War II Army Nurse recruiting poster. The Army had 7,043 nurses when the war began. *National Archives.*

The enormous requirements of the war led to creation of several new corps in the Medical Department as well as changes within existing corps. Dietitians and physical therapists, previously civilian employees, formed the Women's Medical Specialist Corps in 1942 and attained full commissioned officer status along with Army nurses in 1944. In 1943, Congress created the Pharmacy Corps of 72 officers. To free Medical Corps officers for strictly professional work, MAC officers. The MAC grew from 1,048 regulars and reservists on active duty in June 1941 to 19,848 in July 1945. MAC officers took over positions in hospital administration, personnel, medical procurement and logistics, and field units. By 1944, trained MAC officers were replacing medical and dental officers as assistant battalion surgeons throughout the Army.

RESTRUCTURING THE FIELD MEDICAL FORCE

Combat experience in World War I proved the inadequacy of medical support at the regiment and division levels. Beginning in 1920 and continuing through the outbreak of the war, a series of reorganizations reshaped the infantry division and its medical component to provide better medical support under the division surgeon. When finalized in 1942, medical personnel were completely integrated into combat units to provide life-saving medical attention and first aid.

These changes gave infantry regiments organic medical detachments of 10 officers and 126 enlisted men, known as aidmen or medics. In each regiment's three battalions, a battalion surgeon and assistant battalion surgeon commanded medical units of two officers and 36 enlisted men. They set up the battalion aid station during military operations, and directed the work of 13 medics in the battalion's four line companies and anti-tank platoon, plus 12 litter bearers.

During the interwar years, the division's sanitary train became a medical regiment and then a divisional medical battalion aligned to support the new smaller, triangular division. The new battalions consisted of three collecting companies which supported each of the regiments. They transported the wounded and sick from battalion and regimental aid stations to the battalion's fourth company, the divisional clearing station. From there, the wounded were moved to field and evacuation hospitals under corps and Army control.

A similar structure evolved in the new armored divisions, with armored medical battalions providing the divisional medical support. The smaller airborne divisions had a divisional airborne medical company plus organic medical detachments in the parachute infantry and glider infantry regiments.

The evacuation hospital provided critical care in the combat zone. In the rear areas, the 1,000-bed general hospital replaced the former base hospital, offering fixed facilities that provided definitive treatment. Convalescent hospitals with 3,000 beds, under the direction of the field Army surgeon, cared for minor sick and wounded soldiers until they could return to their units.

ADAPTING HOSPITALS TO DEMANDS

Modern mechanized mobile warfare posed new challenges for the Surgeon General's Office in the years immediately preceding American entry into World War II. By 1941, it had developed three types of "mobile hospitals" for the field armies—a surgical hospital, an evacuation hospital, and a convalescent hospital—all of which were able to move rapidly to accompany the mechanized forces.

Pearl Harbor changed everything. In January 1942, the War Department General Staff demanded an "island-type hospital," a smaller and more mobile unit to meet the demands of amphibious warfare and mechanized operations on land. The resulting 400-bed field hospital of February 1942 consisted of a headquarters and three hospital platoons and was transportable by air. When reinforced with surgical personnel, it could support either ground combat forces or an amphibious task force. The 1942 field hospital was more flexible than any existing hospital.

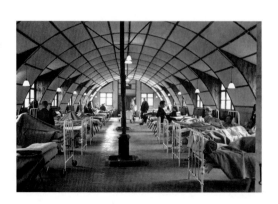

right
Captain W. Lester Henry, Jr., surgeon of the 317th Collecting Station, 92d Infantry Division, stitches the wound of Captain Ezekia Smith, 370th Infantry Regiment. Smith received shell fragments in his face and shoulders in fighting near Querceta, Italy, February 10, 1945. *National Archives.*

bottom left
A typical medical ward of the 2d Evacuation Hospital in Diddington, England, June 3, 1943. *National Archives.*

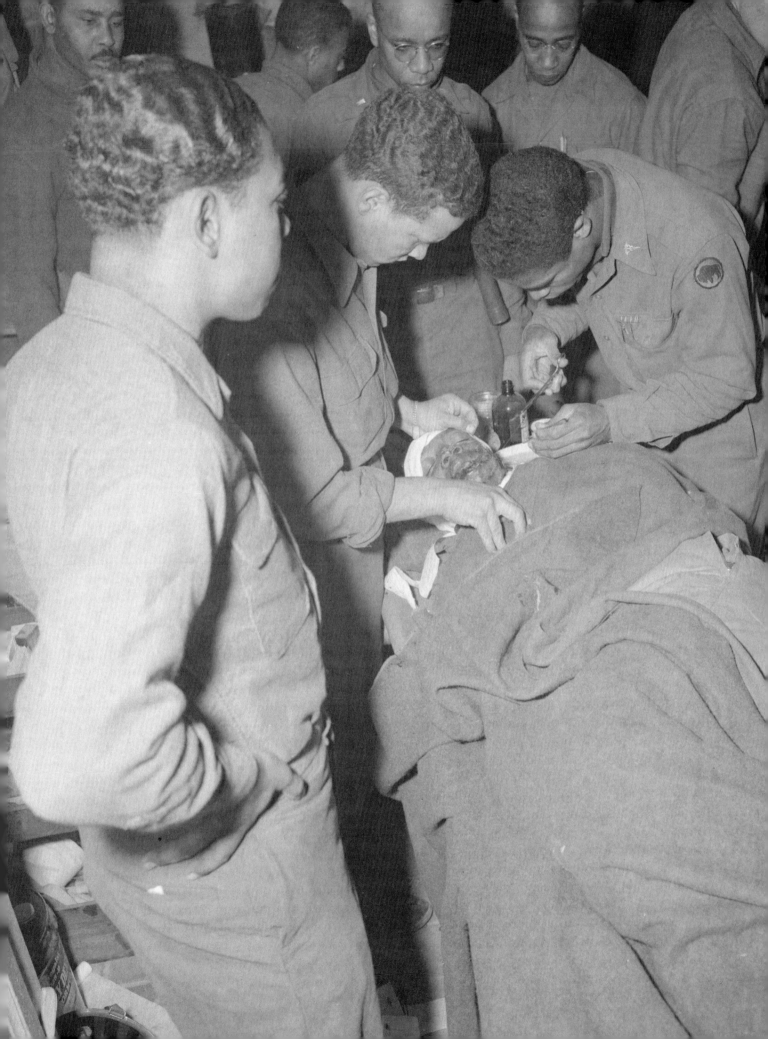

A new evacuation hospital (motorized) was developed in mid-1942. With 36 organic vehicles, the new hospital could move all of its personnel and equipment at one time. By the end of 1942, the Surgeon General's visions of completely mobile field hospitals in the field medical service evaporated. Due to a lack of trucks and shipping spaces, the General Staff cut the number of vehicles. Thus, the evacuation hospital (motorized) became the evacuation hospital (semi-mobile), and the field hospital was also reduced.

Another important unit, the auxiliary surgical group (ASG), was developed within the Surgical Consultants Division of the Office of the Surgeon General in 1942. The ASG was designed as a surgical reserve to be allocated at one per field army to augment the field and evacuation hospital. Six were eventually formed—five served in the European Theater (1st, 3d, 4th, 5th, and 6th ASGs) and the 2d ASG in the Mediterranean. The Surgical Consultants Division handpicked the surgeons based on their surgical experience. Each group had 61 four- to six-person teams in general, orthopedic, maxillofacial, neurological, and thoracic surgery and treatment for shock.

The Consultants Division assembled some of the best medical and surgical men to advise and work with the consultants in each theater and Army. Colonel Edward D. Churchill, from Harvard Medical School and surgical consultant for the Fifth U.S. Army in Italy, analyzed resuscitation and combat surgery from Tunisia onward and developed standardized procedures for use in the Mediterranean Theater. In Washington, surgeon Lieutenant Colonel Michael E. DeBakey realized the value of an Army-wide standardized approach to surgical cases. Working with Churchill, in March 1945 DeBakey produced Technical Bulletin Medical 147 and, for the first time, established Army-wide standards of practice for the surgical care of battle casualties.

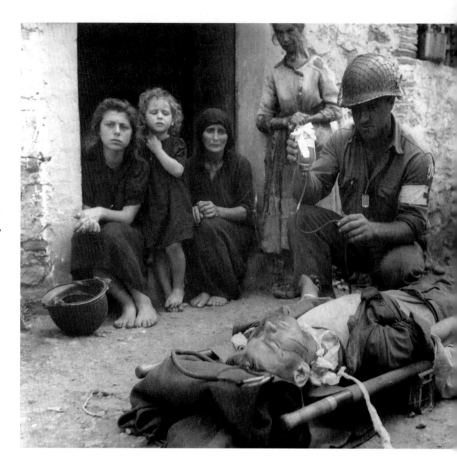

NEW DEVELOPMENTS: SULFA DRUGS, PENICILLIN, ATABRINE, AND BLOOD

For centuries, wound infection was the most persistent problem for combat surgeons. The drugs based on sulfonamide that were developed in the 1930s—sulfanilamide, sulfathiazole, sulfadiazine, and others—controlled some infections, but all had their limitations. Nevertheless, sulfadiazine tablets and sulfanilamide powder were included in each soldier's first aid packet.

The real revolution in infection control came with the introduction of penicillin, which entered large-scale military distribution in 1944. Once available in quantity, penicillin proved extremely effective against a wide spectrum of infections. By the end of the war, this wonder drug had largely eradicated the problem of wound infection. Penicillin also proved to be the most effective weapon in the military's age-old battle against venereal disease. The Army and Navy both adopted penicillin for routine and swift treatment of syphilis in June 1944.

From the outset, it was clear that preventive medicine would be more critical than ever for American forces that would fight in some of the world's most disease-prone places. In

Private First Class Harvey White of Minneapolis, Minnesota, administers blood plasma to Private Roy Humphrey of Toledo, Ohio, who was wounded by shrapnel on August 9, 1943, in Sicily. *National Archives.*

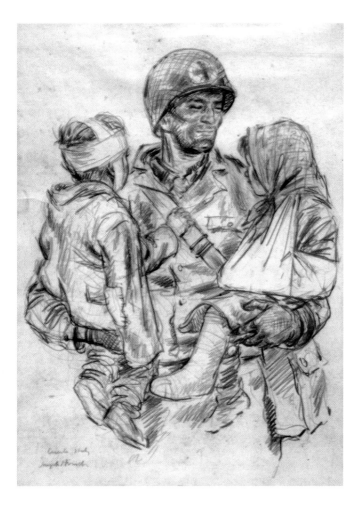

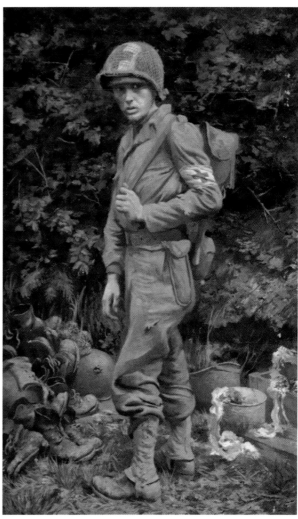

left
"Safe," by Joseph Hirsh.
A World War II medical
corpsman comforts
two orphans at Cassino,
Italy. 1944. *U.S. Army Art
Collection.*

right
"The Man Without a
Gun." A combat medic
shows fatigue and
determination. World
War II. *U.S. Army Art
Collection.*

tropical areas, malaria and other indigenous diseases presented the gravest threats. The Japanese seizure of the Netherlands East Indies early in 1942 deprived the Allies of the largest source of the antimalarial, quinine. Fortunately, the Germans had developed synthetic quinine called Atabrine™ that was effective in suppressing malaria. Atabrine™ was quickly put into mass production and became the standard antimalarial drug during the war.

The Army had used blood transfusions sparingly in World War I. During the interwar years, while studying blood and blood substitutes, the work produced blood plasma, thought to be a remedy to the problems of blood loss and shock resulting from wounding and surgery. Early experience in Tunisia indicated that plasma use was not as effective as first believed, and the medics turned to blood again. The frequent use of plasma and whole blood to maintain blood pressure and to counter shock in wounded soldiers and in subsequent surgeries was one of the most significant developments of the war.

EUROPEAN WAR RECEIVES PRIORITY

The Allies gave overriding priority to defeating Nazi Germany and Italy in Europe. Amphibious and airborne operations in North Africa and the Mediterranean were undertaken before landing on the European continent. The Medical Department was ready but untested for those first operations.

Medical support quickly proved its strengths and weaknesses during the fighting in Tunisia in 1942–43. Mobile hospitals were located too far from the front; thus, the clearing companies absorbed a far heavier surgical load than planned. When plasma was found to be lacking as a substitute for blood in combat surgery, informal blood banks were set up. Critical combat exhaustion and psychiatric problems occurred. A program of rest, sedation, and psychiatric treatment at a frontline hospital was developed that resulted in returning many patients to their units rather than evacuating them as before.

The medics proved highly effective in saving the lives of many wounded men. They stopped bleeding, applied tourniquets, bandaged wounds, administered morphine, gave plasma and later blood, prepared emergency medical tags, and stabilized patients so litter bearers could move them to battalion aid stations. However, the medics suffered a high attrition rate by helping wounded men caught in enemy fire. Soldiers screaming "medic, medic!" caused many a medic to be wounded or killed. Battalion and regimental surgeons advised their medics to wait until the firing stopped before exposing themselves to give aid to the stricken men, but training and human instinct often took over. Due to their high casualty rate, trained medics were increasingly scarce in frontline units toward the end of the war.

Medical support for airborne operations was tested in the invasion of Sicily on July 10, 1943. Medical detachment personnel completed jump training and went in with the paratroopers of the 82d Airborne Division in the combat drop.

The subsequent Italian campaign was difficult due to the mountainous terrain, weather, and tenacious German defense. The landings at Salerno in September 1943 and Anzio in January 1944 required significant medical involvement.

The Anzio beachhead became a story of trial and tragedy for medical personnel. On January 30, 1944, Private First Class Lloyd C. Hawks, a medic with the 30th Infantry Regiment, 3d Infantry Division, received the only Medal of Honor awarded to a medic in the Mediterranean Theater for his heroism at Carano.

The 56th, 93d, and 95th Evacuation Hospitals and 33d Field Hospital were in the beachhead supporting the 3d Infantry Division and the rest of the VI Corps. German shelling and bombing were constant threats. On February 7, 1944, enemy bombs hit the crowded 95th Evacuation

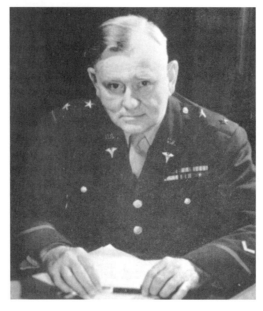

Hospital, wounding 64 and killing 26, including three nurses, two medical officers, a Red Cross worker, 14 enlisted men, and six patients. On February 9, German artillery fire killed Colonel Jarrett M. Huddleston, the VI Corps surgeon, as he left corps headquarters. The next day heavy German artillery fire hit the 33d Field Hospital. First Lieutenants Mary L. Roberts, Rita V. Rourke, and Elaine A. Roe became the first nurses and women to receive the Silver Star Medal for their heroic efforts that day.

THE EUROPEAN THEATER

Major General Paul R. Hawley, MC, the chief surgeon of the European Theater of Operations, was responsible for medical preparations and planning for the Army's campaign on the continent and maintenance of the troops' health. From 1942 on, he and his staff oversaw all medical support for an American ground force that by May 1945 had grown to two Army groups (6th and 12th), five armies (First, Third, Seventh, Ninth, and Fifteenth), 15 corps, and 61 armored, airborne, and infantry divisions.

Medical support for the invasion of France in Operation Overlord was meticulously planned and successfully executed, both in the amphibious landings on Utah and Omaha beaches and the night drops by paratroopers of the 82d and 101st Airborne Divisions. Medics jumped with the paratroopers, and two surgical teams of the 3d Auxiliary Surgical Group flew in on the first gliders of the 101st.

left
Major General Paul R. Hawley, MC, chief surgeon, European Theater of Operations. *National Archives.*

right
Major General John P. Lucas, then Commander, VI Corps, Fifth U.S. Army, presents Silver Star Medals to, left to right, Army Nurse Corps Lieutenants Mary L. Roberts of the 56th Evacuation Hospital, and Elaine A. Roe and Rita V. Rourke of the 33d Field Hospital. They are the first women in the history of the U.S. Army to receive the Silver Star. March 16, 1944. *National Archives.*

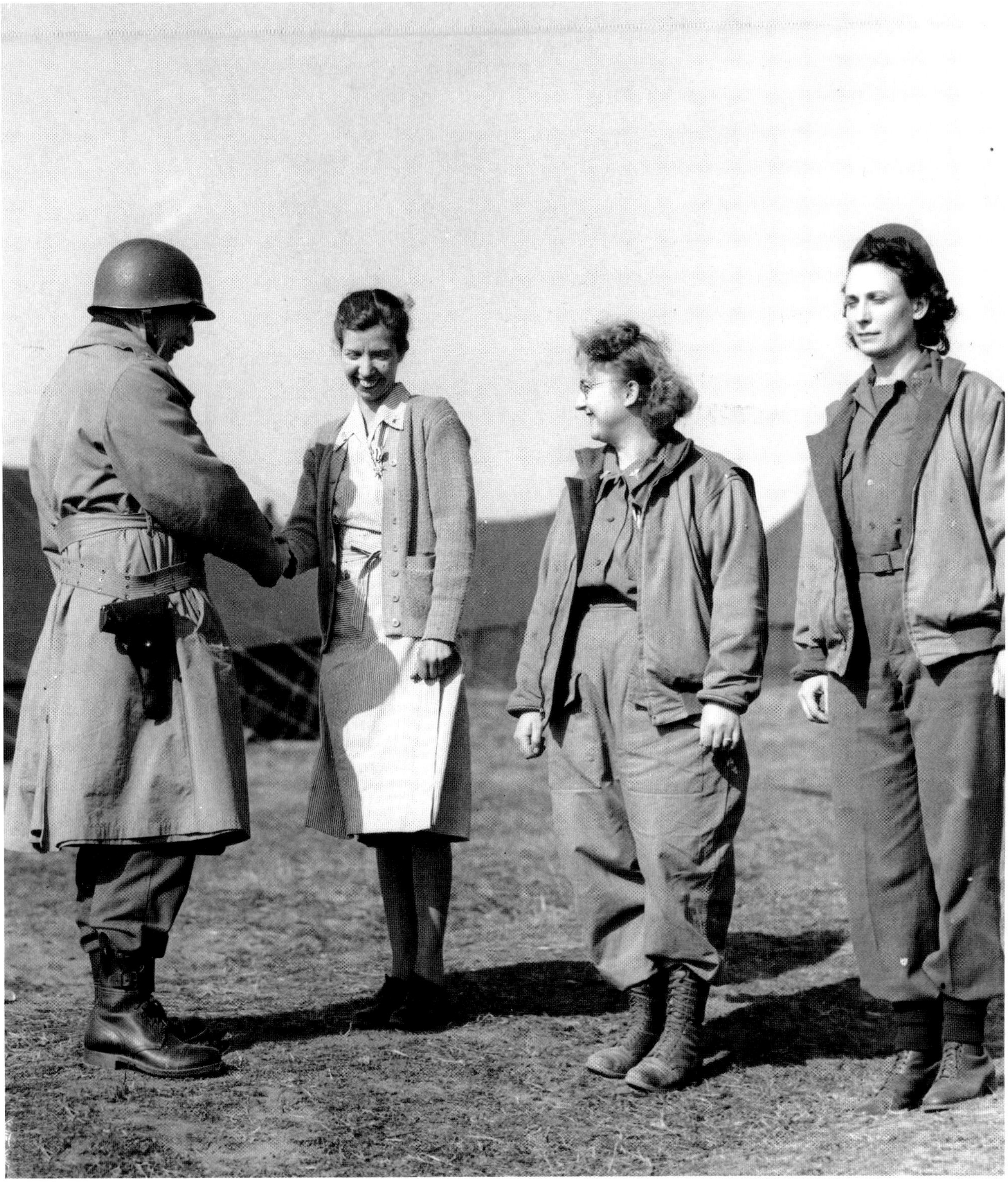

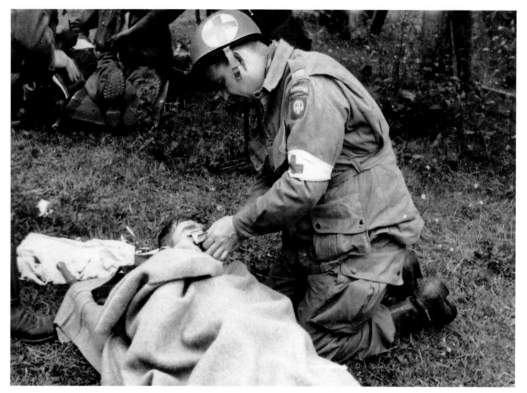

On the fire-swept D-Day beaches regimental and battalion surgeons and enlisted medics of the 1st, 4th, and 29th Infantry Divisions and 5th and 6th Engineer Special Brigades were everywhere. Many were killed or wounded, along with medical personnel of the Navy beach battalions. The Medical Detachment of the 16th Infantry Regiment, 1st Infantry Division, suffered seven medics killed in action and two officers and 25 medics wounded. For their actions that day, the detachment received three Distinguished Service Crosses and 25 Silver Star Medals (two posthumous).

Hospital units followed immediately behind the assault echelons to provide urgently needed surgical care. The 13th and 51st Field Hospitals landed and were operational on Omaha Beach by D + 4 (June 10). The 45th Field Hospital came ashore at Utah Beach on D + 4 (June 10), and the 42d Field and 128th Evacuation hospitals were handling patients on Utah Beach on D + 5 (June 11).

After the breakout from the Normandy Beachhead in July–August 1944, it became standard practice on the continent to attach a field hospital platoon to each division clearing station, and in heavy action to augment them with several general surgery and shock teams from an auxiliary surgical group. When casualty flows became very heavy, such as during the Hürtgen Forest fighting or the Battle of the Bulge, the Army surgeons sent in more teams.

At the next echelon, evacuation hospitals often became overworked when casualties were coming in constantly at 100–150 and more per day. In such situations Army surgeons reinforced them with surgical teams from auxiliary surgical groups and inactive general hospitals.

Surgical teams also augmented organic medical support in operations where the wounded could not be readily evacuated. In addition to Normandy, they participated in airborne operations in Operations Market-Garden in Holland (September 1944) and Varsity across the Rhine River (March 1945). Even during these offensive operations, definitive surgery was performed much closer to the front line than previously believed possible.

By April 1945, more than three million soldiers in Europe were supported by 258,000 medical personnel, including 15,785 medical officers, 17,897 nurses, and 212,655 enlisted men. An imposing medical structure was built—65 evacuation hospitals (22,800 beds), 48 field hospitals (19,200 beds), 146 general hospitals (155,000 beds), 49 station hospitals (27,050 beds), and 10 convalescent facilities (28,000 beds)—a total of 318 hospitals and 252,050 beds.

left
Medical officer of the 82d Airborne Division lights a cigarette for a wounded paratrooper, Ste. Mere Eglise, France, June 12, 1944. *National Archives.*

top right
U.S. Army nurse Second Lieutenant Frances Y. Slanger of Boston, Massachusetts, takes time from her arduous duties at the 45th Field Hospital in Normandy to fix her hair. June 15, 1944. She was one of the first Army nurses to land in France on June 10, four days after the D-Day assault. Second Lieutenant Slanger was the first Army nurse killed in action in the European Theater. An Army hospital ship was named in her honor. *National Archives.*

bottom right
Army nurse administers nighttime transfusion in frontline hospital, France, 1944. *National Archives.*

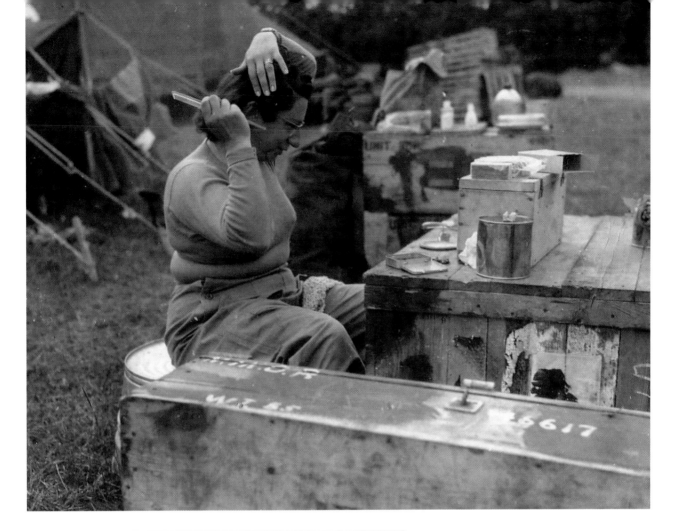

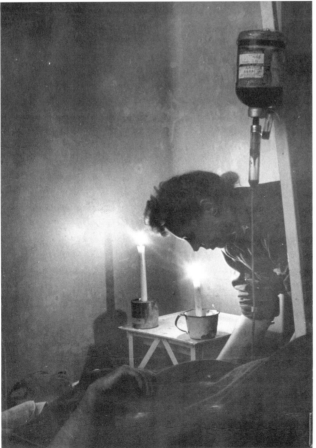

More than 231,000 seriously wounded and sick patients who would not serve again were evacuated to the United States by hospital ship and airplane from the United Kingdom and the continent. From 1942 to 1945, Army medical personnel treated 2,306,734 disease and non-battle injury cases of which only 15,097 died and disease deaths numbered 2,314 for a rate of 0.1 percent. Of 393,987 battle casualties treated, 12,523 died for a rate of 3.2 percent—the lowest yet attained.

Army medics paid a high price for combat success. Medical personnel suffered 14,589 battle casualties, of which 2,265 were killed in action (99 officers and 2,166 enlisted men) and 498 died of their wounds (29 officers and 469 enlisted men), and another 11,826 were wounded. Medics in the European Theater received six Medals of Honor, three of them posthumously. One was awarded belatedly to Technician 5 James K. Okubo of the Japanese-American 442d Regimental Combat Team in 2000, 33 years after his death in 1967.

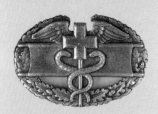

In October 1943, the War Department authorized the Expert Infantryman Badge (EIB) and the Combat Infantryman Badge (CIB) in recognition of frontline service in combat. In June 1944, the Congress awarded an extra $5 pay a month for holders of the EIB and $10 to the CIB. Many in the Medical Department thought that medics who shared the same frontline dangers as the infantrymen should also receive a badge and extra pay. The Surgeon General strongly advocated action on such an award. On January 29, 1945, the War Department authorized a Medical Badge for company grade officers, warrant officers, and enlisted personnel who were "daily sharing with the infantry the hazards and hardships of combat." Congress later in 1945 authorized an additional $10 monthly pay for all wearers of what became the Combat Medical Badge (CMB) except officers. After Operations Desert Shield/Desert Storm, the Army expanded its award provisions to include medics serving in armored and armored cavalry units as well as Navy and Air Force medical personnel assigned to Army units in ground combat. The CMB is one of the most coveted awards that Army medics can receive and testifies to their primary mission in support of the American combat soldier.

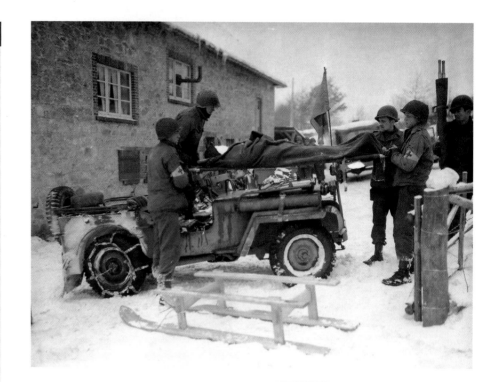

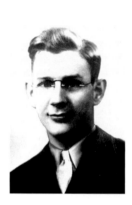

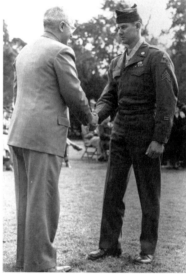

top left
Wounded soldier who was brought in by ski litter is placed on Jeep for evacuation. Medics are from 1st Battalion, 119th Infantry Regiment, 30th Infantry Division. Belgium, January, 1945. *National Archives.*

bottom far left
Private First Class Frederick C. Murphy, a combat medic of the 259th Infantry Regiment, 65th Infantry Division, received the Medal of Honor posthumously for his gallant actions on March 18, 1945. During an attack on the fortified Siegfried Line, although wounded himself, he continued onward to give aid to his comrades. He was mortally wounded by an antipersonnel mine while attempting to treat another soldier. *National Archives.*

The experience of one unit epitomizes the sacrifice of the frontline medics who so often shared the fate of the soldiers they served. The medical detachment of the 60th Infantry Regiment, 9th Infantry Division, landed in Normandy on June 14, 1944, and saw extensive combat thereafter. Through the end of December, it had 25 men killed in action, 125 wounded or injured in action, nine died of wounds, and 23 missing in action.

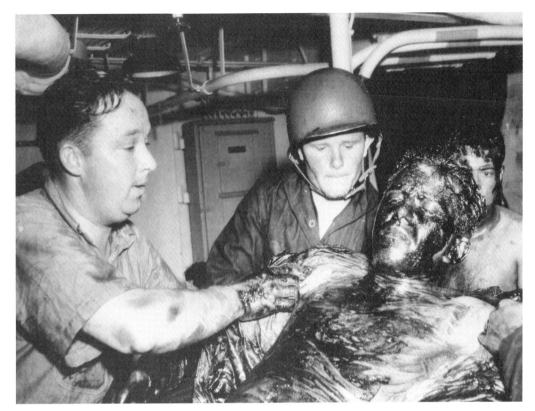

right
Two Coast Guardsmen scrape a thick coating of oil from a U.S. Navy sailor. The survivor's ship, the USS *Lansdale*, was sunk by Nazi planes off the coast of North Africa. April 1944.
U.S. Coast Guard.

NAVY MEDICINE IN THE EUROPEAN THEATER

MAINTAIN THE FIGHTING FORCE

"To keep as many men at as many guns for as many days as possible," was the Navy Medical Department's fighting motto during World War II. The ultimate purpose of military medicine during this conflict was the same as in previous wars; to conserve the strength and efficiency of the fighting forces. Navy medical personnel worked diligently to accomplish that goal.

From an aggregate strength of 13,500 personnel on December 7, 1941, the Navy Medical Department ranks mushroomed to 169,000 personnel in 1945. They staffed 56 hospitals in the continental United States, 12 fleet hospitals, 16 base hospitals, 14 convalescent hospitals, 15 hospital ships, five special augmented hospitals, and many dispensaries.

The enormous commitment to winning the war required all these resources. The nature of conflict between 1941 and 1945 was worsened by the nature of the weapons used by the combatants. World War I had seen the widespread use of machine guns, submarines, airplanes, and tanks. World War II saw these weapons reach unimagined perfection as killing machines.

opposite page
bottom left
President Harry S Truman congratulates Sergeant Thomas J. Kelly after presenting him with the Medal of Honor, earned for exceptional gallantry in Germany on April 5, 1945. Kelly, then a corporal and medic with the 48th Armored Infantry Battalion of the 7th Armored Division, made 10 separate trips through brutal German machine gun fire, each time bringing out a wounded soldier.
National Archives.

The story of Navy medicine in World War II is primarily a story of the Pacific War. However, the Navy played a key role in the liberation of North Africa, Italy, and France, while fighting the U-boat menace in the North Atlantic and escorting convoys to Britain and Russia.

Navy forces' successful participation in the amphibious operations in North Africa and the Mediterranean led to even more significant results in Operation Overlord, the invasion of France that began on June 6, 1944. Navy ships and personnel conveyed the Army soldiers and their equipment from England. Navy battleships, cruisers, destroyers, and rocket-firing amphibious assault vessels pounded German fortifications and cleared the way into the beaches.

Navy personnel were also present on the Normandy shore. These were the men of the 2d, 6th, and 7th Naval Beach Battalions. Their unique skills were essential for the invasion's success. Their mission was to bridge the gap between sea and land and perform other essential functions on the invasion beaches, to include treating and evacuating casualties.

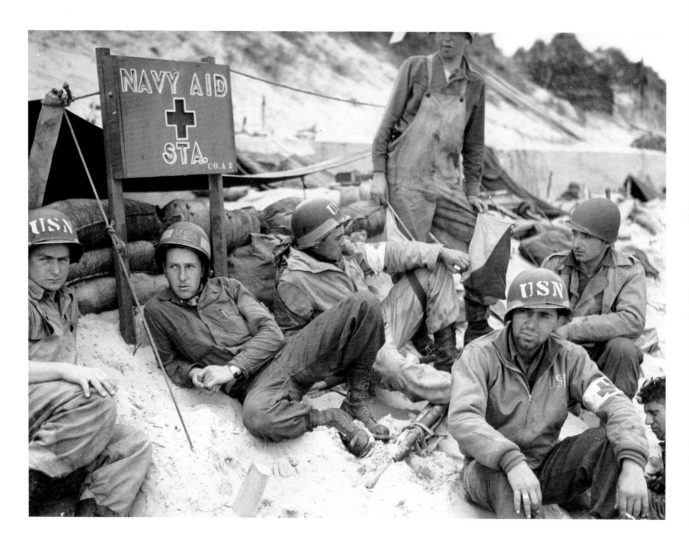

The caregivers—the physicians and hospital corpsmen—coped with penetrating wounds to the head, face, neck, and extremities; fractures; burns; and blast injuries.

As the first American troops went ashore at Omaha and Utah beaches, Navy medical personnel, dressed as soldiers, were indistinguishable from their Army counterparts. They performed bravely and efficiently, rendering first aid to American personnel, whether soldiers or sailors. Physicians provided rudimentary care where possible. Equipped with litters, hospital corpsmen administered first aid—a battle dressing, a tourniquet, a morphine injection, and a casualty tag—and then moved the wounded down to the water's edge to be evacuated aboard empty landing craft heading back to the transports. When that was not feasible, they sought shelter and set up aid stations on the beach above the high tide line.

The Navy also returned the casualties from Normandy to Britain. Once evacuated from the American sectors of Utah and Omaha beaches

aboard landing craft, the wounded were transferred to specially equipped LCTs (landing craft, tank) and LSTs (landing ship, tank) staffed by physicians and hospital corpsmen. Each LST had special brackets to accommodate 147 litters arranged in tiers three high on their tank decks. Two Navy physicians, one Army surgeon, two Army operating room technicians, and 40 Navy hospital corpsmen staffed these versatile ships. They were equipped for providing first aid, stabilization, and an occasional surgery.

Once safely back in Britain, Navy medical personnel, including nurses, triaged patients, conducted emergency surgery, and stabilized the injured until they could be evacuated to other hospitals in Britain or back to the United States for more definitive treatment.

One of the hospitals designated to care for the casualties of the D-Day invasion was Navy Base Hospital No. 12. It occupied the 1,000-bed Royal Victoria Hospital at Netley, adjacent to the major channel port of Southampton. U.S.

top left
Navy Hospital Corpsmen prepared to receive casualties at Navy Aid Station, Utah Beach, D-Day 1944. *U.S. Navy Bureau of Medicine and Surgery.*

top right
D-Day, June 6, 1944. Casualties of the fighting between German and American forces at Omaha Beach have received immediate medical attention and await evacuation to a field hospital. *National Archives.*

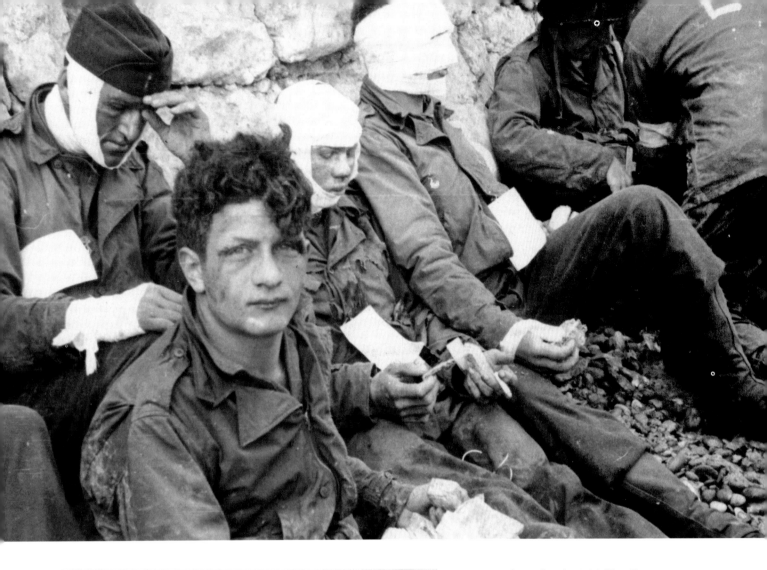

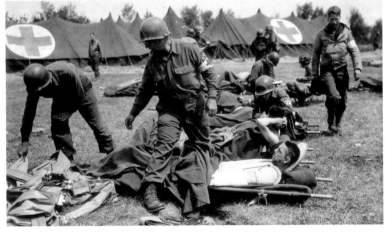

above
U.S. Army medics at a beachhead field hospital in Normandy make patients comfortable and issue life belts to them in preparation to board ships for evacuation to England. June 11, 1944. *National Archives.*

Navy physicians, nurses, and hospital corpsmen operated on patients night and day for the better part of a week after the initial landings. Their dedication and skill guaranteed that 97 percent of the wounded would live—a remarkable statistic.

Seventeen days after the initial landings at Normandy, the casualty evacuation system worked smoothly enough that the naval beach battalions returned to Britain. Although their mission was completed, the cost had been heavy for these brave physicians and hospital corpsmen. Two physicians and 20 corpsmen of the 6th Naval Beach Battalion were killed in action. The 7th Naval Beach Battalion lost a physician and 10 corpsmen. At Utah Beach, the 2d Naval Beach Battalion lost one physician and seven hospital corpsmen. These Navy medical personnel helped ensure the success of what General Dwight D. Eisenhower called the "Great Crusade."

Although Navy medical personnel were also present during the later capture of Cherbourg and August 1944 landings on the French Mediterranean coast, for the most part Navy medicine's contributions to the liberation of Europe were over. The war against Japan remained the major focus of the Navy's attention.

ARMY AIR FORCES MEDICAL SERVICE

AVIATION MEDICINE, RESEARCH, AND TRAINING
During World War II, the doctors, nurses, and other medics assigned to the U.S. Army Air Forces (AAF) practiced aviation medicine in multiple fields. The AAF medical service helped to select the most qualified young volunteers to become pilots of combat aircraft. Both in the United States and abroad, the medical service gave specialized treatment, rehabilitation, and convalescent care to American and Allied aviators. The service ran an aeromedical evacuation system that served the sick and injured on combat fronts. It also trained newly selected AAF doctors, nurses, and medical technicians in the special techniques of military and aviation medicine. And it contributed to aeromedical research.

Aeromedical research was a truly national program, involving even civilian institutions. Among the research studies were those dealing with the physiology of flight and the design of aircraft instrumentation and aircrew support systems. A high priority was assigned to improved oxygen equipment and pressurized cabins for bombers. By the end of the war, the first successful G-suits were produced, safer bailout methods were explored, and a night vision training program was started. Advances were achieved with cooperation of researchers in Allied countries, civilian contract researchers, and specialists of the U.S. Navy.

The Naval Medical Research Institute supplemented work performed by the AAF's School of Aviation Medicine and the Wright Field Aeromedical Research Laboratory. In the field of patient convalescence, the AAF inaugurated treatment that stressed early patient involvement in work-related training programs. AAF patients returned to duty much faster than patients who were less active when recuperating.

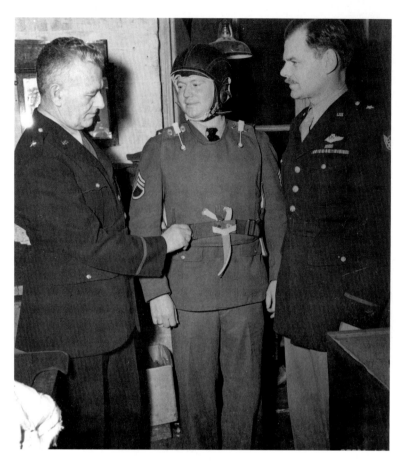

AEROMEDICAL EVACUATION DEVELOPS
In November 1942, at Bowman Field near Louisville, Kentucky, training began for the medics who would form the new AAF aeromedical squadrons. An aeromedical squadron consisted of several flights, each with a surgeon, nurses, and technicians. A squadron had no aircraft of its own. Its members boarded returning Air Transport Command aircraft and helped load them with sick, wounded, and injured casualties. The first squadrons deployed early in 1943. Some went to the Pacific and some to North Africa, where the American and Allied troops soon needed aeromedical evacuation.

Brigadier General Malcolm C. Grow, left, surgeon of the Eighth Air Force, developed flak jackets to protect bomber crews. His jackets saved hundreds of lives. Brigadier General Leon W. Johnson observes. England, 1944. *U.S. Air Force Medical Service.*

Flight nurse First Lieutenant (later Captain) Lillian Kinkella Keil made 250 medical evacuation flights in the European Theater, including 23 transatlantic. She served again during the Korean War, flying 175 aerial evacuations in that conflict. *U.S. Air Force.*

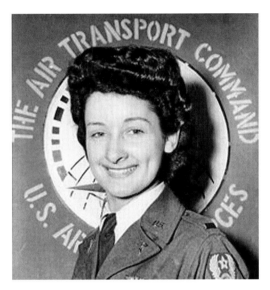

In mid-January 1943, American forces pushed eastward into southern Tunisia where there were few hospitals, roads, or railways. Motor ambulances took 12 to 15 hours to reach the nearest major medical facility in Constantine, Algeria. Hospital trains required 20 to 24 hours. But air evacuation took only one hour, and larger hospitals in Algiers and Oran were only one-and-one-half hours away. In the last push on Bizerte in early May 1943, most patients were evacuated by air. The more serious casualties departed on air ambulances; patients with minor injuries left on transport planes. Although still new and undeveloped in some respects, aeromedical evacuation quickly proved its worth.

The C-47 transport aircraft's success as the aeromedical workhorse in Tunisia and the Allied campaigns in Sicily and Italy was replicated globally. Most C-47 transports carried an evacuation kit containing blood plasma, oxygen, morphine, portable heaters, first aid medicine, and various bandages to control hemorrhages. Flight surgeons selected patients for air evacuation and also accompanied some flights with seriously ill or injured patients.

The standard evacuation flight crew consisted of medical technicians and flight nurses. Many of the nurses had been airline stewardesses before the war. The C-47 usually carried 18 litter patients.

By the end of 1943, the AAF aeromedical evacuation system was ready to assume larger responsibilities in Operation Overlord. The Normandy invasion and the concluding attack on Germany produced the largest, most intense aeromedical evacuation operations of the war. Total AAF aeromedical evacuations more than doubled from June 1944 to May 1945. When European hospitals filled to capacity during the Battle of the Bulge in the winter of 1944–45, patients flew directly to Mitchel Field, New York, only three days after they were wounded.

The benefits of aeromedical evacuation during the campaigns in Europe proved equally invaluable in the Asian and Pacific theaters.

ARMY MEDICAL DEPARTMENT MEDAL OF HONOR RECIPIENTS IN WORLD WAR II–EUROPE

HAROLD A. GARMAN

THOMAS J. KELLY

WILLIAM D. MCGEE

FREDERICK C. MURPHY

JAMES K. OKUBO

ALFRED L. WILSON

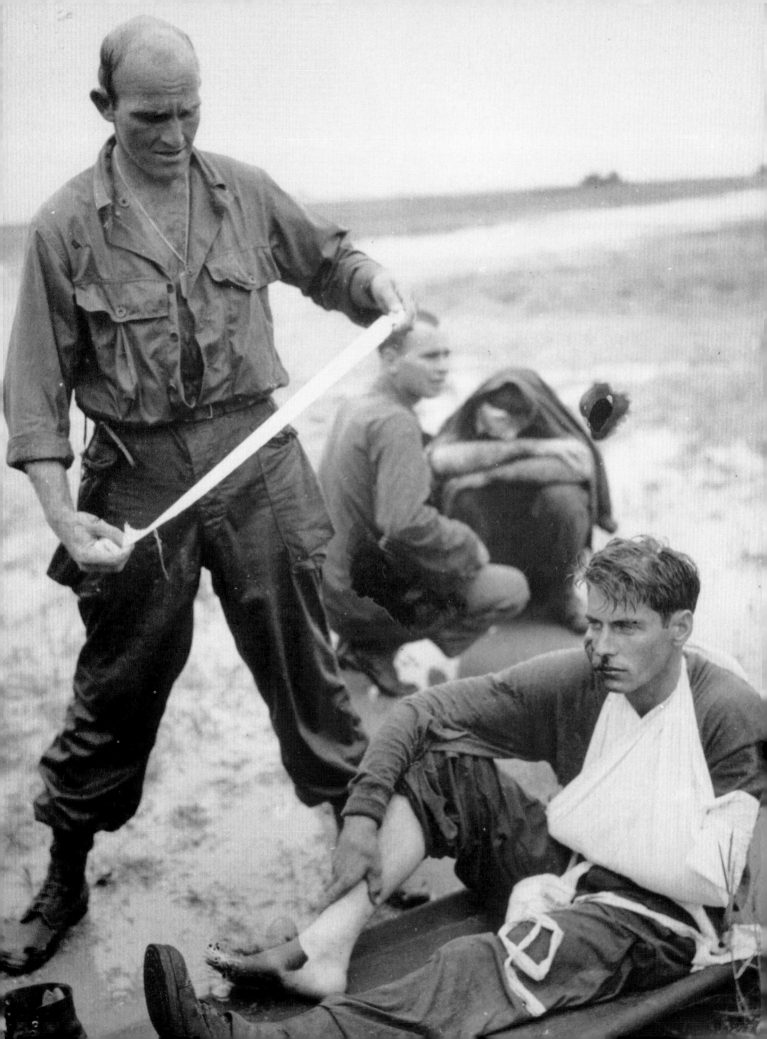

Chapter 6
World War II—The War Against Japan, 1941–45

left
A Coast Guard corps-man bandages a crew member of an American medium tank that hit a Japanese land mine while attacking the Tacloban Air Strip during the early stages of the Philippines invasion at Leyte on October 20, 1944. *U.S. Coast Guard.*

bottom right
This view of Ward 12 of General Hospital No. 2 shows the primitive conditions which Army medics and patients endured on the Bataan Peninsula in February 1942. *Army Nurse Corps Historical Collection.*

DISTANT AND VARIED CHALLENGES

The Japanese attack on Pearl Harbor in Oahu, Hawaii, on December 7, 1941, found the Army Medical Department mobilizing, yet far short of the resources needed for the global conflict ahead. Preparations accelerated while Allied leaders decided upon priorities. Although the Allies soon decided on giving precedence to Europe, combat in the Pacific also demanded immediate attention.

The vast Pacific distances posed considerable disadvantages for American and Allied forces. After the fall of the Philippines early in 1942, the only significant Medical Department presence outside of the continental United States was in Hawaii and Alaska. A major medical infrastructure had to be improvised rapidly in the Pacific region to provide field medical service and hospitalization support.

The Pacific region was exceptionally primitive, undeveloped, unhealthy, and hostile. Allied forces had to cope with vast ocean expanses, thousands of widely scattered islands and coral atolls, rugged mountains, and steamy, impenetrable jungles. Basic facilities required to sustain modern military operations had to be built from scratch. The distances put a premium on control of the air and seas for transport of air and ground combat forces and their logistical and medical support. In all of these actions, Army and Navy medical personnel relentlessly battled hostile environments and diseases, especially the ever-present malaria and dengue fever.

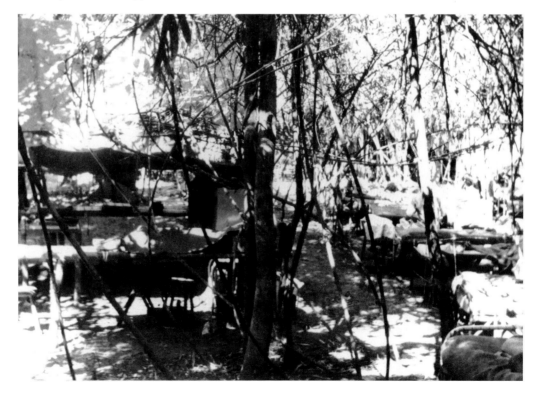

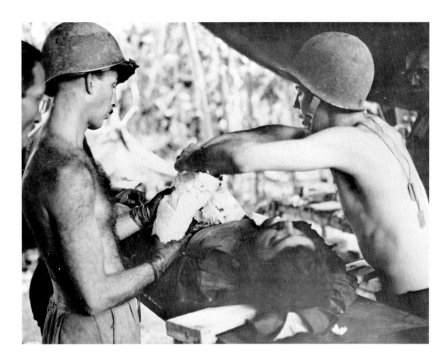

top left
Major George Marks performs surgery on wounded American soldier during the 1943 campaign in New Guinea. *Library of Congress.*

bottom
Two surgical technicians of the 3d Portable Surgical Hospital at Buna, Papua, facing camera, examine a wounded soldier on January 1, 1943. Major William L. Garlick, back to camera, supervises. *National Archives.*

The medics in all Pacific theaters quickly learned that any Red Cross insignias made them targets for Japanese attacks. Imperial Japan had not signed the Geneva Conventions and Japanese forces ignored their provisions. The normal safeguards that protected medical personnel and facilities from attack, including marked hospitals and hospital ships, and that required the proper treatment of prisoners of war (POWs), were nonexistent in this war.

SOUTHWEST PACIFIC AREA

With the establishment of the Southwest Pacific Area (SWPA) Theater under General Douglas MacArthur in March 1942, medical officers built a medical system from the ground up to ensure forces would be fit to conduct military operations. Once again, disease posed a threat. Some of the diseases were familiar, such as syphilis and influenza. Others were more exotic insect-borne diseases such as malaria, dengue fever, and scrub typhus (tsutsugamushi fever), endemic to the tropical areas of northern Australia, Papua, New Guinea, and the nearby Solomon Islands.

Of these diseases, the various malarias spread by mosquitoes were the most dangerous and potentially most destructive to the health of the military forces operating in those areas. Malaria surfaced as a significant health threat when Army forces moved to New Guinea and Papua in September 1942 and launched major ground operations against the Japanese stronghold at Buna. Malaria rates skyrocketed and threatened to incapacitate large numbers of combat soldiers and disrupt operations.

Strongly backed by MacArthur, the Army theater surgeon, Brigadier General Percy J. Carroll, MC, convinced commanders to implement stringent measures to control malaria. During 1943, mandatory daily doses of the malaria suppressants quinine and Atabrine™ were strictly enforced. New programs for malaria survey and control were established. DDT was used extensively to control mosquito populations, and draining and oiling destroyed mosquito breeding areas. By 1944, Carroll's aggressive antimalarial campaign had contained a once threatening health menace.

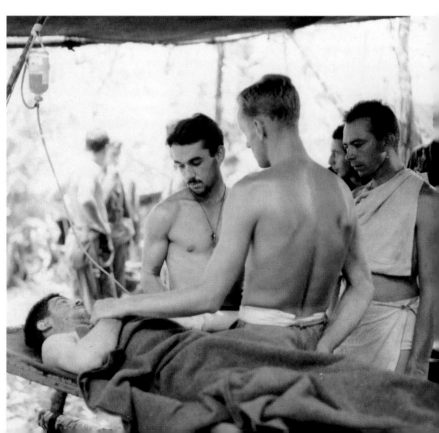

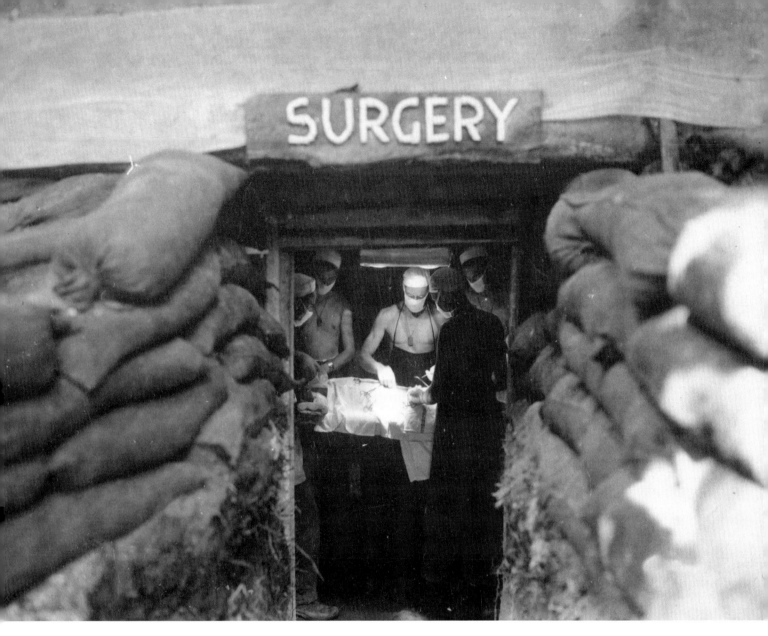

SURGERY

In a surgery bunker behind front lines on Bougainville, an Army surgeon operates on a soldier wounded by a Japanese sniper, December 13, 1943. *National Archives.*

PORTABLE SURGICAL HOSPITALS

In 1942 Carroll also created portable surgical hospitals, one of the most important frontline surgical innovations of the war. He realized that in places like Papua, New Guinea, and adjacent small islands it would be extremely difficult to evacuate seriously wounded soldiers to any hospital unit in time for life-saving surgery. Thus, in September 1942 he organized 25 portable hospitals, units of four surgeons and 25 men that could take surgical care to the soldiers. Attached to regimental combat teams (RCTs), assault landing forces, or infantry divisions, these units worked on the front lines and often performed operations on wounded men within 100 to 200 yards of the Japanese. The SWPA's portable hospitals proved so successful in the Buna campaign of December 1942–February 1943 that within months the War Department adopted their use throughout the Army.

By mid-1944, 47 portable surgical hospitals supported the accelerating pace of MacArthur's offensive operations along the northern coast of New Guinea and northward to the Philippines. During the war, a total of 103 portable surgical hospitals were activated. Of these, 82 served against the Japanese. Carroll's temporary innovation gained significance far beyond SWPA, and the surgical work performed in these hospitals saved the lives of many thousands of critically wounded soldiers and airmen.

By the time MacArthur made his promised return to the Philippines at Leyte on October 20, 1944, the Army's air, ground, and service forces in Australia, Papua, and New Guinea were providing a routinely high level of medical support. Medical strength had grown from 3,330 personnel supporting 62,500 troops in March 1942 to 60,140 personnel supporting more than 670,000 troops in the summer of 1944.

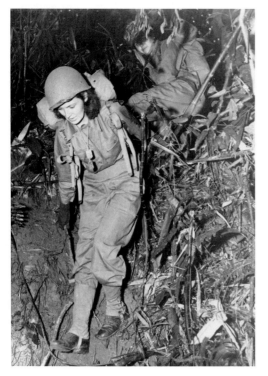

The reconquest of the Philippines that began with Leyte would consume the remaining months of the war, including a major and prolonged struggle from January through August 1945 to retake Luzon and Manila. Determined Japanese resistance combined with exceptionally difficult terrain and poor roads made operations costly and time-consuming. The difficulty of clearing the Japanese from the mountainous areas of northern Luzon and long road evacuation routes put a premium on the use of the mobile hospital units, especially portable surgical hospitals, and air evacuation. Light airplanes such as the Stinson L-5B, and primitive Sikorsky RD-3 helicopters lifted casualties of the 112th Cavalry Regimental Combat Team and 38th Infantry Division to fixed hospitals for treatment.

In the fighting on Luzon near Binalonan and San Manuel on January 18 and 24, 1945, Technician 4 Laverne Parrish, a medic with Company C, 1st Battalion, 161st Infantry Regiment, 25th Infantry Division, was awarded the Medal of Honor. He braved constant enemy fire while treating and rescuing 39 wounded soldiers of his company before Japanese mortar fire mortally wounded him.

CHINA-BURMA-INDIA THEATER

The China-Burma-India (CBI) Theater (split into the India-Burma and China theaters in 1944) operation provided air and logistical support to British Commonwealth and Chinese Nationalist forces. With its minimal commitment of American ground combat forces, the theater's primary objective was to keep China in the war to pin down the Japanese on the Asian mainland.

Aircraft and helicopters were used heavily to evacuate casualties from the remote jungles to hospitals in the rear. On April 23, 1944, Lieutenant Carter Harman of the 1st Air Commando Force picked up casualties near Mawlu, Burma, and completed the first helicopter medical evacuation (medevac) mission flying a Sikorsky RD-3 helicopter.

A medical structure was built up in India and China that by the end of the war numbered 20,025 medical personnel to support about 200,000 American forces. From 1943 onward, 19 portable surgical hospitals served American forces, and also Chinese forces, which had almost no medical support.

top
Army nurses in jungle with full packs, China-Burma-India Theater. *National Archives.*

bottom
Lashio, Burma, April 12, 1945. Surgery team of the 49th Portable Surgical Hospital operates under tropical conditions. *National Archives.*

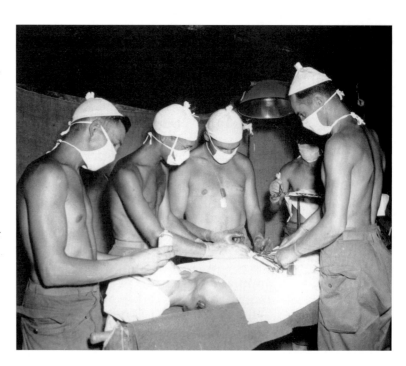

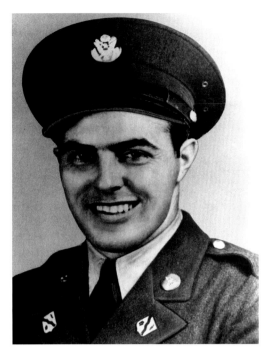

top right
Private First Class Frank J. Petrarca, a medic with the 145th Infantry Regiment, 37th Infantry Division, distinguished himself on July 27, 29, and 31, 1943, in treating and saving his fellow soldiers until he died protecting wounded men with his own body. For his actions above and beyond the call of duty he received the Medal of Honor. *National Archives.*

bottom right
Saipan, 1944. Captain Ben L. Salomon, Dental Corps, then assistant battalion surgeon, 2d Battalion, 105th Infantry Regiment, 27th Infantry Division, was at his battalion aid station when a massive Japanese banzai attack overran the 1st and 2d Battalions on the night of July 6–7. Captain Salomon manned a machine gun to defend his aid station while medics evacuated the casualties. He was later found dead at the machine gun with 98 Japanese bodies littering its field of fire. Captain Salomon's sacrifice was finally recognized when he received the Medal of Honor posthumously in 2002. He was the first member of the Dental Corps to receive it. *University of Southern California School of Dentistry.*

PACIFIC OCEAN AREA

Operating from Hawaii, Army forces worked with the Navy and Marine Corps in the Central Pacific to stave off the Japanese offensive against Midway in June 1942 and then go on the offensive in 1943. Amphibious operations to seize Japanese island strongholds across the Pacific required the Army and Navy to mould medical support on an expeditionary basis that could be put ashore quickly once the beachheads were secured. In these operations, mobility was not as important as holding capacity; once settled, these units usually did not move because the islands were small. This put a premium on division clearing companies and field and evacuation hospitals tailored to landing operations. Division clearing companies were strengthened to operate as hospitals with capacities of 250 to 400 beds.

With Tripler General Hospital as its centerpiece, the Medical Department already had a strong presence in Hawaii. Army station and general hospitals supported Army ground, air, and service forces throughout the theater. The total Medical Department presence reached 35,000 by January 1944 and remained relatively steady thereafter. In contrast to the South and Southwest Pacific and the CBI, the Central Pacific was largely free of malaria and tropical diseases so dangerous to the soldiers' health. In the South Pacific, the push up the Solomon Islands from Guadalcanal was long and tortuous. In a difficult operation, the Army's 37th and 25th Infantry Divisions landed on New Georgia Island in July 1943 and took Munda

Field and the island. Private First Class Frank J. Petrarca, a medic with the 145th Infantry Regiment, 37th Infantry Division, distinguished himself on July 27, 29, and 31 in treating and saving his fellow soldiers until he died protecting wounded men with his own body. For his actions above and beyond the call of duty he received the Medal of Honor.

As the offensive spread westward from Hawaii across the Central Pacific in 1943–44, the islands of the Gilberts (Tarawa and Makin), Marshalls (Kwajalein and Eniwetok), and Marianas (Saipan, Tinian, and Guam) were taken in hard fighting. In these operations, new portable surgical hospitals played prominent roles in coordination with divisional medical battalions and field hospitals.

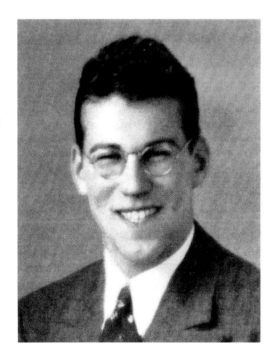

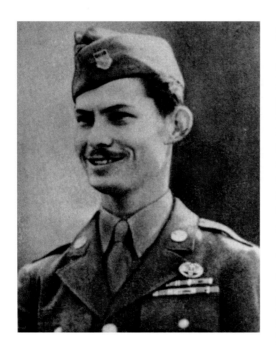

NAVY OPERATIONS IN THE PACIFIC

DAY OF INFAMY

December 7, 1941, remains the U.S. Navy's greatest catastrophe. In little more than two hours, much of the Pacific Fleet was destroyed or seriously damaged. The pride of the fleet—seven battleships that once projected U.S. might and prestige—either lay on the bottom or were too crippled to be of any immediate use. Bombs, torpedoes, and machine guns had taken a terrible toll, with the Navy alone losing 2,008 men.

The badly burned and wounded survivors required immediate treatment and Navy medical personnel were there to provide it with a naval hospital, a partially assembled base hospital, and the USS *Solace* (AH-5), the newest Navy hospital ship. The men and women who staffed these facilities began heroic round-the-clock efforts to save lives minutes after the first Japanese bomb dropped and never waned until the last casualty was attended.

Physicians, nurses, and hospital corpsmen on duty at the Pearl Harbor Naval Hospital performed emergency surgery, treated burns, and comforted the dying. The same scene played out aboard USS *Solace*, which lay at anchor just beyond "Battleship Row." Oil-soaked sailors plucked from the harbor were rushed to the hospital ship for treatment.

If the ferocity of the Japanese onslaught that followed Pearl Harbor left American forces reeling, isolated, and with scant hope of reinforcement, as an institution Navy medicine was equally stretched. Possessing limited resources and with a presence only in Hawaii, the Philippines, Guam, a few small installations, and aboard the few vessels of the Asiatic Fleet, Navy medical personnel were hard pressed to treat patients as the Japanese rolled through the Pacific conquering everything in their path.

Okinawa, 1945. During bitter fighting from April 29 to May 21, Private First Class Desmond T. Doss, a company medic with the 1st Battalion, 307th Infantry Regiment, 77th Infantry Division, repeatedly risked his life to treat and evacuate wounded men until his own wounds forced his evacuation. This humble Seventh Day Adventist saved the lives of many soldiers, and for his selfless heroic actions received the Medal of Honor. *National Archives.*

Following the capture of Iwo Jima in early 1945, Okinawa was the next step toward the assault on the Japanese home islands. The Okinawa campaign lasted from April until June and was a prolonged and costly struggle that claimed thousands of American, Japanese, and Okinawan lives.

By the end of the war, the Medical Department had 120,000 personnel in the western Pacific readying for the final assault of the Japanese home islands. Thankfully, that assault never took place. In all of the Pacific campaigns, medical personnel contributed significantly to victory and also suffered commensurate losses. A total of 5,574 medical personnel were battle casualties or injuries. The number included 1,474 dead (139 officers and 1,335 men) of which 858 were killed in action (58 officers and 800 men). This brought total Army Medical Department battle casualty deaths for World War II to 3,690 killed in action (196 officers and 3,494 men) out of 4,665 battle deaths (293 officers and 4,372 men and women).

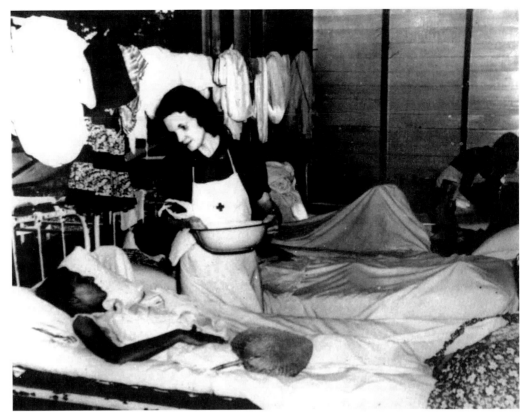

Navy Nurse Margaret Nash, captured by Japanese forces, attends a fellow internee in Santo Tomás Prison in the Philippines, during World War II. *U.S. Navy Bureau of Medicine and Surgery.*

STRETCHED THIN IN THE PHILIPPINES

On December 8, 1941, the war came to the Philippines when Japanese bombers blasted Clark and Nichols fields. Enemy bombers returned two days later, destroying the Cavite Navy Yard and killing and maiming scores of Americans and Filipinos. Personnel at the nearby Cañacao Naval Hospital worked frantically to treat the wounded.

Japanese soldiers landed on Philippine beaches a few days before Christmas 1941, and swept aside the ill-equipped Americans and Filipinos. As the Japanese entered Manila on January 1 after General MacArthur declared it an open city, its battered defenders quickly retreated to makeshift positions on the Bataan Peninsula.

Meanwhile, disease ran rampant as supplies dwindled. Without sufficient quinine, many men came down with malaria. Nearly everyone suffered debilitating weakness from dysentery. Overwhelmed, Bataan's 75,000 defenders finally surrendered in April 1942.

Out in Manila Bay, the island fortress of Corregidor remained defiant. But soon food and ammunition ran out, and the power of the enemy was too great. After a month of heavy bombardment, followed by landings by Japanese forces, Corregidor surrendered on May 6,

1942. American power in the Far East had been extinguished. Yet despite the new reality, the hundreds of medical professionals captured in the Pacific were still "Doc" or "Nurse" to their fellow POWs. Without hospitals or supplies, they continued to practice their healing art, often under unimaginable circumstances.

Although some 10,000 surrendered at Corregidor, thousands of captured Americans and Filipinos had already died on the infamous Bataan Death March. Those who survived Japanese brutality and neglect now faced Japanese prison camps. For the approximately 17,000 Americans and 12,000 Filipino scouts who surrendered in the Philippines, the real ordeal had barely begun. Atrocities, forced labor, starvation, and boredom became the norm in Japanese POW camps throughout the Far East.

Even though physicians and corpsmen did the best they could to provide health care in these camps, they lacked drugs and medical instruments. Malaria and dengue fever were endemic. Sanitation was nonexistent and almost everybody had dysentery. Many came down with deficiency diseases like scurvy, optic neuritis, and beriberi. By the summer of 1942 the Japanese held more than 50,000 prisoners, 20,000 of them Americans.

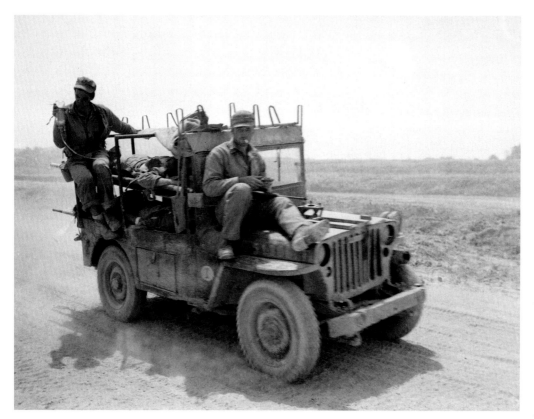

top left
Navy corpsman gives transfusion to a wounded Marine as Jeep careens along a road on Okinawa. *National Archives.*

bottom left
Navy corpsmen give transfusion to wounded Marine on landing craft off Peleliu. *National Archives.*

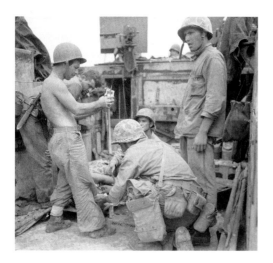

Eleven of these were Navy nurses from the Cañacao Naval Hospital. They spent the war in internment camps at Santo Tomás in Manila and then at Los Baños in the Philippine countryside, where they were liberated in February 1945. Many of their male colleagues never made it home, either succumbing to disease, starvation, brutal treatment by their captives, or dying by "friendly fire" when the so-called hell ships in which they were being transported to Japan were sunk by American submarines or aircraft.

STEPPING-STONES TO TOKYO

Despite the fate of these unfortunate POWs, the war against Japan was in full swing by the summer of 1942. Reconquering territory held by the enemy became the priority and it meant fighting island by island, each one a stepping-stone to Tokyo.

The Navy Medical Department undertook the major task of organizing care for the thousands of Navy and Marine Corps casualties generated by opposed amphibious landings, treating them, and then returning them to duty. Navy medicine faced its greatest challenge in the Pacific War by having to cope with the aftermath of intense, bloody warfare fought far from fixed hospitals. This put enormous pressure on medical personnel closest to the front and forced development of new approaches to primary care and evacuation.

A Navy hospital corpsman's most dramatic and demanding duty was that of supporting Marine Corps units in the field. Since the Marine Corps had always relied upon the Navy for medical support, corpsmen accompanied the leathernecks and suffered the brunt of combat themselves. Many of them went unarmed, reserving their carrying strength for medical supplies.

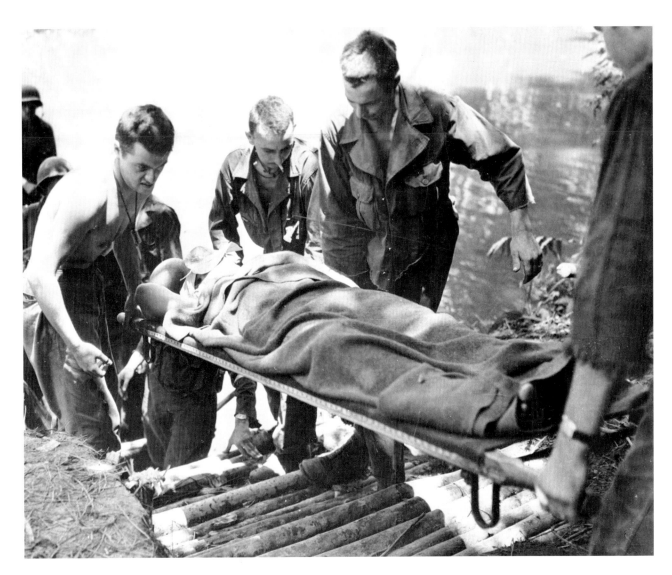

Unloading wounded soldier from an assault boat in the Southwest Pacific Area Theater. Soldiers wounded at the front are moved to the hospital in this manner. *Library of Congress.*

Navy corpsmen were the first critical link in the evacuation chain. From the time a Marine was hit on an invasion beach at Guadalcanal, Tarawa, Saipan, Iwo Jima, Okinawa, and a host of other Pacific islands, the corpsman braved enemy fire to render aid. He applied a battle dressing, administered morphine, and tagged the casualty. If he were lucky, the corpsman might commandeer a litter team to move the casualty out of harm's way and onward to a battalion aid station or a collecting and clearing company for further treatment. This care would involve stabilizing the patient with plasma, serum albumin, and, later in the war, whole blood. In some cases, the casualty was then moved to the beach for evacuation. In others, the casualty was taken to a divisional hospital, where doctors performed further stabilization, including surgery, if needed.

Four Navy corpsmen received the Medal of Honor for exceptional gallantry during the tough campaign to take Iwo Jima in February and March 1945: Francis Pierce, Jr., George E. Wahlen, Jack Williams, and John H. Willis.

In the bitter fighting to seize Okinawa in May and June 1945, three Navy corpsmen earned the Medal of Honor: Robert E. Bush, William Halyburton, and Fred F. Lester.

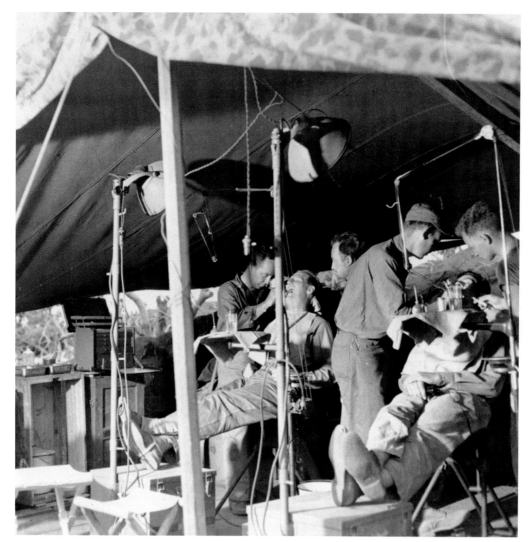

top left
In the midst of battle on Iwo Jima, March 1, 1945, Navy dentists tend to the oral health of the troops. *U.S. Navy Bureau of Medicine and Surgery.*

bottom
Coast Guardsmen transfer a wounded Marine from his amtrac damaged by Japanese fire to a landing craft for evacuation and care. Iwo Jima, February 19, 1945. *U.S. Coast Guard.*

Supporting the Navy and Marine Corps in their effort to defeat the enemy also meant recognizing that disease more often than enemy action threatened this goal. During the battle for Guadalcanal in the Solomon Islands, malaria was responsible for more casualties than Japanese bullets. Shortly after the landings, the number of patients hospitalized with malaria surpassed all other diseases. Some units exceeded a 100 percent casualty rate, with personnel being hospitalized more than once. Only when malaria and other tropical diseases could be brought to heel, could the Pacific War be won.

Navy medical personnel moved quickly to reduce the impact of malaria and other tropical diseases. Personnel trained in preventive medicine oiled mosquito breeding areas and sprayed DDT. Physicians and corpsmen dispensed quinine and Atabrine™ as malaria suppressants.

Navy hospital ships, employed mainly as seagoing ambulances, provided first aid and some surgical care for the casualties' needs while ferrying them to base hospitals in the Pacific or back to the United States for definitive care. As the war continued, air evacuation helped carry the load. Trained Navy nurses and corpsmen staffed the evacuation aircraft.

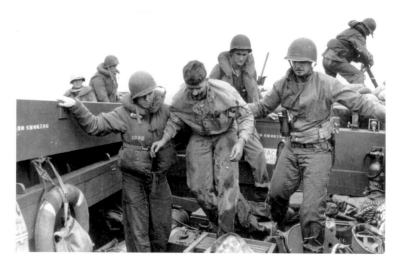

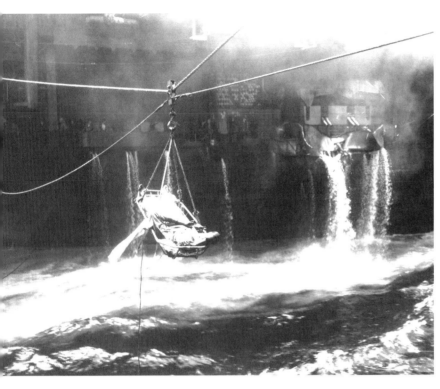

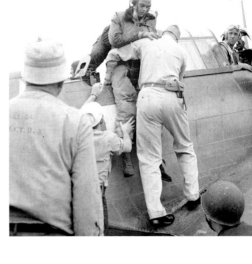

During routine operations, physicians and corpsmen serving aboard vessels in the South Pacific encountered and treated heat and humidity related maladies exacerbated by confinement without air conditioning—heat exhaustion and stroke, fungus infections, heat rash, and breathing disorders.

The encounters between Japanese and American fleets were most often brutal affairs with many casualties generated in both brief and sustained actions. Torpedoes, bombs, and armor-piercing shells produced horrendous wounds. When the Japanese launched their kamikaze terror campaign, medical personnel were often overwhelmed. A single suicide plane plunging through the flight deck of an aircraft carrier and igniting fueled and armed aircraft produced hundreds of burn victims within seconds. As the fighting drew ever closer to the Japanese home islands in early 1945, thousands of sailors were killed and wounded by these human-guided missiles.

above
Casualties are transferred via lifeline from the aircraft carrier USS *Bunker Hill*, background, to USS *Wilkes Barre*. They were injured during fire aboard the carrier following a Japanese suicide dive-bombing attack off Okinawa in the Ryukyus on May 11, 1945. *National Archives.*

top right
Navy aircrewman wounded during a raid on Rabaul is helped from his SBD Dauntless aircraft aboard USS *Saratoga* (CV-3), November 5, 1943. *National Archives.*

bottom right
Navy chaplain comforts wounded patient aboard the battleship USS *Wisconsin* (BB-64), 1945. *National Archives.*

PRACTICING SHIPBOARD MEDICINE

The Pacific War was massive in scale, fought over vast stretches of ocean. Fleets engaged one another while separated by many miles of water. Carrier-based aircraft were surrogates that sought out the enemy and delivered the ordnance. United States Navy task forces consisting of carriers, battleships, cruisers, destroyers, and destroyer escorts required their own medical support. The crews of each of these vessels included corpsmen and physicians. Dentists served aboard the larger vessels.

By October 1945 the fleet in the Pacific numbered more than 7,000 vessels. They ranged from small landing craft and auxiliaries to the Essex class carriers and Iowa class battleships. The hundreds of vessels smaller than destroyers had corpsmen assigned. The larger vessels rated physicians, corpsmen, dentists, fully equipped sick bays, battle dressing stations, and usually an operating room.

The standard medical complement for a 7,250-ton escort carrier was one medical officer, a flight surgeon for the embarked air group, a dentist, and about 13 corpsmen. A much larger 27,100-ton Essex class carrier like the USS *Franklin* (CV-13) boasted four physicians augmented by a flight surgeon, three dentists, and 31 corpsmen.

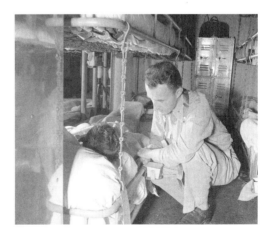

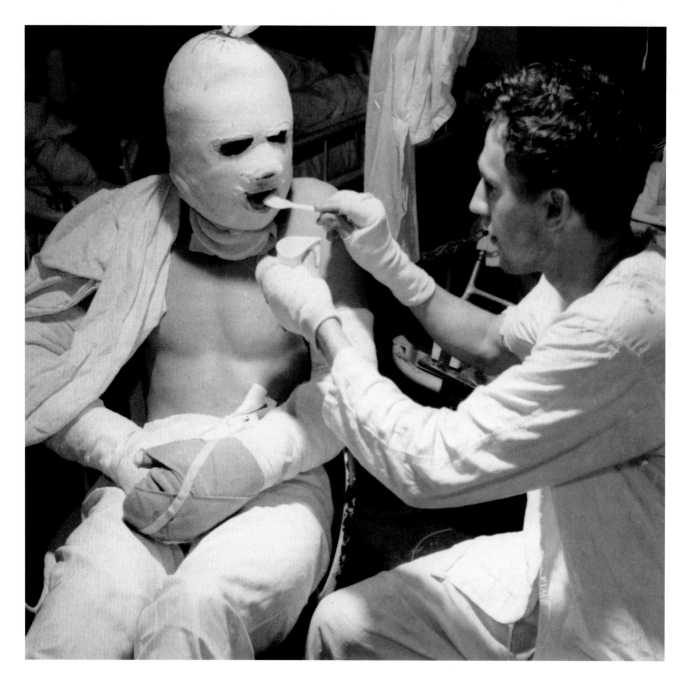

Navy medical personnel also served aboard the submarines that prowled the Pacific Ocean destroying thousands of tons of Japanese shipping. Among its crew, each submarine carried one highly trained corpsman or pharmacist's mate, as they were then called, because physicians were not assigned to submarines. One of the most dramatic stories to come out of World War II recounted an emergency appendectomy performed by a 23-year-old corpsman as his submarine, USS *Seadragon*, cruised submerged in enemy waters. The corpsman, Wheeler B. Lipes, successfully removed a badly infected appendix and saved his patient. This heroic story highlighted the skill and resourcefulness of Navy corpsmen, and also buoyed the nation's

spirits early in the war when news from the Pacific was anything but encouraging.

When World War II finally ended with the Japanese surrender aboard the USS *Missouri* in Tokyo Bay on September 2, 1945, the U.S. Navy had become the largest maritime force the world had ever known. And the Medical Department which supported that Navy would itself never again have as many personnel, or staff as many hospitals, dispensaries, and hospital ships as it did on that day.

Pressure bandaged after they suffered burns when their ship was hit by a Japanese kamikaze attack, sailors are fed aboard the hospital ship USS *Solace* (AH-5), May 1945. *National Archives.*

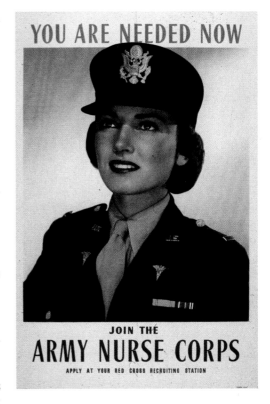

top
Army Air Forces nurses were imprisoned by the Japanese during World War II. These nurses from Bataan and Corregidor, Philippine Islands, were freed after three years' imprisonment. They are wearing new uniforms with flight nurse badges to replace their worn-out clothes. Manila, Luzon, Philippine Islands, February 1945. *National Archives.*

bottom
"You are needed now." Army Nurse Corps recruiting poster, World War II. At war's end, 55,702 Army nurses were serving on active duty. *National Archives.*

What followed victory was rapid demobilization as soldiers, sailors, airmen, and Marines in the Pacific Theater headed home. Helping get them there were aircraft carriers, battleships, LSTs (landing ship, tank), and Navy hospital ships—all of which became troop transports in what was called Operation Magic Carpet.

WARTIME ACCOMPLISHMENTS

The Army Medical Department saw extraordinary wartime achievements. Army hospitals worldwide admitted 16,744,724 patients. Better surgical care, sulfa drugs and penicillin, medics on the frontlines, far forward surgical units, plasma and whole blood, sound preventive medicine practices, and speedier evacuation all contributed to a historically low died of wounds figure of 26,309 out of 599,724 wounded in action (4.4 percent compared with 8.1 percent in World War I). Of 14,345,000 disease admissions, only 14,904 died for a rate of 0.1 percent.

Aeromedical evacuation had proved its benefits in both Europe and the Pacific. It was at least as safe as ground and sea evacuation. It saved sick or wounded patients many painful, uncomfortable hours en route to a hospital. Speedier arrival at definitive medical care reduced deaths and hastened recovery. Aeromedical evacuation also saved money. When patients were moved by air, ground transportation for nonmedical items and troops became more efficient. General Dwight D. Eisenhower, Supreme Commander, Allied Expeditionary Forces and

YOU ARE NEEDED NOW

JOIN THE
ARMY NURSE CORPS
APPLY AT YOUR RED CROSS RECRUITING STATION

Commander, U.S. Army European Theater of Operations, said that aeromedical evacuation was as important as other World War II medical innovations—sulfa drugs, penicillin, blood plasma, and whole blood—in reducing the fatality rate of battle casualties.

WORLD WAR II SERVICE AND CASUALTIES 1941–45

Total U.S. Service Members (Worldwide)	16,112,566
Battle Deaths	291,557
Other Deaths in Service (Non-Theater)	113,842
Non-Mortal Woundings	671,846

Source: Department of Veterans Affairs from Department of Defense.

ARMY MEDICAL DEPARTMENT MEDAL OF HONOR RECIPIENTS IN WORLD WAR II–PACIFIC

FRANK J. PETRARCA

LAVERNE PARRISH

DESMOND T. DOSS

BEN L. SALOMON

NAVY MEDICAL DEPARTMENT MEDAL OF HONOR RECIPIENTS IN WORLD WAR II–PACIFIC

ROBERT E. BUSH

WILLIAM HALYBURTON

FRED F. LESTER

FRANCIS PIERCE, JR.

GEORGE E. WAHLEN

JACK WILLIAMS

JOHN H. WILLIS

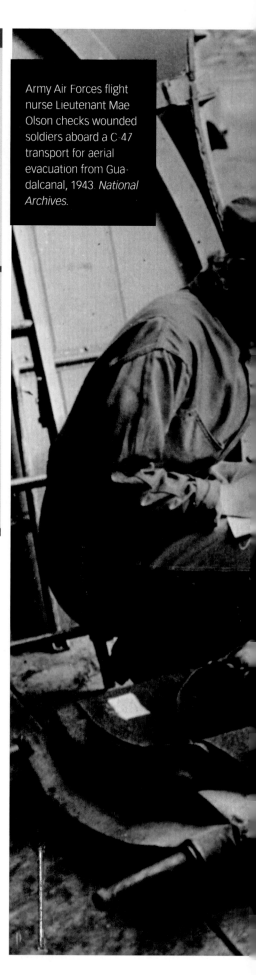

Army Air Forces flight nurse Lieutenant Mae Olson checks wounded soldiers aboard a C-47 transport for aerial evacuation from Guadalcanal, 1943. *National Archives.*

Unfortunately, accidents from mechanization of the Army and aircraft training and operations were responsible for a large number of non-battle injury fatalities, accounting for 61,503 deaths out of 1,800,000 cases for a rate of 3.4 percent—significantly higher than World War I.

Wartime service in the Army and Navy medical departments provided inestimable experience for thousands of health care professionals. Their experience greatly benefited postwar American medicine and surgery when they returned to civilian practice and to teaching in medical schools. Dr. Michael DeBakey noted that a combat surgeon at a frontal hospital would perform as much trauma surgery in one day as he would in several years of peacetime civilian practice. The four years of war significantly affected the development of American medicine, surgery, dentistry, nursing, and veterinary medicine as well as the careers and contributions of those who served.

Despite deteriorating relations with the Soviet Union and start of the Cold War, dwindling military budgets resulted in drastic reductions in resources and manpower for all services. The Army and Navy Medical Departments and Army Air Forces Medical Service shrank accordingly.

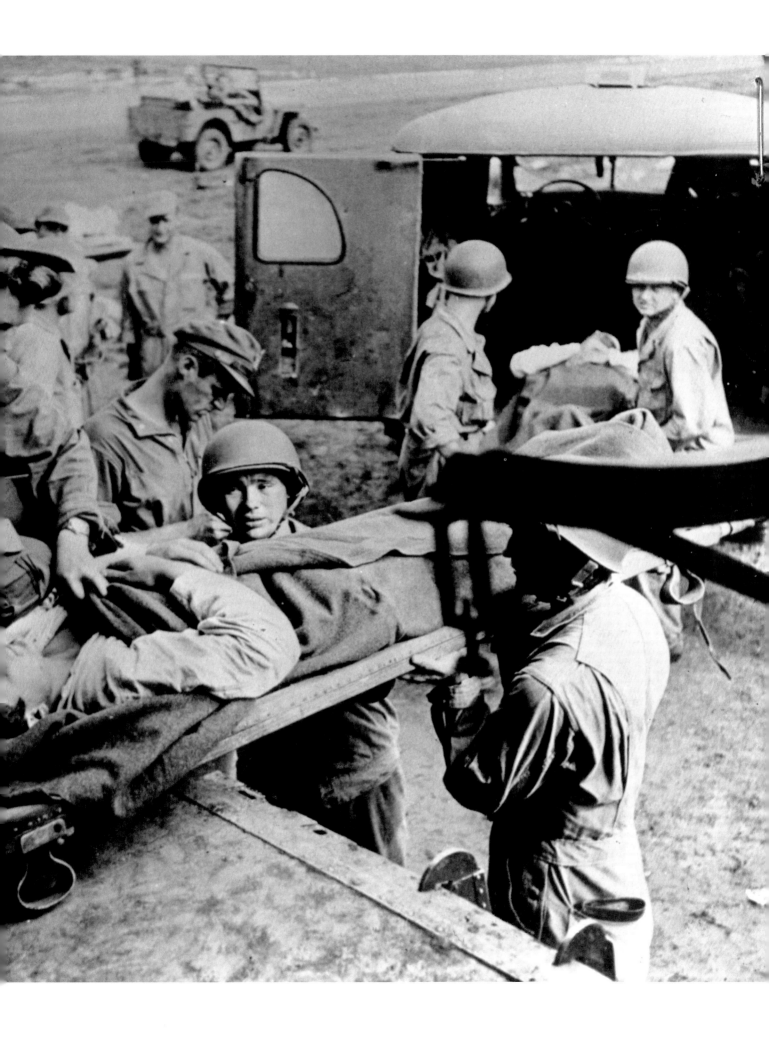

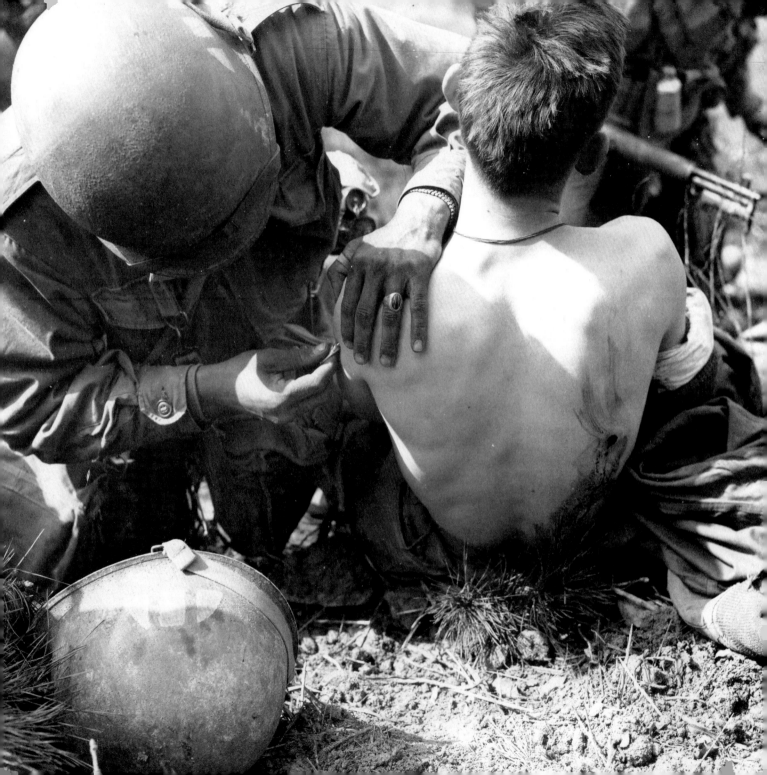

Chapter 7
Postwar and Korean War Era, 1945–53

left
Korea, March 8, 1951. Army medic administers a morphine injection to a paratrooper of Company E, 187th Airborne Regimental Combat Team (ARCT), Eighth Army, wounded with a bullet in his back. Five days earlier the 187th ARCT made a combat jump at Munsan-ni, Korea, to cut off retreating Communist forces. *National Museum of Health and Medicine.*

right
Major General Malcolm C. Grow, first Surgeon General of the Air Force Medical Service, July 1, 1949. He served with Russian forces in combat during World War I. During World War II, he was surgeon of the Eighth Air Force in Europe. *Air Force Medical Service.*

DEMOBILIZATION AND SURPRISE

Within a year after the Japanese surrender on September 2, 1945, the impressive medical structures that the Army, Navy, and Army Air Forces medical departments had built during World War II were torn asunder. The familiar cycle of demobilization and the American penchant for "return to normalcy" dismembered the wartime organizations.

The Navy Medical Department shrank swiftly. Hospitals were decommissioned; hospital ships were mothballed; and reserve physicians, dentists, nurses, and hospital corpsmen returned to civilian life.

The Army Medical Department experienced similar cutbacks. By the end of 1945, 24 of the 66 wartime general hospitals had closed or were transferred to the Veterans Administration. In 1946, another 30 shut their doors. By March 1946, 29,924 medical officers and 39,311 nurses had departed from active duty and more moved out daily. By February 1947, the Medical Department was down to 72,835 personnel. Among that total were 7,850 physicians (about 5,000 serving out wartime educational commitments) and 6,675 nurses.

These drawdowns occurred as the entire U.S. defense structure was being reshaped. The National Security Act of 1947, signed by President Harry S. Truman on July 26, established the Office of the Secretary of Defense, the National Security Council, the Central Intelligence Agency, and the United States Air Force as a separate military branch. The new organizations became reality on September 18, 1947.

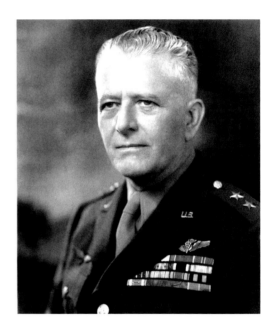

Although the new United States Air Force was no longer a part of the Army, its medical service remained under control of the Army Surgeon General. Major General Malcolm Grow, who became the Air Surgeon in 1946, campaigned for medical independence from the Army. The campaign bore fruit with the establishment of the Air Force Medical Service on July 1, 1949, with personnel and facilities transferred from the Army Medical Department. General Grow served as its first Surgeon General.

AIR FORCE MEDICAL SERVICE BECOMES INDEPENDENT

The Air Force Medical Service was created on July 1, 1949. Air Force General Order No. 35 established a medical service with the following officer personnel components:

a. Medical Corps
b. Dental Corps
c. Veterinary Corps
d. Medical Service Corps
e. Air Force Nurse Corps
f. Women's Medical Specialist Corps

The order stated, "The above listed corps shall consist of those personnel transferred from corresponding corps of the Department of the Army, and personnel subsequently commissioned in the respective corps of the Medical Service, United States Air Force. Personnel appointed in the above corps will be carried on separate promotion lists."

Each officer corps also received a contingent of enlisted medics.

Significant medical support was needed to provide public health services to millions in postwar-occupied Austria, Germany, Japan, and Korea. To retain as many medical professionals as possible, Major General Norman T. Kirk and his successor, Major General Raymond E. Bliss, stressed both graduate and continuing medical education programs and board certification. To attract new physicians, they emphasized internship and residency opportunities in Army general hospitals.

In 1947, officers in the Army Nurse Corps and Women's Medical Specialist Corps became commissioned officers in the regular Army, a major achievement they had long sought. That same year, the Medical Service Corps (MSC) was created from the Pharmacy, Sanitary, and Medical Administrative Corps. The new corps comprised an amazing variety of health care specialists and allied scientists. They included pharmacists, sanitary engineers, entomologists, psychologists, audiologists, optometrists, medical logisticians, personnel officers, resource managers, laboratory officers, hospital administrators, and company and battalion officers in field medical units. MSC officers were essential to the efficient functioning of the modern Army Medical Department in peace and war.

The Berlin Blockade (June 1948–May 1949) and ensuing freezing of relations with the Soviet Union after 1948 further strained an overcommitted and undernourished Army. By early 1950, just when the Cold War was growing hotter with the Communist takeover in China and the Soviet nuclear advances, the Medical Department faced such serious shortages of professional personnel that it closed general hospitals. Moreover, its most critical shortages were in Medical Corps officers in the Far East.

BIRTH OF THE MASH

Near the end of World War II, the Surgeon General's Office used wartime experience to analyze the Army's future field medical requirements and organization. The successes of the portable surgical hospital, field hospital augmentation by teams from the auxiliary surgical group (ASG), and the ASG itself were clear. However, they represented differing approaches to the initial medical treatment of critically wounded soldiers. None of them was completely adequate, and none were retained in the postwar Army. In their place, a new hospital unit was created based largely on the European experiences of the field hospital platoon augmented with surgical teams from an ASG. On August 23, 1945, the War Department issued the blueprint for the new 60-bed "mobile army surgical hospital," better known by its acronym, MASH.

The new MASH had 16 officers (14 Medical Corps, six of them surgeons), 12 nurses, one warrant officer, and 95 enlisted personnel (a total of 124 persons) with 13 trucks and 11 trailers. The MASH was an Army-level medical asset allocated at one per division and to be located adjacent to the division's clearing station. It was intended to handle the seriously wounded, provide life-saving surgery, and care for non-transportable patients. With such a unit nearby, the division's clearing station could handle all of the other wounded, sick, and injured, and be prepared for rapid movement with the division if required.

The MASH was indeed a good idea, but was not implemented promptly. By January 1950, only five MASH units were established: three in the United States and two in Europe. Not one was fully staffed or operational.

KOREAN WAR, 1950-53

The outbreak of the Korean War on June 25, 1950, changed the MASH and frontline surgery forever. Faced with a catastrophic collapse of the Republic of Korea's army before the North Korean Peoples' Army, General Douglas MacArthur's U.S. Far East Command (FECOM) struggled into action. The main ground component of FECOM was the Eighth U.S. Army, then scattered on occupation duty throughout the Japanese islands.

The Eighth Army's Chief Surgeon, Colonel Chauncey E. Dovell, MC, realized that ground operations would be difficult on the Korean peninsula due to its rugged terrain and lack of modern roads and railroads. Field medical operations in this environment presented an enormous challenge to a medical organization that was already seriously short in virtually every professional medical category.

Dovell saw the MASH as an answer to some of his most urgent problems. They were small units (126 persons as of October 1948), so they consumed fewer of his limited medical resources. They were mobile and had organic transportation, so they could move on their own, even on Korea's poor road system. Their presence could commit surgical skills close to the front line, where they would be most urgently required.

On July 1, 1950, he organized the first MASH in the Eighth Army. Major Isaac "Ike" Tender commanded the new 8055th MASH at the 155th Station Hospital in Yokohama, staffed with medical personnel from all over Japan. Just barely organized, the 8055th sailed from Sasebo, Japan, to Pusan, Korea, and entrained northward to Taejon. On July 9, it went into operation in support of the 24th Infantry Division.

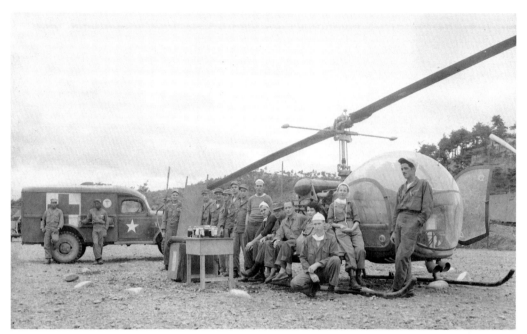

8225th Mobile Army Surgical Hospital Korea. The medical personnel and equipment needed to save a soldier's life are assembled for this photo. October 14, 1951. *National Archives.*

The second MASH, the 8063d, was formed on July 7 at Camp Coe, Yokohama, and arrived at Po'hang-dong, Korea, on July 18. The 8076th was the third MASH established in Japan that summer. On July 17, personnel from throughout Japan began arriving at the 155th Station Hospital, Yokohama, to form the unit and were joined by 10 medical officers just flown in from the United States. Major Kryder E. Van Buskirk commanded the 8076th. He was an urologist who had been closing down Valley Forge General Hospital near Philadelphia less than three weeks before. He activated the 8076th on July 19 with little or no idea of what a MASH even was. On July 21, the 8076th sailed for Korea. It arrived at Pusan on July 25 and moved north to Taegu before being driven back to Miryang by the North Korean advance.

MASH UNITS IN ACTION

As in the World War II fighting against the Japanese, the medics quickly learned that the Geneva Conventions meant nothing to the North Koreans who intentionally targeted any person or vehicle bearing a red cross. From early in the fighting, medics were armed to protect themselves and their patients from North Korean soldiers and roving bands of Communist guerrillas operating behind American lines.

During the hard fighting on the Pusan Perimeter during July, August, and September and following the breakout and pursuit north, the three MASHs were severely tried. Even at full strength, they could not meet their operational requirements in Korea. The MASHs were rou-

tinely handling 150 to 200 patients daily and often exceeded 400 per day. From August 2 to October 5, 1950, the 8076th alone admitted 5,674 patients. The greatest numbers logged in a single 24-hour period were 244 surgical patients and 608 dispositions.

Being completely mobile, the MASHs were totally involved in the ebb and flow of combat operations once the North Koreans were driven past Seoul, north of the 38th Parallel, and back toward the Yalu River, in the fall of 1950. The limited use of evacuation hospitals and the fluid nature of operations after the Inchon landing and breakout from the Pusan Perimeter in September 1950 made the mobility of the MASH and the daily removal of most of its casualties absolutely mandatory.

In November 1950, the Eighth Army modified the MASH in response to the demands placed on it during the early months in Korea. An orthopedic surgeon, 24 enlisted personnel (12 of them surgical technicians), and more nurses were added. Bed capacity was increased to 200. An additional 11 trucks and 10 trailers made it fully mobile.

Another MASH, the 1st (later redesignated the 8209th MASH) from Fort Benning, Georgia, arrived in August and was assigned to the 7th Infantry Division of the X Corps for operations at Inchon and Seoul. It remained with the 7th Infantry Division for operations in northeast Korea, including the bloody Chosin Reservoir fighting in December.

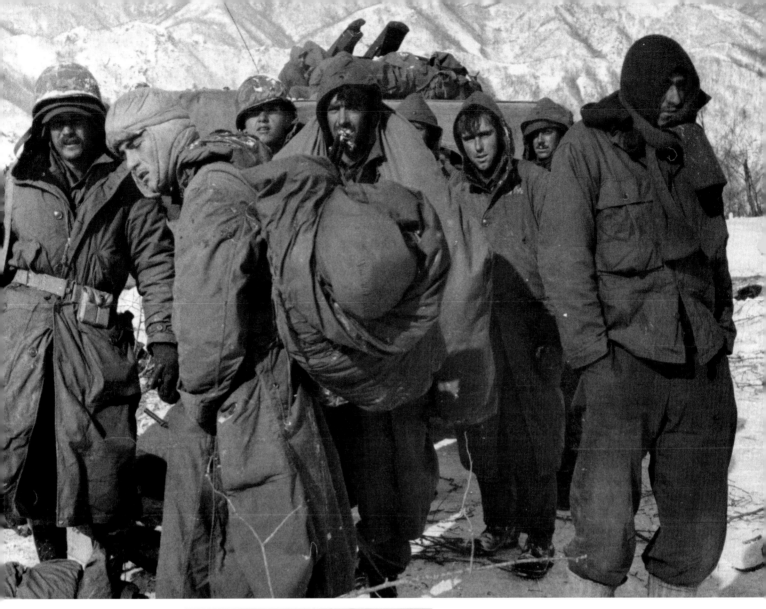

above
Frostbite casualties
of the 1st Marine
Division and the Army's
7th Infantry Division
from Chosin Reser-
voir withdrawal await
evacuation aboard
aircraft of U.S. Air Force
Far East Combat Cargo
Command. *National
Archives.*

right
Surgery is performed
on a wounded soldier
at 8209th Mobile Army
Surgical Hospital, 20
miles from front lines.
Korea, April 8, 1952.
National Archives.

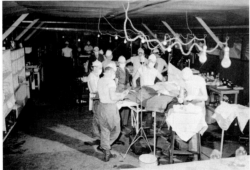

From July to December 1950, the 8055th, 8063d, and 8076th MASHs moved 50 times as operations surged up and down the peninsula. During their first six months in Korea, the three MASHs demonstrated their great value in admitting 22,758 patients and would go on to admit a total of 127,496 patients during their three years at the front.

Massive intervention of Chinese Communist Forces (CCF) in October–November 1950 drove U.S. and United Nations Command (UNC) forces back below Seoul. Divisional medical units, especially those of the 1st Cavalry and 2d and 7th Infantry Divisions, were hit hard and lost a number of soldiers who were killed, wounded, missing, or taken as POWs. The MASHs all escaped, just barely in some cases, and proved that their own mobility was an invaluable and life-saving asset in certain situations.

The bitter cold winter weather that hampered the American soldiers struggling to hold against the Chinese onslaught also claimed a growing number of unprepared soldiers. As World War II experience had shown, cold injuries were very disabling, but entirely pre-ventable, and demanded command attention. It took a year to bring the cold injury problem under control. Cold injuries accounted for 8,255 admissions during the war, 6,350 (77 percent) of them between November 1950 and March 1951.

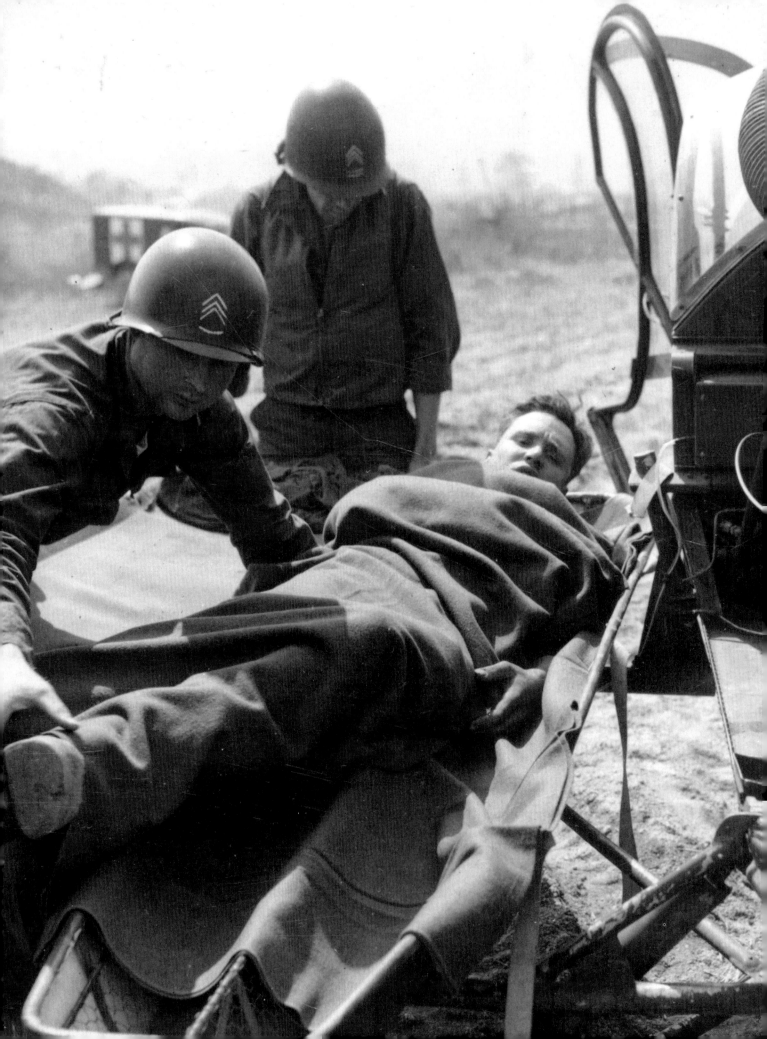

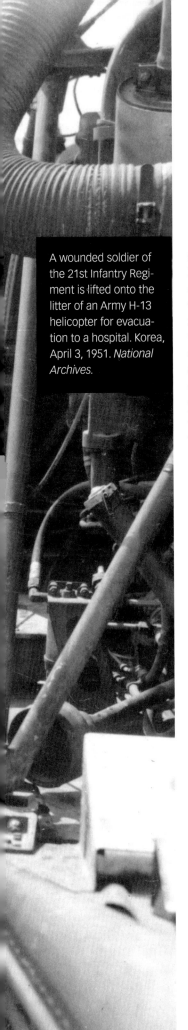

A wounded soldier of the 21st Infantry Regiment is lifted onto the litter of an Army H-13 helicopter for evacuation to a hospital. Korea, April 3, 1951. *National Archives.*

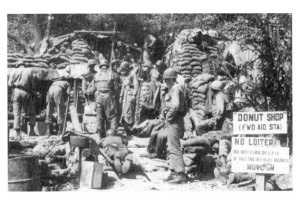

EVACUATION IMPROVISATIONS

From the outset of combat in Korea, medical evacuation was hampered by dangerous tactical situations at the front and Korea's mountainous terrain and poor roads. During the chaotic operations of 1950–51, evacuation of the wounded from the front lines was slow and difficult, even after limited helicopter evacuation began. Approximately 40 percent of the evacuees reached MASHs or evacuation hospitals the same day they were wounded. As the fighting front and medical support stabilized in 1951, from 60 percent–85 percent of the casualties reached medical treatment facilities the same day they were wounded and 80 percent–100 percent reached medical care within the first day after wounding.

Almost anything that moved, from Army motor ambulances to local gasoline-powered Korean railroad cars, affectionately known at "doodlebugs," was pressed into service to haul casualties. Rapid evacuation was critical because the time between wounding and professional medical attention was still the most crucial factor in saving the soldier's life.

Evacuation from Korea was simplified because the large Army hospital structure in Japan supporting the occupation forces was quickly switched to caring for the sick and wounded from the Korean fighting. No large fixed hospitals were sent to Korea; instead, a shifting mix of field, evacuation, and station hospitals met the demand. From July 1950 onward, U.S. Air Force and Navy air transports evacuated patients to Japan where they were treated. If necessary, air evacuation transported them to the U.S. for additional specialized care and rehabilitation. During the war, more than 39,000 patients were evacuated from Japan

above right
Forward aid station near Old Baldy (Hill 487), Korea, 1951. *National Archives.*

to the United States, and 95 percent of them moved by air, continuing the trend begun in World War II.

MORE PHYSICIANS AND INNOVATIONS

In the late 1940s, the Army and Navy medical departments had confronted a serious shortage of physicians, which only grew more critical with the outbreak of the Korean fighting. With the reserves tapped out, both services had few inducements to lure physicians to the colors in the summer of 1950.

The critical shortage of military physicians led Congress to pass legislation nicknamed the "Doctor Draft Law" in September 1950. It provided for drafting physicians who had gone to medical school at government expense during World War II but who graduated after the war was over and had not been called to service. Now they were required, and many physicians were recalled to active duty. Older physicians who had served as reservists during World War II, many with combat experience, were not high on the priority list and would not see action in the new war.

The first of the draft physicians reached Korea in January 1951 after brief orientation and field training courses. By 1952, 90 percent of the medical officers that the Army required for service in the Far East were procured through the "doctor draft." The Army would continue to rely on this draft, which became extremely unpopular with medical students and young physicians during the Vietnam years, until the All-Volunteer Force was established in the early 1970s and the doctor draft was abolished.

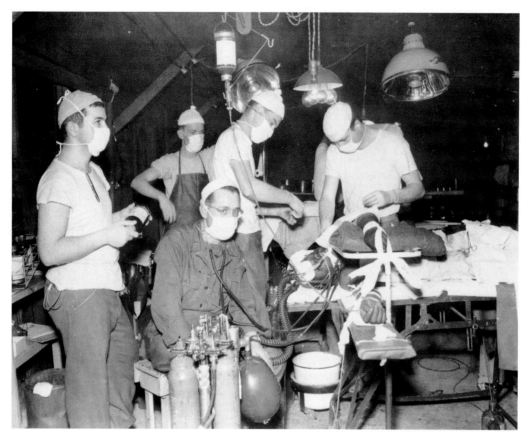

A patient at the 47th Mobile Army Surgical Hospital in Korea receives blood in preparation for an operation, February 25, 1953. *National Archives.*

The young physicians and surgeons who staffed the MASHs were courageous and innovative. Operating on the edge, they were willing to take chances to save the lives and limbs of the wounded. Arterial wounds of the extremities typically led to amputation. With assistance from surgical teams from Walter Reed General Hospital, frontline surgeons began to perform vascular surgery to replace the damaged arteries with vein grafts from the patient himself. Much was learned, and by 1953 arterial repair was a successful procedure that saved many damaged limbs.

In 1951, two additional MASHs were added to the lineup—the 2d MASH (redesignated the 8225th MASH) from Fort Bragg, North Carolina, and the 8228th MASH activated on June 8, 1951, in Chungju specifically to treat hemorrhagic fever victims and research the disease. In addition, the Norwegians manned a MASH equipped by the United States that served in Korea from June 1951 to the war's end. These additional units brought the total number of MASHs to seven, a number that would remain unchanged for the rest of the war.

Special surgical teams or detachments could be added to the MASHs to enhance their capabilities. During 1951, neurosurgical detachments were collocated with MASHs to handle all head and brain wounds. The 140th Medical Detachment (Neurosurgical) supported the 8209th and the 3d Neurosurgical Detachment (Provisional) served with the 8063d MASH.

During early 1952, Colonel L. Holmes Ginn, Eighth Army Surgeon, decided to use the MASHs as the Army Medical Department planners had originally envisioned before 1950. Out of necessity, the Eighth Army had evolved the MASHs into half-scale, semimobile, 200-bed evacuation hospitals. They were supporting multiple combat divisions, and helicopter evacuation had allowed them to move 10 to 20 miles behind the front. In the positional war and stalemate after the fall of 1951, the MASHs had stabilized their locations and begun to look more like semipermanent facilities with prefabricated buildings and even Quonset™ huts. (The tents were stored away for future use.) While such an evolution provided much better conditions for the patients and units' personnel, it also made them immobile. The transition back to mobility was completed in early 1953, and as the war drew to a close in July 1953, the MASH returned to its original 60-bed, tented, highly mobile structure.

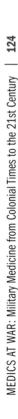

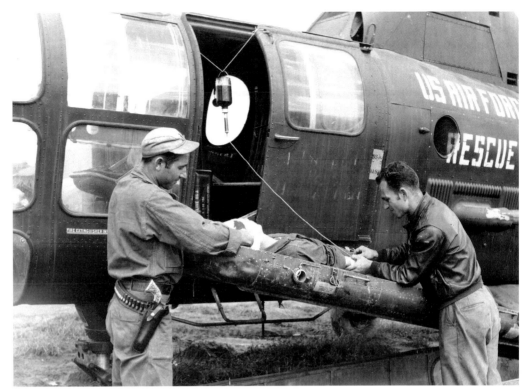

3d Air Rescue Squadron helicopter crew members administer whole blood and prepare a casualty for flight to a hospital behind the lines in Korea, 1950. Air Force helicopters evacuated many of the first casualties in the Korean War. *Air Force Medical Service.*

HELICOPTERS REVOLUTIONIZE THE CHAIN OF EVACUATION

Although U.S. Air Force and Marine Corps helicopters had conducted some special medical evacuation missions in July 1950, it was not until late that month that Dovell initiated the greatest revolution ever to occur in Jonathan A. Letterman's chain of evacuation. He asked the U.S. Air Force's 3d Air Rescue Squadron (Helicopter) if, when they were not otherwise engaged, he could use their Sikorsky H-5 helicopters to transport seriously wounded soldiers from the frontline clearing stations to the MASHs for treatment. When they agreed and provided the helicopters on a regular basis, standard helicopter medical evacuation (medevac) was born. Finally, the solution to the dilemma of moving the surgeon forward to the front lines or the patient back to the rear for life-saving surgery was found in a flying machine.

The rotary-wing aircraft could fly vertically as well as horizontally, operate even in the worst possible terrain with a minimal landing area, and swiftly move the seriously wounded soldier to surgeons waiting in a fully equipped field hospital no farther from the front lines than the division clearing station.

The slow, dangerous, and often deadly ground evacuation for the critically wounded from the front lines to the battalion aid station and then back to definitive surgical treatment would soon be a thing of the past. The development of an operational helicopter configured as an air ambulance and linked directly to the newly developed MASH and the rear area hospitals opened the way for a revolutionary approach to medical evacuation that would save many thousands of military and civilian lives in the years and wars to come.

In September 1950 during a visit to Korea, Major General Bliss, Army Surgeon General, supported Dovell's request for 50 rotary-wing aircraft and Army helicopter units. In October and November the Army activated four helicopter detachments. Each detachment had four pilots (after Korea they would be Medical Service Corps personnel) and four Bell H-13 helicopters, each capable of carrying two litter patients. The 2d Helicopter Detachment arrived in Korea in late November 1950, completed familiarization training, and was attached to the 8055th MASH near Seoul on January 1, 1951. It flew the first official U.S. Army medical evacuation mission of the Korean War the next day.

In 1952, the helicopter detachments were transferred to the Army Medical Department and came under the full control of the Army and corps surgeons in the combat zone to prevent their diversion or misuse.

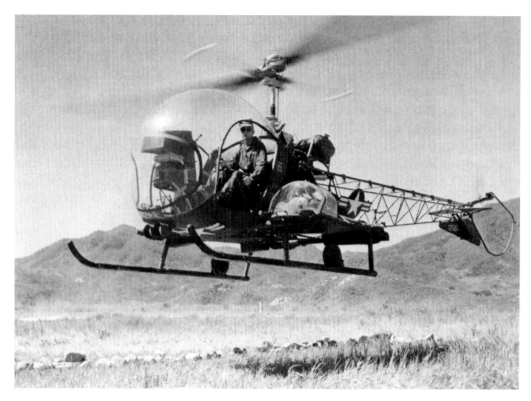

top
U.S. Army H-13 mede-
vac helicopter arrives
with two patients,
Korea, 1953. *National
Archives.*

bottom
Medics of the 5th
Cavalry Regiment give
first aid to a wounded
soldier north of the Im-
jin River, Korea, June 5,
1951. *National Archives.*

The MASHs quickly understood the importance of the helicopter to their missions. In 1951, Major Van Buskirk of the 8076th wrote: "Too much cannot be said in praise of the helicopters stationed at the hospital who brought seriously wounded patients from inaccessible areas and evacuated seriously wounded casualties from forward medical installations, thereby providing a quick, smooth, comfortable evacuation from forward areas to the hospital with a minimum of shock and delay."

From the first medical evacuation missions, until the end of the fighting in Korea on July 27, 1953, Army helicopters evacuated 21,658 casualties. The helicopter evacuation contributed substantially to achieving the lowest mortality rate for wounded (2.4 percent) in any war to that time. In Korea, the Medical Department's frontline surgery reached a new level of lifesaving efficiency with the introduction and maturing of the MASH and its union with the medical evacuation helicopter.

However, the medic was still the point man of the Medical Department. Medics once again carried the heaviest burden in supporting the fighting man on Korea's jagged and barren hills and through its frigid winters and sweltering summers. Sergeant David B. Bleak and Privates First Class Richard G. Wilson and Bryant E. Womack (both posthumous) received Medals of Honor for their selfless work.

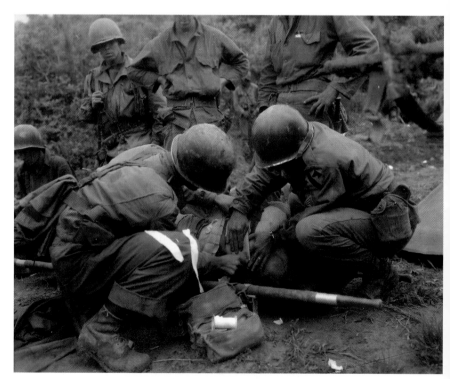

Private First Class Bryant E. Womack, of the Medical Company, 14th Infantry Regiment, 25th Infantry Division, displayed conspicuous gallantry above and beyond the call of duty in action against the enemy on the night of March 12, 1952, and earned the Medal of Honor posthumously. He was the only aidman accompanying a night combat patrol when it encountered a numerically superior enemy force and suffered numerous casualties. Womack went immediately to their aid and was wounded by the heavy enemy fire. Refusing aid for himself, he continued to minister to his comrades and was hit again, losing his right arm. He directed other soldiers in first aid techniques to succor the wounded. He was the last man to withdraw, and died of loss of blood while being carried by his comrades. He was born in Mill Springs, North Carolina. His memory is honored through Womack Army Medical Center at Fort Bragg, North Carolina. *National Archives.*

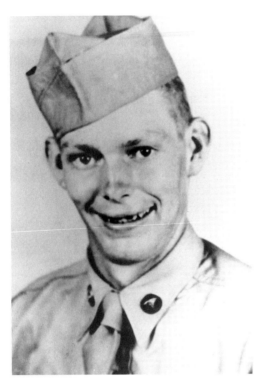

The performance of the MASHs in Korea confirmed that treatment should be conducted as far forward as possible to reduce the loss of strength through medical channels. The earliest possible treatment and the least possible evacuation rearward came to define Medical Department thinking on all aspects of battlefield medicine from surgery to maintenance. The creation of the MASH brought definitive surgery to the division area and had returned 35 percent–40 percent of battle casualties to duty without evacuating them beyond the division clearing station. The MASH had also helped to reduce the death rate, cut disability, and shortened later hospitalization for those severely injured who required definitive surgery prior to further evacuation.

The helicopter and MASH combined to resolve the dilemma that had so long dominated battlefield medicine by swiftly taking the wounded soldier to the surgeon. Time, the oldest and most formidable enemy of the critically wounded, had at last begun to lose its deadly grip.

NAVY MEDICINE IN KOREA, 1950-53

HARSH REALITY OF A NEW WAR

For many Americans in the 21st century, the Korean War is fictional, defined by a novel, a movie, and *M*A*S*H*, the popular television show that still survives in re-runs. But the Korean War was not the fiction of *M*A*S*H*; it was reality of the most brutal sort.

It was a war in which helicopters swiftly airlifted casualties from the battlefield to medical care; where the first large-scale use of antibiotics during wartime saved many from slow death by infection; and where the new practice of vascular surgery salvaged many limbs. It was a conflict in which well-equipped hospital ships began providing definitive care for patients, and an advanced aeromedical evacuation system transported large numbers of seriously ill or injured patients from the battlefield to naval hospitals where their illnesses and wounds could be treated effectively.

When North Korean troops invaded South Korea on June 25, 1950, only five years had elapsed since the end of World War II. The condition of the U.S. armed forces had so deteriorated in numbers and training that those troops who were dispatched to Korea to stem the tide were initially overwhelmed by the Communists.

DRAFTING PHYSICIANS

The military medical services charged with caring for these troops were also not up to the task. The Navy Medical Department was a shadow of its wartime self. Whereas the number of naval hospitals had reached 83 during World War II, by 1950 this number had decreased to 26. Bed capacity had plummeted from 138,000 beds to less than 23,000. Medical personnel numbers shrank from 170,000 at the end of 1945 to 21,000 in the summer of 1950. The "doctor draft" mentioned earlier brought physicians into uniform to meet their obligations.

Few, if any, of the new doctor draftees had experience in combat medicine. The most seasoned may have had three years of residency. As a result, those with the least training and background ended up in Korea. More often than not, pediatricians, gynecologists, and even dermatologists became surgeons once they reported to their units.

With only brief exposure to surgery during their internships, many of these doctors found themselves debriding frostbitten tissue, amputating shattered limbs, suturing lacerated kidneys and perforated intestines, and extracting shrapnel and bullets from every part of the human body. Ending up in a new field hospital as the first patient was a scenario few troops joked about. Yet despite the inexperience and shortages of medical equipment and supplies during the early months of the war, many of these neophytes quickly learned the skills they needed to save lives and return many Marines and sailors back to their units.

COPING WITH CLIMATE AND DISEASE

With a rugged, inhospitable terrain and climate that seesawed between very hot and extremely cold, Korea was a bad place to fight a war. Late fall and winter of 1950 in North Korea was the coldest in memory. In late November, temperatures began plummeting. During the fighting at the Chosin Reservoir, improperly clothed troops had to fight their way out of Chinese encirclement in temperatures as low as 35 degrees below zero Fahrenheit. Keeping alive, must less functioning, became anything but routine. For Marines fighting off hordes of Chinese, everything appeared hopeless. Weapons ceased to function. C-rations froze in their cans as did canteen water. Unable to drink, men sucked snow to relieve their thirst, further lowering body temperature and making them more susceptible to hypothermia.

With inadequate clothing and the harsh conditions, frostbite downed more men than Chinese bullets. Removing clothing to treat a wound was impossible. Lieutenant (Junior Grade) Henry Litvin, attached to the 2d Battalion, 5th Marines, described just how difficult practicing medicine in such an environment could be:

> If you were treating a wound, you'd cut through the clothing to where the wound was, or you'd put a battle dressing over the clothes and make sure the wound wasn't leaking blood. It seemed that the intense cold inhibited bleeding. The wounds we saw had already been wrapped by corpsmen in the companies. If the battle dressing was in place, even over their clothing, and there was no leaking blood, we just checked the battle dressing and left the wounds alone.

As an exotic and underdeveloped nation, Korea presented a host of diseases many American doctors had only read about in medical school. Smallpox was endemic, as were typhus, cholera, malaria, tuberculosis, and Japanese B encephalitis. Poor sanitation and polluted water accounted for the more common maladies such as dysentery and other diarrheal diseases.

Despite these overwhelming challenges, by the second year of the war, Navy physicians, dentists, nurses, Medical Service Corps officers, hospital corpsmen, and dental technicians held their own in Korea. They practiced their professions in four medical companies ashore; aboard three Navy hospital ships; and in sick bays of aircraft carriers, cruisers, destroyers, and other vessels patrolling offshore. Unlike Army nurses who staffed the MASHs and field and evacuation hospitals in Korea, Navy nurses were assigned only to hospital ships, aeromedical evacuation squadrons, and the naval hospital in Yokosuka, Japan.

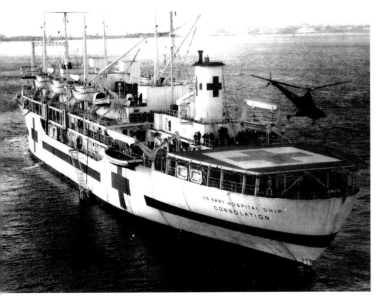

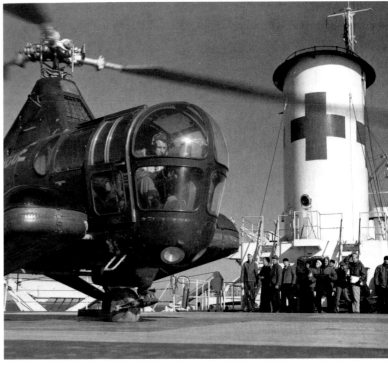

left
USS *Consolation* (AH-15), the first Navy hospital ship to be fitted with a helicopter deck. The first patient to arrive by helicopter flew aboard on December 18, 1950.
U.S. Navy Bureau of Medicine and Surgery

right
Marine Corps HO3S helicopter delivers casualties from fighting in east central Korea to medical care aboard USS *Consolation* (AH-15). January 19, 1952.
U.S. Navy Bureau of Medicine and Surgery.

APPLYING ADVANCES IN MEDICINE

The five years that separated Korea from World War II represented a modest leap in the practice of military medicine. New so-called "miracle" antibiotics such as Aureomycin™, chloramphenicol, streptomycin, and Terramycin™ were now available; penicillin and the sulfas had been used since World War II. Other drugs that advanced the healing art included the antimalarials, such as chloroquine and primaquine; the sedative, sodium pentobarbital (Nembutal™); the anticoagulant, heparin; and serum albumin and whole blood to treat shock.

During World War II, some surgeons experimented with repairing severed blood vessels as a means of restoring damaged limbs that routinely required amputation. As previously mentioned, in Korea surgeons advanced this art of vascular repair, which restored circulation and thereby saved many limbs.

Mobile army surgical hospitals and Navy medical companies deployed near the front enabled rapid surgical intervention. Evacuating the sick and wounded to MASH units or to hospital ships offshore by helicopter, often within an hour after they were wounded, resulted in mortality rates dropping well below those of World War II. In that war, 4.5 percent of the wounded who reached hospitals did not survive. In Korea, the proportion of patients surviving evacuation during the Inchon landing alone reached the remarkably high rate of 99.5 percent.

During World War II, amphibious landings in the Pacific required a fleet of hospital ships, which were often employed as ambulances to evacuate the wounded back to hospitals at island bases for more definitive treatment. In Korea, well-staffed and fully supplied hospital ships, as modern as the most advanced back in the states, provided definitive treatment. Rather than being evacuated to the naval hospital at Yokosuka, Japan, or to stateside hospitals, many Marines, sailors, and United Nations (UN) troops were returned to duty.

By 1951, the hospital ships *Consolation, Haven,* and *Repose* were either on station as base hospitals pierside in Pusan, anchored offshore, or cruising within range of UN operations ashore. Before long, all had been retrofitted with helicopter landing decks so patients could be flown aboard. The marriage of hospital ship and helicopter truly revolutionized wartime health care.

When the Korean War began in June 1950, few could have predicted that it would drag on for three years or that Communist Chinese troops would change the dynamics of the conflict. Few anticipated the brutal combat conditions that service members faced. Navy medicine had adapted quickly to crisis during World War II. In Korea, its practitioners were put to the test. Through innovation and skill, they performed heroically.

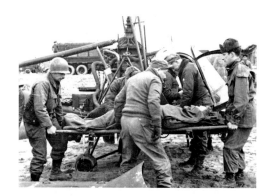

AIR FORCE MEDICAL SERVICE IN THE KOREAN WAR

INNOVATE TO EVACUATE

When North Korean troops invaded South Korea in June 1950, Far East Air Forces (FEAF) had only about 30 doctors, 30 nurses, and 25 Medical Service Corps officers. They supported the entire Air Force population in Korea, Japan, Guam, Okinawa, and the Philippines. Within two months, heavy U.S. and UN casualties almost overwhelmed the meager resources of the Allied medical services in the Far East. But the FEAF medical service soon increased to 236 physicians, 210 nurses, and 161 dentists. Just one-fourth of FEAF medics actually served in Korea itself, because the Air Force could operate effectively from other Far Eastern bases, safe from the dangers of the ground war.

In the first months of the Korean War, the U.S. Army and U.S. Marines still preferred rail and sea evacuation for most of their casualties. But the war soon showed that aeromedical evacuation, which had already proved valuable in World War II, was the ideal method of evacuation for all U.S. casualties. Army and Air Force helicopters and Air Force C-47s and C-54s evacuated most of the Korean War's casualties.

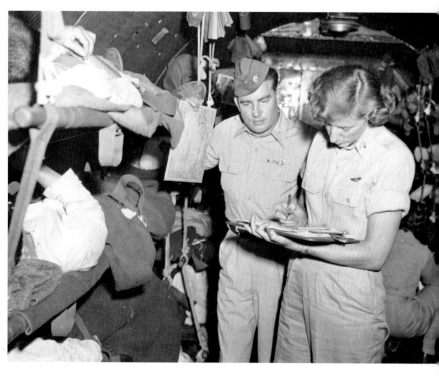

In the summer of 1950, to cope with the rush of casualties, Air Force H-5 rescue helicopters of the 3d Air Rescue Squadron went into action with the Army as frontline medical craft. C-47 transports of the 315th Air Division, carrying aeromedical crews, also flew into the most forward airstrips, even under enemy fire, and saved many American lives. The Air Force's 801st Medical Air Evacuation Squadron (MAES) was one of the first units to receive a Distinguished Unit Citation, for evacuating more 4,700 casualties from the Chosin Reservoir. Many 801st flights originated from Sinanju airfield in late November, where 2,700 patients were evacuated. The 801st MAES helped the embattled soldiers and Marines make a successful fighting withdrawal from the Chosin Reservoir to the port of Hungnam on the northeast coast of Korea.

The other services contributed to the development of combat aeromedical evacuation. The Army soon set up its own helicopter evacuation service, and by late 1951 aeromedical helicopters enabled the U.S. Navy's hospital ships to serve as floating hospitals off Korea rather than as medical transports.

left
Wounded unloaded from U.S. Air Force Captain Eliasson's helicopter, March 1951. Next stop: a mobile army surgical hospital at a Fifth Air Force fighter strip. *National Archives.*

right
Flight nurse, First Lieutenant Victoria Malokas, of Cleveland, Ohio, checks a patient's progress chart in flight aboard a U.S. Air Force C-54 transport aircraft en route from Korea to Japan. Aircraft commander Major George E. Cichy, of San Pedro, California, observes. *National Archives.*

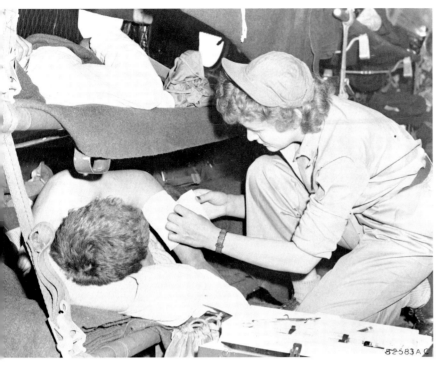

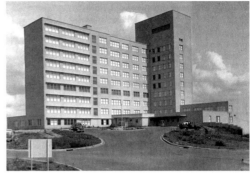

left
Second Lieutenant Pauline Kircher, of Saginaw, Michigan, a member of the 801st Medical Air Evacuation Squadron, changes the dressing on a wounded man's arm during the aeromedical evacuation from Korea to Japan. *National Archives.*

right
Wilford Hall Medical Center at Lackland Air Force Base, Texas, in 1957. Three years later its capacity was doubled to 1,000 beds. *U.S. Air Force Medical Service.*

At the start of the Korean War, the Army and Air Force still had not reached agreement on a division of aeromedical responsibilities. By December 1951, however, Air Force Headquarters agreed that the U.S. Army and the U.S. Marines should assume primary responsibility for forward medical evacuation and acquire their own aeromedical helicopters. The Air Force would supply longer-range aeromedical evacuation. In December 1953, the Air Force was also given responsibility in forward combat areas for organizing and staffing aeromedical staging facilities. In response to new aeromedical evacuation duties, specially designed C-131 Samaritan joined the Air Force's aeromedical fleet in 1954.

While dealing with the special duties of the Korean War, the Air Force Medical Service (AFMS) began to construct its own hospital facilities at each Air Force base around the world. In the 1950s, the Surgeon General's Office helped design the first major U.S. Air Force hospitals at Elmendorf, Travis, Andrews, and Lackland Air Force bases. In 1957, the Lackland Air Force Base Hospital became the Air Force's largest medical facility, with 500 beds. Three years later another 500 beds were added to it. In March 1963, this Lackland hospital was renamed after Major General Wilford Hall, USAF, MC.

The Korean War also demonstrated the Air Force's need for better field hospitals. The medical facilities in Korea, although clinically adequate, were constructed out of shells and Quonset™ huts, with no common plan or design. In response, the AFMS in August 1953 tested a standard 50-bed field hospital that could be flown 1,000 miles by C-119 cargo airplanes. The first Air Force airborne medical assemblages, containing 36 beds, were procured in 1955, and these early air transportable hospitals became operational in 1959. In the decades to come, the AFMS continued to develop ways to modularize and tailor portable medical assemblies to meet the precise needs of each deployment.

ARMY MEDICAL DEPARTMENT MEDAL OF HONOR RECIPIENTS IN KOREAN WAR

DAVID B. BLEAK
RICHARD G. WILSON
BRYANT E. WOMACK

NAVY MEDICAL DEPARTMENT MEDAL OF HONOR RECIPIENTS IN KOREAN WAR

EDWARD C. BENFOLD
WILLIAM R. CHARETTE
RICHARD DEWERT
FRANCIS C. HAMMOND
JOHN E. KILMER

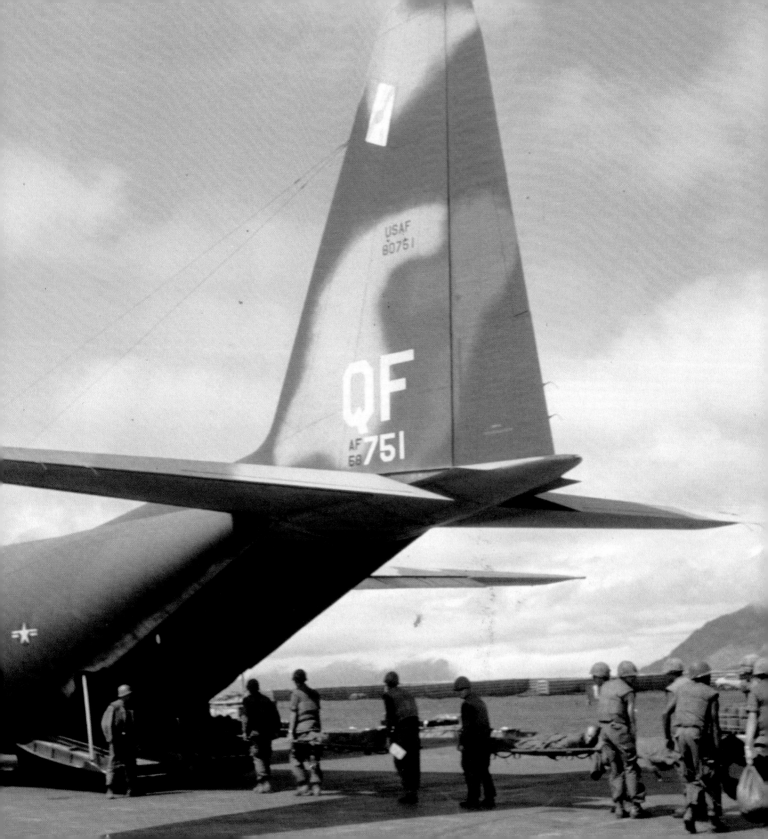

Chapter 8
Cold War and Vietnam War, 1954–75

left

Khe Sanh, South Vietnam, February 4, 1968. Wounded Marines are loaded aboard a U.S. Air Force C-130 transport for evacuation from the besieged base. *U.S. Air Force.*

bottom right

UH-1 Huey air ambulance of the 15th Medical Battalion, 1st Cavalry Division, evacuates a wounded soldier from combat action. *Henry M. Jackson Foundation for the Advancement of Military Medicine.*

COLD WAR AND THE NUCLEAR BATTLEFIELD

In the early 1950s, the U.S. Army and the North Atlantic Treaty Organization (NATO) joined forces in Europe to confront the Soviet Union and its Warsaw Pact allies. The vastly expanded Army required a larger Medical Department to care for the nearly 300,000 American troops, dependents, and civilian employees stationed there. With the exception of Vietnam, Europe remained the most heavily committed area for the U.S. Army and its Medical Department until long after the collapse of the Soviet Union and Warsaw Pact.

The use of helicopters to evacuate the wounded had shown great promise in Korea. After 1953, the Medical Department elected to use only Medical Service Corps pilots and to develop new equipment. In 1960, the Bell UH-1A "Hueys" began replacing the Sikorsky H-19Ds in helicopter ambulance units. The Huey could carry two litters or five ambulatory patients, along with a flight crew of two, the crew chief,

and flight medic. The medical air ambulance company, a new tactical unit with 25 helicopters in four platoons, was set up. The 45th Medical Company (Air Ambulance) at Fort Bragg, North Carolina, was the first of these new units.

The Modern Mobile Army divisions of 1960 and the Reorganization Objective Army Division of 1961 contained a division support command that included a medical battalion. The new air assault and airmobile divisions of the mid-1960s retained the support command and its medical battalion. Each division eventually had its own helicopter ambulance platoon of UH-1 Iroquois medical evacuation helicopters. The 1st Cavalry Division (Airmobile) became the first division with an organic air evacuation capability with creation of an air ambulance platoon in its 15th Medical Battalion.

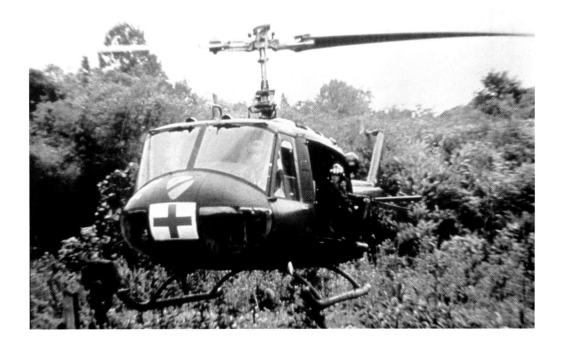

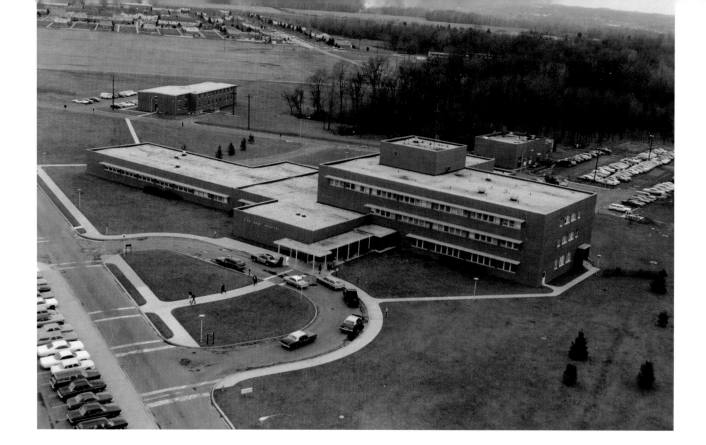

MAINTAINING MEDICAL CARE

In June 1959, Major General Leonard D. Heaton, MC, became the Army Surgeon General. In September, he was promoted to Lieutenant General, the first Army Surgeon General to reach three-star rank. In his 10-year tenure, which lasted through four presidents, he accomplished remarkable achievements.

Heaton's position was "Modern medicine can be practiced adequately only in modern facilities." He emphasized the urgent need for new medical facilities to raise the standard of medical care in the Army. Heaton's modern hospitals used an "expansible chassis" design, which featured a central core of facilities to which beds could be added as needed. Through his efforts, 15 new Army hospitals were opened with four more under construction by 1969.

In 1961, the Army Health Facility concept was introduced which grouped a hospital, outpatient service, dental clinic, and troop dispensary together. The first of these new medical treatment facilities, the Kirk Army Hospital, named after the Army Surgeon General of World War II, opened at Aberdeen Proving Ground, Maryland, in July 1964. Many of today's Army health clinics are patterned on this 1961 concept.

The general hospitals remained the core of the Medical Department. They included Walter Reed in Washington, D.C.; Brooke in San Antonio, Texas; Letterman in San Francisco, California; Fitzsimons at Aurora, Colorado; Madigan at Fort Lewis, Washington; William Beaumont at Fort Bliss, Texas; and Tripler at Fort Shafter, Hawaii. Heaton encouraged Congress to appropriate funds to design and build a new Walter Reed hospital that opened in 1977. Appropriately, in 1994 the building was designated the Heaton Pavilion.

Other significant advances took place in the 1950s and 1960s. In 1951, the first female dentist was commissioned in the Dental Corps. The first female physician was commissioned in the regular Army Medical Corps in February, 1953, although women had received temporary reserve commissions in World War II. In 1955, men were first commissioned in the previously all-female Army Nurse Corps and Women's Medical Specialist Corps, which became the Army Medical Specialist Corps. In May 1966, the first doctors of osteopathy were commissioned in the Medical Corps.

Kirk Army Hospital, at Aberdeen Proving Ground, Maryland. It was one of the first examples of the Army Health Facility concept. *U.S. Army.*

ACQUIRING AND RETAINING MEDICAL PROFESSIONALS

After the Korean War, the services relied on the draft to obtain many of their medical officers. To soften the draft's impact in 1954, Dr. Frank B. Berry, Deputy Assistant Secretary of Defense (Health and Medicine), created what became known as the "Berry Plan." It allowed medical school students to sign up for reserve commissions and defer their service until after they completed their residencies. The "Berry Plan" provided the services with much needed physicians and medical and surgical specialists until the end of the doctor draft in 1973.

By 1960, the actual commissioned officer strength of the Medical Department had eroded to 13,052 from its Korean War peak of 18,887. The number of Medical Corps officers dwindled from 5,714 in 1953 to 3,676 in 1960. However, the Army's expansion during the Vietnam years raised the Medical Department's strength to its postwar high of 22,012 commissioned officers, including 7,131 medical officers.

BROADER MISSIONS

The Army provided extensive opportunities for essential postgraduate education and continuing medical, dental, and nursing training. General hospitals specialized and offered residencies in their fields of expertise. Fitzsimons General Hospital specialized in heart surgery, and became well known when President Dwight D. Eisenhower suffered a heart attack while on vacation in Colorado on September 24, 1955. He spent seven weeks there under the care of Army heart specialists.

The Medical Department encountered increased responsibility in caring for dependents and military retirees in the postwar era. In the 1950s, the Department of Defense began the Dependent Medical Care program to cover 2.8 million of these beneficiaries. This program expanded as the number of married military personnel with families increased. In 1968, an enlarged Civilian Health and Medical Program of the Uniformed Services emerged. It covered civilian health care costs for active duty military, dependents, and retirees. By 1972, 6.2 million persons were eligible for benefits under the program whose operating costs had reached $455.4 million. The Army Medical Department had become one of the world's largest health care maintenance organizations.

Medical research and development was critical to progress in field and clinical medicine. The Medical Department's research and development program supported both internal and external research projects that produced numerous new drugs, surgical procedures, and other advances. During the 1950s and 1960s, the U.S. Army Medical Research and Development Command (MRDC) had programs at 14 research institutes and 15 Army hospitals, plus the Armed Forces Institute of Pathology.

At the Walter Reed Army Institute of Research (WRAIR), 300 doctoral-level researchers worked on all aspects of military medicine, especially infectious diseases. Its major contributions included chloroquine, which replaced Atabrine™ as the basic antimalarial drug, and development of a new drug for chloroquine-resistant malaria. Other WRAIR products were an adenovirus vaccine and use of Camolar for leishmaniasis treatment.

Another MRDC laboratory, the U.S. Army Medical Research Institute for Infectious Diseases at Fort Detrick, Maryland, researched defenses against the deadly biological warfare agents then under development in the Soviet Union. The Institute of Surgical Research at Brooke General Hospital specialized in research and treatment of burn victims, earning a worldwide reputation. It developed a new topical antibacterial preparation, Sulfamylon™, which reduced burn deaths due to infection by 50 percent, and is still in widespread use.

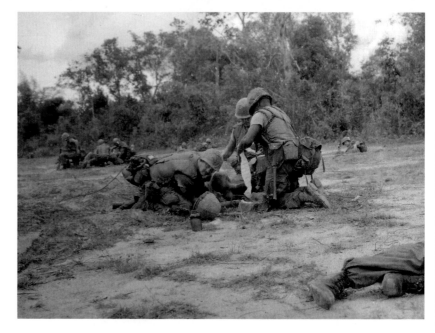

MEDICAL READINESS IN HOT SPOTS

After the Korean War, significant efforts were devoted to ensuring medical readiness and field support for an ever-changing Army. A combat support hospital with 200 beds was developed in the early 1960s as an all-purpose hospital, smaller and more manageable than the standard 400-bed evacuation hospital. To support armored operations in Europe, the Medical Department modified the M577 command post version of the standard M113 armored personnel carrier into an advanced battalion aid station, still operational in 2005.

Army medical units supported American forces in Cold War hot spots worldwide. Two hospitals from Europe were sent to Lebanon from July to October 1958. The Lebanon experience demonstrated the importance of having preventive medicine personnel and surgical capability with the first troops to deploy in a crisis, because medical problems were most significant early in any operation.

The erection of the Berlin Wall in August 1961 and the Cuban Missile Crisis of October–November 1962 provided major tests for the Medical Department. In 1965, the 15th Field Hospital, 54th Medical Detachment (Helicopter Ambulance), and other medical elements deployed with the 82d Airborne Division to the Dominican Republic. Two field hospitals and two helicopter ambulance detachments, each with the new UH-1A Hueys, were dispatched to Chile in May–July 1960 in response to an earthquake. In July 1963, the 8th Evacuation Hospital from Germany was airlifted to Yugoslavia to assist after the Skopje earthquake disaster. Medical units also played important relief roles in the Alaskan earthquake of March 1964 and undertook a number of minor disaster relief missions in Italy, Morocco, and Somalia that honed their skills for potential combat action. The major combat came in Vietnam.

COMBAT MEDICINE IN VIETNAM

American involvement in the fighting in the Republic of Vietnam began in the late 1950s and early 1960s with military advisors who assisted the Army of the Republic of Vietnam (ARVN). A medical capability accompanied the advisors. In April 1962, the 8th Field Hospital arrived at Nha Trang, with dental, thoracic, orthopedic, and neurosurgical detachments. The 57th Medical Detachment (Helicopter Ambulance) also arrived with five UH-1A Hueys.

Early American military support emphasized helicopters to give the ARVN greater capability to attack the Vietcong in their jungle and mountain bases. The 57th Medical Detachment soon began flying medevac missions, which would continue for the next 11 years. Early in 1964, the 57th adopted the tactical call sign "Dustoff," which came to stand for a medevac mission throughout the Vietnam fighting and ever since.

In January 1964, Major Charles L. Kelly assumed command of the 57th Medical Detachment then based at Soc Trang south of Saigon. Kelly and Major Patrick H. Brady became well known for their willingness to go just about anywhere against Vietcong fire to pick up wounded American advisors and ARVN soldiers. On July 1, 1964, Kelly was called for a "Dustoff" mission near Vinh Long. As he descended under exceptionally heavy enemy fire, an advisor on the ground told him to get out of the area. Kelly answered, "When I have your wounded." Enemy fire hit the aircraft, killing Kelly, and the aircraft crashed. Charles Kelly set the standard not only for "Dustoff" pilots, but for all Army medical personnel during the Vietnam conflict.

above
Medics of Company B, 4th Battalion, 23d Infantry Regiment, 25th Infantry Division, care for soldiers wounded in a Vietcong ambush near Cu Chi, Vietnam, May 18, 1966. *National Archives.*

right
"Dustoff" medical evacuation of wounded soldiers of the 173d Airborne Brigade north of Nha Trang. *Henry M. Jackson Foundation for the Advancement of Military Medicine.*

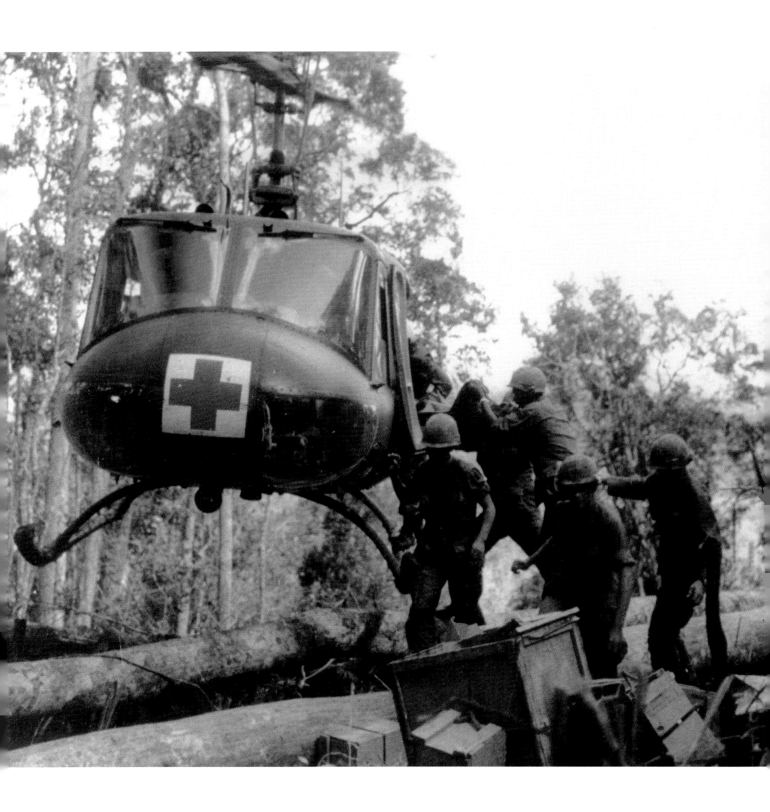

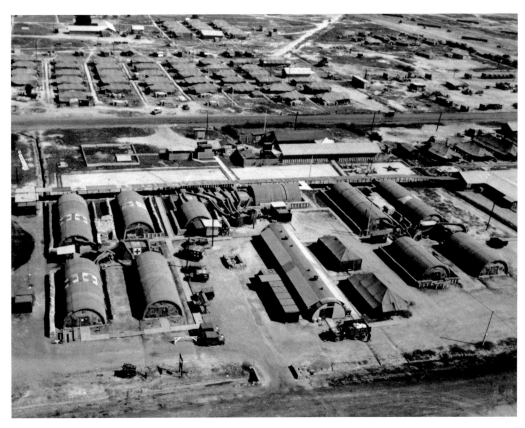

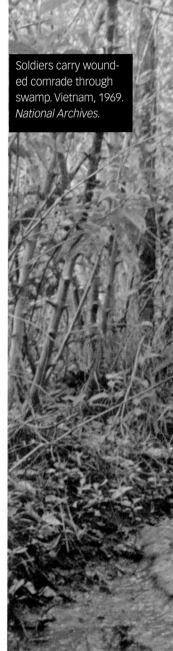

Soldiers carry wounded comrade through swamp. Vietnam, 1969. *National Archives.*

The massive American buildup in South Vietnam that began in 1965 required an equally large medical presence. Heaton directed the deployment of a Medical Unit, Self-Contained, Transportable (MUST) hospital to Vietnam in 1965. Of modular design and intended for the battlefields of Europe, the MUST was highly transportable. Its major components, which traveled in shipping containers, could be immediately converted into functional operating rooms and laboratories. Inflatable rubber shelters that were air conditioned, heated, and fully provided with electrical power served as wards and quarters.

The 45th Surgical Hospital (Mobile Army) was the first MUST hospital deployed to Vietnam. It arrived at Tay Ninh in late October 1966 and was functioning by early November, supporting the 196th Light Infantry Brigade, 25th Infantry Division, and Special Forces teams operating nearby. Tragically, Major Gary Wratton, MC, its commander, was killed in a mortar attack before the hospital was operational. Six MUST hospitals eventually served in Vietnam.

DISEASE AND COMBAT

Tropical diseases in Vietnam presented the greatest threat to and drain on American combat and support troops. Indigenous virulent strains of malaria (*Plasmodium falciparum*) could hospitalize a soldier for five weeks or longer. During the years of U.S. involvement, disease accounted for about 70 percent of all admissions to Army medical treatment facilities. Building on previous work on tropical diseases and malaria, the Army fielded strong preventive medicine programs that were critical to maintaining the health of the troops. As a result, disease admissions were only one-third of those recorded in the China-Burma-India and Southwest Pacific Area theaters during World War II.

Influenced by the monsoon seasons, Vietnam's climate produced skin diseases. Among them were fungal and bacterial infections as well as immersion foot or "paddy" foot.

above left
Aerial view of the 45th Surgical Hospital (Mobile Army) at Tay Ninh, Vietnam, early 1967. The hemispheric structures contain the wards. They are inflatable and air-conditioned. *National Archives.*

bottom right
Patients who could return to their units within 30 days were accommodated at the 6th Convalescent Center at Cam Ranh Bay, Vietnam, established in April 1966. *National Archives.*

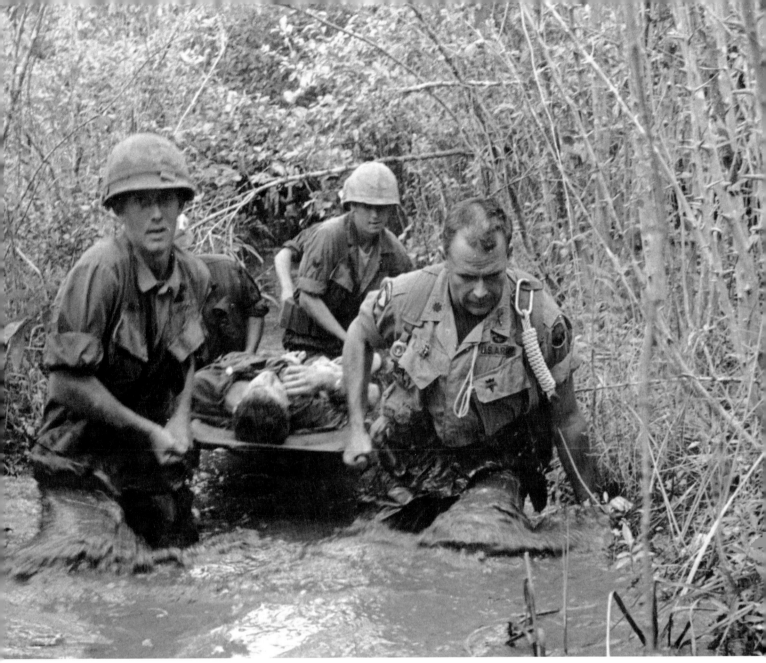

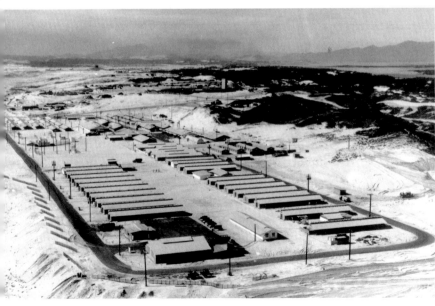

The surgical, evacuation, and field hospitals in Vietnam were fixed in semipermanent and fully equipped facilities on installations. Instead of moving around as in earlier wars, they provided area support to tactical and logistical units. These fixed installations were subject to rocket and mortar attacks, which accounted for many of the Medical Department's personnel losses. By December 1965, the Army had eight hospitals in Vietnam with 1,627 beds. The expansion in American forces that occurred over the next two plus years saw the addition of 15 hospital units to bring the total to 23 hospitals with 5,283 beds. In April 1966, the 6th Convalescent Center opened at Cam Ranh Bay for medical and surgical patients who could return to their units within the theater's 30-day evacuation policy.

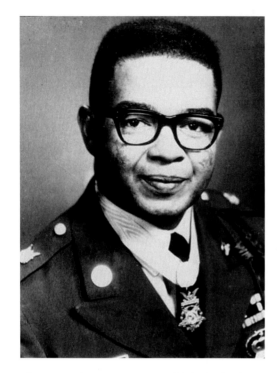

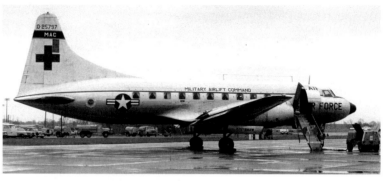

The Medical Department established a high standard of care for the wounded in Vietnam. It was a dirty war, due to the heavy use of mines, booby traps, and high-velocity small arms. The Soviet AK-47 and American M-16 rifles caused serious wounds and severe tissue damage. Mines and booby traps especially presented major surgical challenges. The blast not only destroyed tissue and bones, but further contaminated the injury site with dirt, debris, and secondary missiles.

Medics at the front line provided immediate care for the injured even under the worst conditions. They bandaged wounds, controlled bleeding, provided plasma expanders and fluids, and sedated the patient to await evacuation. More than 1,100 enlisted medics were killed in action and many others were wounded. Of the 17 Medals of Honor awarded to Army medical personnel, the most ever awarded to the Medical Department in any war in American history, 15 went to frontline medics and eight of these were posthumous. The two others went to "Dustoff" pilots Major Patrick H. Brady and Chief Warrant Officer Michael J. Novosel.

"Dustoff" and medical evacuation were critical to wounded soldiers' survival. With flight medics and medical supplies onboard, the medevac helicopters were on call and quickly lifted the wounded to the nearest available medical facility. By 1966, the medevac force in Vietnam had grown to one company, four detachments, and a platoon with the 1st Cavalry Division.

By 1969, two companies (45th and 498th) and 11 detachments with 116 UH-1D and H model Hueys operated in Vietnam. The D and H models could carry six litters or nine ambulatory patients versus the UH-1B's two litters or five sitting. Medevac missions in 1965 carried 13,004 American, Vietnamese, and Free World Forces evacuees. By 1969, that number had increased geometrically to 206,209. Medevac helicopters flew an average of two missions per day in 1965 and four per day in 1969.

From the 57th Medical Detachment's first mission on May 12, 1962, until it flew the last American medevac mission on March 11, 1973, air ambulances carried an estimated 850,000 to 900,000 allied military personnel and Vietnamese civilians. These accomplishments came with a high cost. More than 208 pilots and crew were killed by hostile fire and another 545 wounded; 48 pilots were killed and 200 injured in non-battle crashes. A total of 199 air ambulances were lost, and 1,635 were hit by hostile fire. Despite enemy fire and flying conditions, they never faltered from Charles Kelly's promise, "When I have your wounded."

At forward hospitals (and in Vietnam, all hospitals were forward), blood was readily available along with skilled surgical, medical, and nursing staffs and the most advanced medical technology. Possibly only second to medevac, blood was most critical to survival. The Military Blood Program Agency orchestrated blood collection, processing, shipment, and distribution to and within Vietnam. From 100 units monthly in 1965, blood supplies increased to 38,000 units monthly in February 1969.

Complex operations, including vascular surgery and neurosurgery, were performed routinely. Specialty surgical teams as well as teams composed of different specialties were used in all hospitals.

left
Specialist Fifth Class Lawrence Joel earned the Medal of Honor for exceptional gallantry in combat in Vietnam on November 8, 1965. As a medic in the 1st Battalion (Airborne), 503d Infantry, 173d Airborne Brigade, Joel treated many wounded comrades during an intense 24-hour battle in which he was himself wounded. *National Archives.*

right
The C-131 Samaritan aircraft joined the Air Force's aeromedical fleet in 1954. It was the first aeromedical evacuation aircraft with a pressurized cabin. Configured as an airborne ambulance, it carried 27 stretchers or 37 ambulatory patients. *U.S. Air Force.*

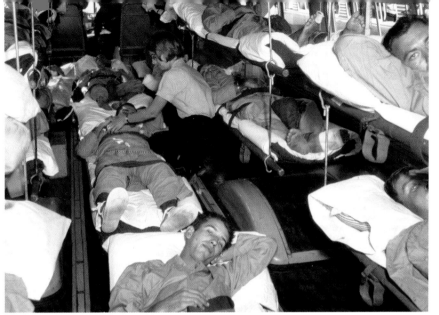

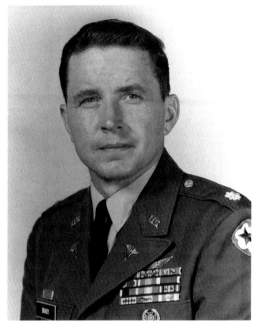

left
U.S. Air Force Second Lieutenant Patricia Hines, 21st Casualty Staging Flight, checks the safety belts of patients aboard an ambulance bus taking them to an aircraft for evacuation to Japan. Tan Son Nhut Air Base, South Vietnam, February 1968. *U.S. Air Force.*

right
Major Patrick H. Brady, Medical Service Corps, earned the Medal of Honor on January 6, 1968, during a series of hazardous medical evacuation missions under heavy enemy fire. The citation says, "Throughout that day Maj. Brady utilized three helicopters to evacuate a total of 51 seriously wounded men, many of whom would have perished without prompt medical treatment." *National Archives.*

Initially, the U.S. Air Force air evacuation flights moved sick and wounded soldiers who required more than 30-day care to Clark Air Base in the Philippines and then onward to Okinawa, Japan; Tripler General Hospital in Hawaii; or the continental U.S. Hospital facilities in the Pacific were limited; many patients were sent to the U.S. to make space for new arrivals. To reduce the drain of manpower from Vietnam, in 1967 a large hospital complex (three-and-one-half general hospitals) was opened in Japan to take evacuees who could return to action within 60 days. Patients who required additional or specialized care were evacuated to the continental U.S. when they were stabilized. From 1965 through 1969, a total of 116,179 patients were evacuated from Vietnam. To cope with this flow, the general and post hospitals in the U.S. expanded their bed capacities to handle the large increases in patients.

The Army and its medical units were largely gone from Vietnam by the end of 1972. The 57th Medical Detachment (Helicopter Ambulance), one of the first medical units to arrive in Vietnam in April 1962, was one of the last to leave in March 1973.

From January 1965 to December 1970, 97,659 wounded were admitted to Army hospitals with a mortality of 2.6 percent. This rate was slightly worse than Korea's 2.5 percent because helicopter evacuation was so swift that mortally wounded patients who would have died on the battlefield in prior wars now died in the hospitals. If those soldiers who died within the first 24 hours were counted in this class, the mortality rate is closer to 1 percent. By any measure, this was an astonishing achievement—the promise of Korea became the reality of Vietnam.

**ARMY MEDICAL DEPARTMENT
MEDAL OF HONOR RECIPIENTS
IN VIETNAM WAR**

GARY B. BEIKIRCH
THOMAS W. BENNETT
PATRICK H. BRADY
DONALD W. EVANS, JR.
CHARLES C. HAGEMEISTER
LAWRENCE JOEL
KENNETH M. KAYS
JOSEPH G. LAPOINTE, JR.
THOMAS J. MCMAHON
EDGAR L. MCWETHY, JR.
JAMES H. MONROE
MICHAEL J. NOVOSEL
ALFRED V. RASCON
LOUIS R. ROCCO
CLARENCE E. SASSER
DANIEL J. SHEA
DAVID F. WINDER

**NAVY MEDICAL DEPARTMENT
MEDAL OF HONOR RECIPIENTS
IN VIETNAM WAR**

DONALD E. BALLARD
WAYNE M. CARON
ROBERT R. INGRAM
DAVID RAY

NAVY MEDICINE, POST-KOREA THROUGH VIETNAM

TRANSPORTING REFUGEES

The signing of the Korean armistice at Panmunjom in July 1953 ended hostilities without a permanent peace. Nevertheless, the pattern of demobilization that had characterized the end of all American wars continued. The authorized ratio of medical officers to active duty troop strength was cut in half. During the 1953–54 fiscal years, the Navy lost more than 1,000 physicians—a 25 percent reduction. Several naval hospitals were closed or downgraded to infirmaries.

Many of the Navy's "small boys"—destroyers, submarines, LSTs (landing ship, tank), and other amphibious craft—had minimal or no medical staff aboard. For the larger vessels, the reduction meant battleships were reduced from two medical officers to one, aircraft carriers from three to two, and LST squadrons from two physicians to one.

When French colonial rule in Indochina came to a chaotic end in 1954 after the climactic defeat at Dien Bien Phu, the U.S. Navy helped evacuate 721 French troops and transport them to metropolitan France and North Africa. The hospital ship *Haven*, which had already seen action in World War II and four tours during the Korean War, was again pressed into service for Operation Repatriation.

One of the Legionnaires died en route. As Navy nurse Anna Corcoran later recalled, "They offloaded the body in a casket with the French flag draped over it. That was very, very emotional to watch. Of course, at that time, we didn't know how many of our own would be going home that way from Vietnam. We couldn't have imagined back in 1954 that ten years later we would be involved just like the French were."

The Navy was again called upon to spearhead another humanitarian operation shortly after completing Operation Repatriation. Under the terms of the 1954 Geneva Accords, which ended the war between France and the Communist Viet Minh, the people of Vietnam could decide where they wished to settle. Few in the south chose to go north. However, with the collapse of French rule, hundreds of thousands of refugees streamed south to escape the Communists. In Operation Passage to Freedom, Navy ships evacuated more than 860,000 refugees to South Vietnam.

In Operation Passage to Freedom, Navy physicians and hospital corpsmen provided medical care for the refugees, many of whom were already very debilitated by their ordeal. Skin diseases, dysentery, and intestinal parasites were common as was the highly contagious eye affliction—trachoma. As the refugees were brought to Haiphong—the port from which they would embark for South Vietnam—the Navy set up temporary camps for them complete with tents, potable water, food, and medical care. Preventive medicine teams worked diligently to control the rodent and insect population, spray for malarial mosquitoes, and purify water. Men, women, and children were vaccinated, deloused, and treated for their illnesses. When they boarded transports and LSTs for the journey south, Navy medical personnel accompanied them, dressing wounds, treating fractures and fevers, and delivering an average of four babies per trip.

NAVY MEDICAL PRESENCE ESTABLISHED ASHORE

In the late winter of 1963, Navy physicians and nurses began arriving in Saigon. By that fall, they began setting up what became known as Station Hospital Saigon. It was a five-story concrete building which at that time served as the only Navy hospital receiving American combat casualties directly from the field. The 100-bed hospital was established to meet the need for

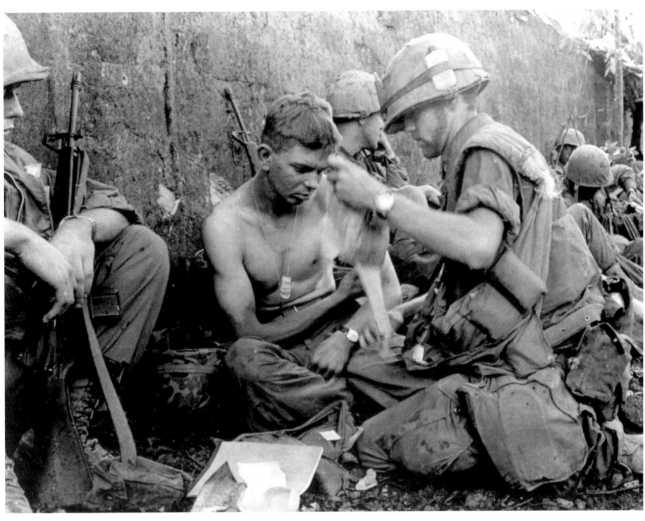

Hospital Corpsman D. R. Howe, right, treats wounded Private First Class D. A. Crum of Company H, 2d Battalion, 5th Marines, during the fighting at Hue City, February 6, 1968. *U.S. Navy Bureau of Medicine and Surgery.*

an inpatient facility in the southern portion of South Vietnam. Also, increased terrorist activity in Saigon itself supported the need for a hospital in or near the capital city. Vietcong terrorists were rampant, exploding bombs in the Central Market and in bars and theaters frequented by Americans. On Christmas Eve 1964, a Vietcong agent parked a bomb-laden car in the underground garage of the Brink Hotel, used as American bachelor officer quarters. The bomb detonated with devastating results. Many casualties resulted, including an Army dentist killed. Four Navy nurses among the wounded became the only Navy nurses to be awarded the Purple Heart during the Vietnam War.

The Gulf of Tonkin Resolution passed by Congress on August 7, 1964, gave the president the power "to take all necessary measures to repel any armed attack against the forces of the United States and to prevent further aggression." Escalation of the war in Vietnam ensued.

Winning the hearts and minds of the South Vietnamese people was crucial to keeping the

Communist insurgency at bay. Medical care of any kind was a luxury few Vietnamese in the impoverished countryside could afford. Therefore, medical aid programs became a high priority. In response, the Department of State, the U.S. Agency for International Development (USAID), and the Department of Defense co-sponsored Military Provincial Health Assistance Program teams or MILPHAP, with the Department of Defense providing military personnel to staff the teams. These teams practiced medicine in South Vietnamese civilian hospitals alongside their Vietnamese counterparts. By the spring of 1969, the Navy fielded seven MILPHAP teams that operated in many of South Vietnam's provinces.

The Navy and the other services also began what were called civic action or "people to people" programs whose primary aim was to enable the Vietnamese to help themselves. These programs also embraced English and technical training classes and on-the-job instruction. In addition, they provided medical and dental assistance.

The Medical Civil Action Program (MEDCAP) was one of the first civic action programs to be implemented. MEDCAP provided emergency care for civilian casualties and refugees in combat areas, offered sick call and limited dispensary care in populated areas not yet secure, and provided professional medical assistance in secure areas and local hospitals.

COMBAT MEDICINE ASHORE

The 3d Marine Division was the first major U.S. combat unit to arrive in Vietnam. It came ashore in March 1965 to defend the Danang airfield. Marines were soon deployed to Chu Lai, about 50 miles south of Danang, to protect the airstrip and also to Phu Bai, about 40 miles north, near the city of Hué, to defend another airfield. Medical support of the force became a high priority, and the 3d Medical Battalion provided that support.

The 3d Medical Battalion had a collecting and clearing company for each of the infantry regiments and one at the division headquarters. The collecting and clearing company was intended to be mobile so it could move within the infantry regiment to which it was attached. Because the war in Vietnam was essentially a "frontless" conflict with little movement, the collecting and clearing companies were in fixed locations. These companies traditionally were not designed as definitive treatment facilities but were the only companies then available to assign to Danang, Chu Lai, and Phu Bai, where airfields needed protection.

Despite their limitations at the outset, within a few short months, these collecting and clearing companies became real hospitals. Charlie Company organized at Danang, Bravo at Chu Lai, and Alpha at Phu Bai. Before long, Delta Company was also operational.

A wounded soldier was brought to the medical company, admitted, and treated. If he could recover from disease or wounds within 120 days and return to duty, he was kept in theater. If additional care was required, he was shipped back to the United States.

As troop buildups continued and the war became more violent and widespread throughout South Vietnam, the demands on Navy medical personnel increased. The types and severity of the injuries were those typically inflicted by the weapons of war—mines, high-velocity small arms, artillery, grenades, mortars, rockets, and booby traps. In time, the medical battalions were well staffed and equipped to handle the large influx of casualties. Skilled surgeons, anesthesiologists, orthopedists, and oral surgeons, many hailing from some of the United States' finest medical schools and hospitals, performed definitive surgery. Many of the mine-inflicted injuries required vascular repairs, and skilled surgeons saved many limbs from amputation.

Navy anesthesiologist William Mahaffey recalled that Charlie Med of the 3d Medical Battalion saw mostly "massive soft tissue injury and those which had utterly destroyed femurs, tibias, fibulas, and ankles—things that I had never seen in a civilian setting." His hospital also treated many patients suffering from malaria and disabling diarrhea and dysentery.

The first caregiver a wounded Marine encountered was his "Doc," the ubiquitous Navy hospital corpsman attached to his outfit. This Vietnam-era corpsman was very special to the Marines he served and highly protected by them. They knew he was there to take care of them and had the skills to save their lives if they were hit.

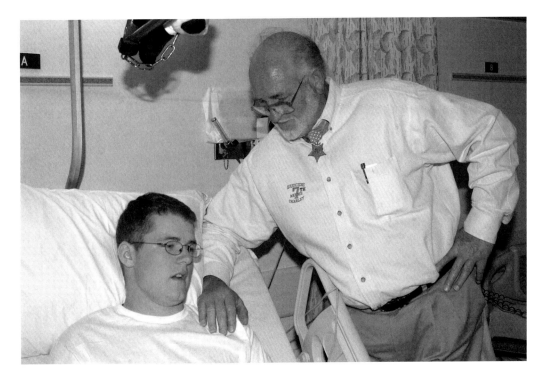

Medal of Honor recipient Robert R. "Doc" Ingram visits with a patient from combat in Iraq at the National Naval Medical Center, Bethesda, Maryland, in April 2003. Ingram, former Navy Hospital Corpsman Third Class, earned the Medal of Honor for conspicuous gallantry in Vietnam on March 28, 1966, with Company C, 1st Battalion, 7th Marines. *U.S. Navy Bureau of Medicine and Surgery.*

As in other wars, corpsmen were trained to accomplish the four basic resuscitative techniques: stop the bleeding; clear the airway; protect the wound; treat and prevent shock. To accomplish this, the corpsman's Unit 1 medical kit typically contained battle dressings and other bandages plus morphine syrettes, a wire splint, atropine, adhesive tape, scissors, casualty tags, iodine, bacitracin ointment, aspirin, and sometimes a small surgical kit containing a forceps and scalpel blades.

The corpsman in Vietnam practiced medicine in a particularly hostile environment. The extreme heat and humidity and the necessity of living in the field for long periods meant that disease and injury were constant companions. During the summer, heat exhaustion and heat stroke were common.

Colonel Michael Holladay, a former Marine Corps platoon commander who served near the Demilitarized Zone (DMZ), recalled: "We had only the clothes we were wearing, which were the old green jungle utilities. We spent so much time in the bush that your clothing stayed wet damn near all the time. Because we went through the old tiger grass, which had a razor edge on it, the crotch of the utilities wore out. A lot of Marines had groin infections and boils. The corpsman spent much of the time trying to deal with some of the health issues that came up with men who were constantly living in a muddy, wet environment."

That constant wetness also contributed to foot problems and jungle rot. Leeches were common; occasionally a corpsman was called upon to render first aid to a snakebite victim. A testimony to their valor, four Navy hospital corpsmen in Vietnam were awarded Medals of Honor, two posthumously.

HOSPITALS AND HOSPITAL SHIPS

In the Korean War, Navy nurses were relegated to duty aboard hospital ships or in naval hospitals far from the front. Navy nurses in Vietnam served at Station Hospital Saigon; as part of MILPHAP teams working in Vietnamese civilian hospitals; aboard the two hospital ships, *Sanctuary* and *Repose*; and at the Naval Support Activity (NSA) hospital in Danang.

By the summer of 1966 there was a functioning hospital at Danang with a highly skilled staff and a range of specialties not seen anywhere else in Vietnam except aboard the two hospital ships. In addition to general and orthopedic surgeons, NSA Danang had the luxury of urologists, neurosurgeons, and even plastic surgeons. And even though frozen blood technology was still experimental at the time, NSA Danang maintained a blood bank with a frozen blood capability. Units donated, processed, and frozen in the United States were shipped to NSA where they were thawed, processed, and used when needed.

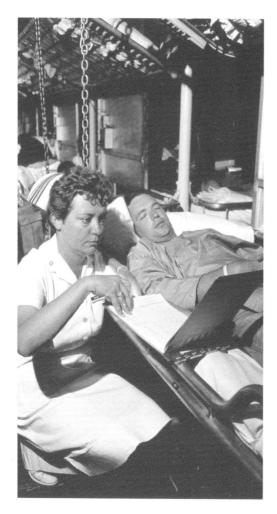

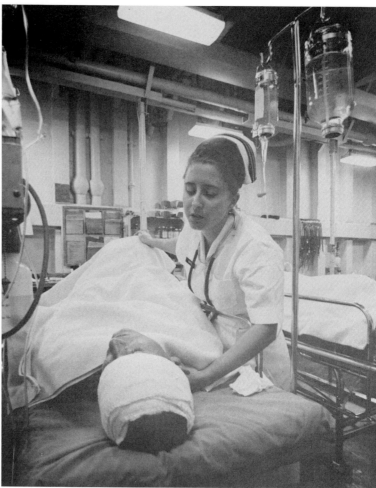

By 1967, two hospital ships augmented the Medical Department's assets in theater. USS *Repose* had been recommissioned in the fall of 1965 and arrived on station off Chu Lai in February of the following year. *Sanctuary* had arrived in Vietnam in April of 1967. Both vessels were once part of the World War II Navy hospital ship fleet and all were of the *Haven* class built near the end of that conflict. The medicine practiced aboard these vessels was as state of the art as any practiced at the finest hospitals in the United States. But, most importantly, both ships had helicopter landing decks allowing for patients to arrive aboard ship, some within an hour of having been injured. In addition, their mobility allowed them to cruise off the Vietnamese coast and render aid in areas where combat operations were under way.

Although helicopters had been used extensively during the Korean War, the helicopter realized its fullest potential in Vietnam. In a country of few roads, little infrastructure, and a topography of jungle, highlands, and delta, helicopters handily transported troops and airlifted supplies. The omnipresent UH-1 Hueys, employed so effectively to airlift Marines, soldiers, or ARVN troops, doubled as ambulances, evacuating the wounded from where they had been injured to medical company hospitals, NSA Danang, or to the hospital ships.

Rear Admiral Almon Wilson, who commanded Charlie Med shortly after it was established, recalled the speed with which the system worked: "We had people always available to take patients from the helicopters. Standard procedure was for somebody to take the stretcher under an arm and rush out to the helicopter with another stretcher bearer, get the patient out of the helicopter, put the fresh stretcher in, and move the patient into the shock and resuscitation area. The helicopter could then leave, and this was a matter of 20 seconds if just one patient was involved."

left
Navy nurse Lieutenant Commander Dorothy Ryan checks chart of Marine Corporal Roy Hadaway aboard USS *Repose*, April 22, 1966. *National Archives.*

right
Navy nurse tends to patient just out of surgery on hospital ship USS *Repose*, October 1967. *National Archives.*

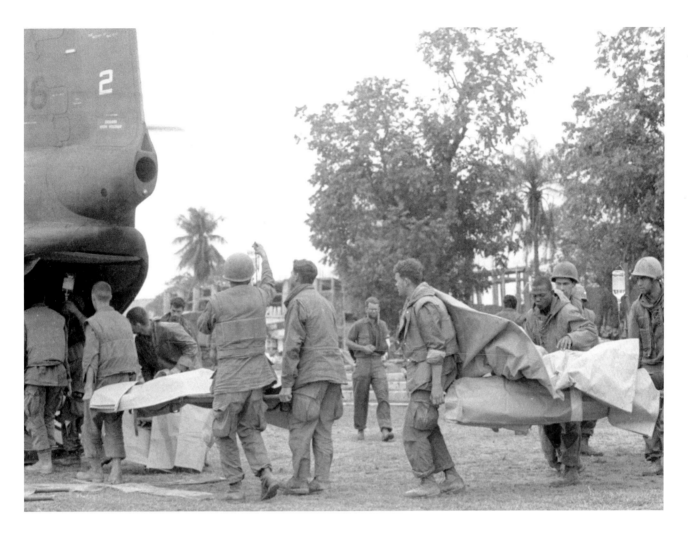

Marines wounded during combat in Hue City are loaded aboard a CH-46D helicopter of Marine Air Group 36 for evacuation. February 14, 1968. *U.S. Navy Bureau of Medicine and Surgery.*

SHIPBOARD MEDICINE

The Marine Corps did not hold a monopoly on Navy medicine during the Vietnam War. Navy medical personnel were represented elsewhere in Vietnam serving aboard the battleship USS *New Jersey*, on cruisers, destroyers, and aircraft carriers. Beginning in August of 1964, carrier-based aircraft began the long air campaign against North Vietnam, hitting enemy roads, rail yards, bridges, and antiaircraft missile sites. They also provided close air support to ground forces fighting south of the DMZ.

The continuing presence of Navy ships in North Vietnamese waters occasionally generated casualties when shore batteries scored hits on American destroyers and other vessels patrolling offshore. But, for the most part, those staffing sick bays treated colds, sore throats,

minor injuries, sprains, fractures, and the occasional appendectomy. However, everything could change in an instant. In October 1966 and July 1967, fire erupted aboard two carriers, USS *Oriskany* and USS *Forrestal*, generating many casualties. Aboard the *Forrestal* alone, 134 sailors lost their lives and many more were badly injured. Medical personnel aboard both vessels responded to these tragedies rendering care until the casualties could be medevaced.

During the Vietnam War, 771 American military personnel were taken prisoner of war (POW), most of them aviators. In 1973, 658 were returned to U.S. military control; 113 died in captivity. The POWs who were freed returned with debilitating physical and psychological issues. Navy orthopedists confronted the aftermath of torture and maltreatment—broken bones that had not mended properly, and the ravages of osteoarthritis that sometimes resulted. Treatment for these conditions is ongoing in some former POWs more than 30 years later.

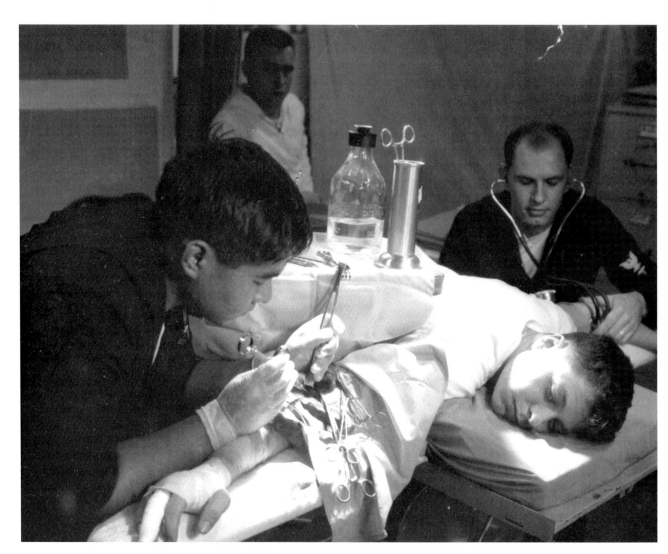

When the war ended in 1975 with a Communist victory, Navy medical personnel suddenly had a new constituency: Vietnamese refugees fleeing their homeland. Navy ships rescued these so-called "Boat People" at sea and took them to special refugee camps set up in Guam and the United States. Medical personnel at the camps provided care until the refugees could be resettled into a new life. The story of Navy medicine in Southeast Asia had come full circle. Two decades after 1954, Operation Passage to Freedom was repeated.

Hospital Corpsman T.C. Miyahira, left, closes wound in Seaman J. Romine's arm as Corpsman D.M. Friend takes the patient's blood pressure in sick bay of USS *Constellation* (CVA-64) June 24, 1965, off the coast of Vietnam. *U.S. Navy Bureau of Medicine and Surgery.*

VIETNAM WAR SERVICE AND CASUALTIES 1964–75

Total U.S. Service Members (Worldwide)	9,200,000
Deployed to Southeast Asia	3,403,000
Battle Deaths	47,415
Other Deaths (in Theater)	10,785
Other Deaths in Service (Non-Theater)	32,000
Non-Mortal Woundings	153,303

Source: Department of Veterans Affairs from Department of Defense.

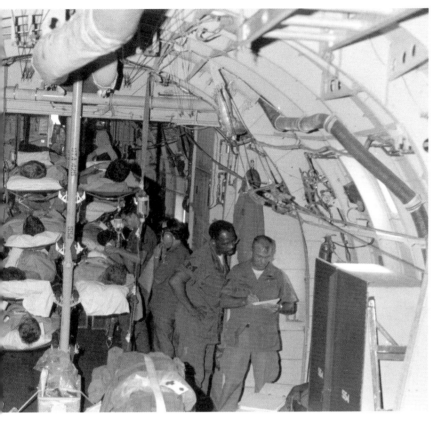

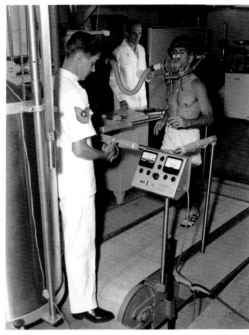

left
Cam Ranh Bay, South Vietnam, May 1970. Wounded personnel await airlift aboard a U.S. Air Force medical evacuation aircraft. *U.S. Air Force.*

right
Aerobic fitness research conducted at Wilford Hall Hospital at Lackland Air Force Base stimulated new physical fitness programs in the Air Force and popularized aerobic fitness training nationwide. *U.S. Air Force.*

U.S. AIR FORCE MEDICAL SERVICE

VIETNAM

In the mid-1960s, Air Force flight surgeons and other physicians, dentists, nurses, and medical technicians established a presence in Vietnam and Thailand. At first, the Vietnamese and Thai hosts were unable to supply suitable medical buildings, and the Air Force itself had none to deploy. By mid-1966, however, the Air Force Medical Service (AFMS) purchased modular steel container express (CONEX) boxes, 10 feet X 10 feet X 40 feet, and shipped them to Southeast Asia, where they were connected and equipped as medical units.

By 1968, the 12th USAF Hospital at Cam Ranh Bay Air Base was the largest Air Force facility in Vietnam, and the second largest hospital in the Air Force, with 475 operating beds and a 100-bed casualty staging facility. The Cam Ranh Bay airfield was also the main aeromedical evacuation hub for Southeast Asia. In the summer of 1968, at the peak of the Vietnam War, about 1,900 Air Force medics were deployed to Southeast Asia.

Advances in aeromedical evacuation improved medical care during the Vietnam War. Rapid evacuation from Vietnam's battlefield by helicopter, followed by airplane transport to advanced surgical hospitals, saved many lives. Helicopters picked up most battle casualties shortly after they were wounded. Pacific Air Command operated a scheduled aeromedical service in Vietnam and also a transoceanic jet service to the hospitals at Clark Air Base, Philippine Islands, and Yokota Air Base and Tachikawa Air Base, Japan. Military Airlift Command helped evacuate many casualties out of Vietnam, and handled patient movement to the United States. The Air Force also acquired its first specially designed aeromedical jet, the C-9A Nightingale, in August 1968.

During the Vietnam War, the AFMS began to strengthen its efforts to ensure a healthy and fit fighting force. The Air Force adopted a new physical fitness program developed at Wilford Hall USAF Hospital in January 1970. It eventually helped popularize aerobic fitness training—running, swimming, and bicycling— throughout the United States.

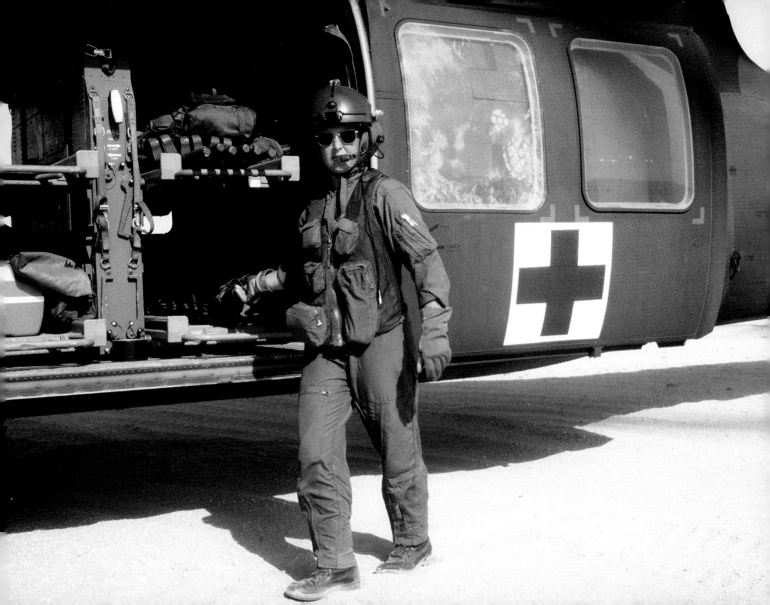

Chapter 9
Post-Vietnam to End of
20th Century, 1975–2000

The crew chief of a 45th Medical Company UH-60A Black Hawk helicopter stows a folded-up stretcher aboard the helicopter during Operation Desert Shield. Saudi Arabia, January 23, 1991. *Department of Defense.*

ESTABLISHMENT OF THE UNIFORMED SERVICES UNIVERSITY OF THE HEALTH SCIENCES

GENESIS OF THE UNIVERSITY

The Uniformed Services University of the Health Sciences (USU) was chartered in 1972 by act of Congress. It was the brainchild of Representative F. Edward Hébert (D-LA). The medical school, later named for Hébert, opened in 1976. A Graduate School of Nursing was added in 1993. In the 1970s, the USU focused on accession of fully qualified officers into the uniformed services' medical departments; development of career officers to lead the services' health activities in the future; and generation of new knowledge, particularly with regard to combat medical care.

Congressman Hébert first advocated a military academy for doctors in 1947. Through the 1950s and 1960s, the U.S. military acquired physicians primarily by drafting them. The medical departments were chronically short of experienced specialists. From 1961 onward, Congressman Hébert introduced bills to create a military medical academy. Both organized medicine and the Department of Defense (DOD) were opposed. DOD was wary of the time and expense involved. The American medical establishment questioned a military medical school's commitment to free inquiry and advancement of knowledge.

COMPROMISE AND ESTABLISHMENT

In 1970, President Richard M. Nixon ended the draft. DOD planners believed that scholarships and compensation enhancements were the best means to attract physicians. Congressman Hébert became chairman of the House Armed Services Committee in 1971, and again introduced his military medical academy bill. Secretary of Defense Melvin R. Laird was not keen on the proposal. Hébert was skeptical about the all-volunteer force. They compromised. Laird would re-examine the academy idea and testify about it before Congress, and Hébert would hold hearings on the all-volunteer force concept. Both won.

In 1972, the Health Professions Revitalization Act became law. It expanded special pays, established the Health Professions Scholarship Program, and chartered the USU. A board of regents was appointed and academic leadership recruited: a mix of civilian medical educators of national reputation, some promising young scholars, and some military medical department officers. A curriculum was shaped.

The USU chartering legislation required an accredited medical school with a "Professor of Military, Naval or Aerospace Science," but did not specify how the new school should differ from other medical schools.

The faculty faced the challenge of modifying traditional medical education to create the leadership cadre needed for effective future military health care. Congress mandated that professional military education be part of the curriculum. This requirement was met by creating an expanded curriculum and a new academic unit headed by a Commandant and Professor of Military Medicine. Second, deployed military physicians needed knowledge and skills beyond that necessary for civilian medical practice. This material was added to the curriculum. Finally, the largely operational aspects of military medicine, not directly related to any traditional medical school, required an additional department.

The first students reported in October 1976 to the interim location at the Armed Forces Institute of Pathology in Washington, D.C., while the Bethesda, Maryland, campus was being built. The Bethesda buildings were completed and the first class graduated in 1980.

REALIZING THE IDEAL
The USU provided about 10 percent of accessions over the closing years of the 20th century. The preponderance of graduates became career officers, fulfilling the need for senior leadership. About 25 percent of active duty military medical officers are USU graduates. The development of joint military medical thinking fulfilled the USU's mission of generating new combat medicine knowledge.

Before 1975, the use of "military medicine" rarely meant a joint or combined thought process at the strategic or operational level. Army medicine, and naval and aviation medicine, were generally discussed separately in American medical literature and doctrinal publications. The USU faculty combined these fields. It assembled textbooks from those different traditions. It prepared and ran joint exercises for its fourth-year students. Most important—and

hardest to document—the faculty and students increasingly wrote about and talked about military medicine as a joint ideal.

The ideal was given practical reality by USU alumni in combat and other deployments of the late 20th and early 21st centuries. Hypothetically, a Marine wounded in action could receive initial care from a Navy shock trauma platoon, then transfer to an Army Combat Surgical Hospital, and then be cared for by an Air Force combat casualty evacuation team on a C-17 aeromedical transport to definitive care in the United States. At any level, the wounded Marine might encounter a USU medical or nursing graduate.

ARMY MEDICINE ADAPTS

CREATION OF THE ALL-VOLUNTEER FORCE
After Vietnam, during the 1970s and 1980s, the Army and its medical support were entirely reshaped. An essentially new Army emerged with an all-volunteer force, new doctrine of AirLand Battle, a new organization, and new equipment.

The Medical Department's first responsibility was to meet the wartime operational needs of the new field Army. At the same time, it had to manage an increasingly complex system of military health care that confronted the same challenges of quality care, integration of new technologies, and cost containment as in the civilian world.

The legislation that established the USU also contained the Uniformed Services Health Professional Scholarship Program (USHPSP). The program continues in 2005. It pays for medical, dental, veterinary medicine, and other schooling in return for a specific service commitment.

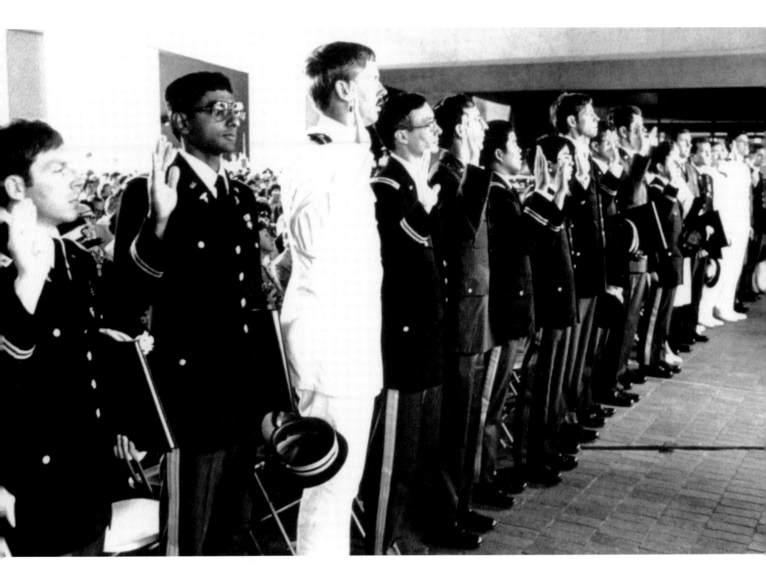

The 28 members of the first class of physicians from the Uniformed Services University of the Health Sciences take the Hippocratic Oath at graduation on May 24, 1980. *Uniformed Services University of the Health Sciences.*

Until the USU began producing graduates in 1980, the Medical Department relied upon USHPSP participants and volunteers. Their numbers did not always cover requirements. However, the graduate medical education specialty programs offered at the Army's teaching hospitals attracted many medical students.

In 1978, as the last of the "Berry Planners" completed their obligations, the Army had 4,140 physicians handling a workload requirement that called for more than 5,800 physicians. By 1980, this situation eased somewhat with the USHPSP supplying 400 physicians per year. By 1986, 77 percent of the Army's new physicians came from this program.

DEVELOPMENT OF "PHYSICIAN EXTENDERS"
Studies over the years emphasized that military physicians could achieve maximum efficiency if they were relieved of routine duties by "physician extenders." Physician assistants (PAs) and nurse clinicians or practitioners were the most likely physician extenders who could replace or supplement physicians in tactical units, troop clinics, and outpatient care.

For many years, the Army and other services relied heavily on general medical officers (GMOs) or general practitioners for duty in troop clinics and as battalion surgeons. With the supply of GMOs also dwindling, the Army decided that the available physicians would be much more valuable serving in the medical treatment facilities in peacetime. Only when tactical units deployed would they take up their assignments as battalion surgeons.

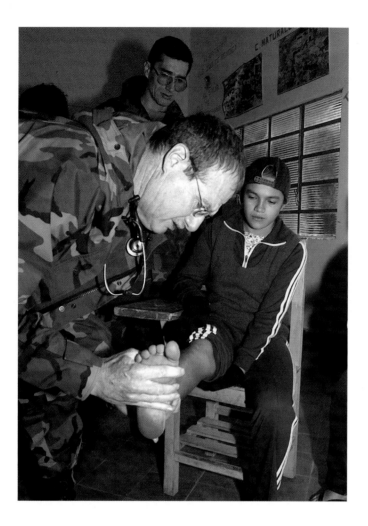

The Army's maneuver battalions required significant medical support as part of their organizations. Hence, the PA program was established in 1972 to train warrant officer physician assistants and to relieve medical officers of many of their former functions. By 1980, 400 PAs were authorized in the Army. Physician assistants continue to play a significant role in Army health care. In February 1992, more than 300 PAs then serving in the Army were converted from warrant officers to commissioned officers and became part of the Army Medical Specialist Corps.

Clinical nurse practitioners were also added in increasing numbers to assume duties formerly performed by physicians. They were trained to supplement or replace physicians, and new nurse practitioner training programs were added in ambulatory care, obstetrics and gynecology, pediatrics, psychiatric and mental health, intensive care, and Army health. Both PAs and nurse practitioners have increasingly assumed greater roles than originally envisioned in the early 1970s.

Additional programs were also implemented to attract and retain physicians, dentists, and other health care professionals or to relieve them of routine administrative duties. From the variable incentive pay program of 1974 through the Medical Officers Retention Bonus of 1989, incentive pay initiatives provided significant annual bonuses linked to specialties and experience. Where possible, contract physicians were also used to offset the shortages. To relieve medical officers for clinical duties, Medical Service Corps (MSC) officers received more "branch immaterial" command and staff positions, including the command of divisional medical battalions. In coming years such positions would increasingly be opened to MSC officers, nurses, and others.

During these years, major hospital construction and modernization programs strove to keep Army medical facilities as modern as possible. In 1975, the Surgeon General established the Health Facilities Planning Agency to manage all design, construction, and budgeting of Army health facilities worldwide. By 1980 the Army Health Facility Modernization

U.S. Army Major Gene Nuse, Family Nurse Practitioner from the Army Reserve, 21st General Hospital, St. Louis, Missouri, examines a Paraguayan girl's foot during cooperative engineer and medical operations in Paraguay. May 4, 2001. *Department of Defense.*

Program had 90 projects valued at $500 million under way to replace all World War II and older medical and dental facilities. More than in Leonard Heaton's day, modern quality health care facilities were absolutely essential to the recruitment and retention of both soldiers and health care professionals, and to the practice of modern medicine.

ARMY AND MEDICAL DEPARTMENT REORGANIZATION

Planning for the all-volunteer Army emphasized the total Army, which combined the active Army, the Army National Guard, and U.S. Army Reserve. A large part of the "go to war" combat support and combat service support units, including many medical units, were placed in the Army National Guard and Army Reserve. Any sustained combat operations required their recall.

The Army reshaped itself by splitting the former Continental Army Command into two new major commands, the Forces Command and the Training and Doctrine Command. A third new major command, the U.S. Army Health Services Command (HSC), emerged from this reorganization in 1972–73, along with a restructuring of the Army Medical Department.

The new HSC set up at Fort Sam Houston, Texas, and assumed control of all Army health and dental care systems in the continental United States on April 1, 1973. (Those in Alaska, the Canal Zone, and Hawaii were added later.) It assumed responsibilities for all Army hospitals, medical centers, dental and veterinary activities, and Medical Department Activities (MEDDACs).

HSC also assumed control of all officer and enlisted medical education and training programs through the Academy of Health Sciences at Fort Sam Houston, which became the largest medical training institution in the world.

The MEDDAC concept was introduced in the late 1960s to provide better and faster care for the sick and wounded returning from Vietnam. All Army medical, dental, and veterinary activities in the area of an installation with an Army hospital were integrated under that hospital commander. However, from 1978, dental activities were removed from MEDDAC control to form Dental Activities (DENTACS) that functioned under the Chief of the Dental Corps, responsible for all dental care in the Army.

HSC emphasized new programs to improve ambulatory care, family practice, and primary care. Those benefits were vital to a volunteer Army with more married personnel and families than the old draftee Army. The first family practice residency was set up at Martin Army Hospital at Fort Benning, Georgia, in 1971. By 1979, 15 residency programs were producing 90 family practice physicians annually to support the changing face of Army health care.

A major challenge for the Medical Department was to create a system of medical treatment facilities (MTFs) and tactical medical units under the constraint of severely limited resources. The solution was to embed clinical personnel and even tactical units in MTFs, including the general hospitals and medical centers. The personnel and units had mobilization or wartime assignments that required deployment, which meant that they would be "carved out" of the facility.

This system, known as the Professional Filler System (PROFIS), was set up in 1980. It proved ineffective in Operation Urgent Fury in Grenada in October 1983. Improvements were made in the practical training and familiarity of PROFIS personnel with their assigned tactical units. The replacement of the PROFIS personnel in hospitals remained a significant problem. The adopted solution recalled reservists to fill positions vacated by deploying personnel and aligned reserve hospital units to replace the deployed unit.

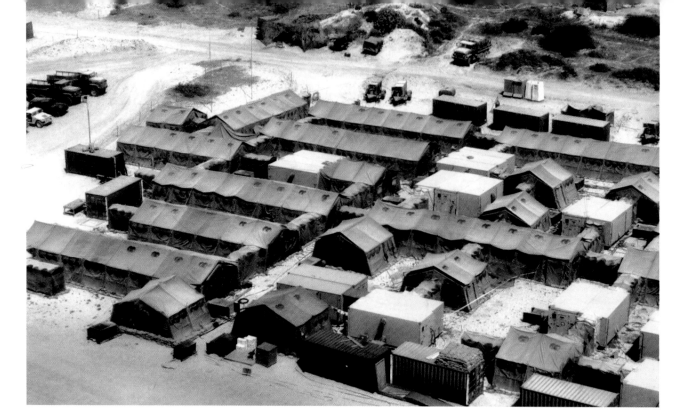

RESTRUCTURING FIELD MEDICINE

The Army updated its utility helicopters in the late 1970s, choosing the UH-60A Black Hawk to succeed the UH-1 Huey. The medevac version was capable of carrying four litters or 14 ambulatory patients. The first UH-60A medevac helicopters arrived at Company D, 326th Medical Battalion, 101st Airborne Division, at Fort Campbell, Kentucky, in January 1982. The Army adapted its combat support hospital (CSH) and the mobile army surgical hospital (MASH) to the new AirLand Battle requirements. The CSH was reduced to 120 beds, and a new 60-bed MASH of 224 personnel was created in 1979. Each division now had a MASH, a CSH, two evacuation hospitals, and a helicopter ambulance detachment allocated for support and evacuation. By 1986, the Army had 106 hospital units in the active Army and Reserve components.

At the same time, the Department of Defense was developing standardized deployable medical systems (DEPMEDS) for use by all services. The systems had standard functional medical modules and non-medical support equipment with fabric-wall, extendable, modular tents and rigid-wall shelters replacing the Medical Unit, Self-Contained, Transportable hospital's inflatable tents and expandable shelters. The DEPMEDS initiative to reconfigure the medical equipment sets went hand-in-hand with the development of new modular medical support concepts to support AirLand Battle doctrine and Army redesign.

HEALTH SERVICE SUPPORT FOR AIRLAND BATTLE

The Academy of Health Sciences at Fort Sam Houston had been rethinking combat medical support for some years. Historical lessons going back to World War II provided important data for the Health Systems Program Review of December 1984. This review shaped the Medical Department's operational concept for the modern battlefield.

Health Service Support for AirLand Battle (HSSALB) appeared in April 1986. HSSALB stressed six primary pillars and a continuum of care from the individual through the unit and division and the corps and communications zone to the continental United States. The six primary pillars were:

- wellness or fitness,
- prevention,
- immediate far-forward care,
- a deployable and mobile hospital structure,
- a dedicated evacuation system, and
- a U.S. support base.

The new modular medical support system was based on self-aid, buddy-aid, combat lifesaver, and combat medic care far forward on the battlefield. At the next levels came treatment squads and platoons, forward support medical companies of forward support battalions in the brigades, and medical treatment and evacuation assets in the main support battalions in the divisions.

86th Evacuation Hospital at Mogadishu Airport, Somalia, 1993. *U.S. Army.*

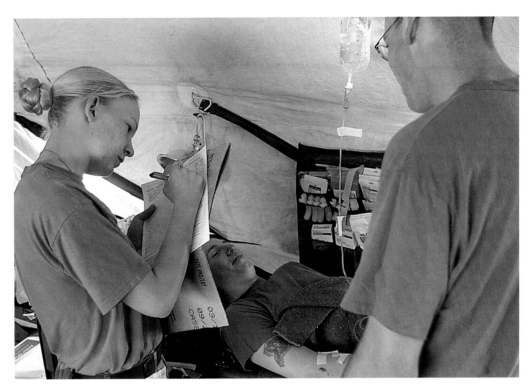

right
U.S. Army Captain
Joseph Chapman, right,
and Corporal Heidi
Eddy, of Company C,
782d Forward Surgi-
cal Team (FST) of Fort
Bragg, North Carolina,
tend to a patient during
a multinational exercise
in Kazakhstan, Septem-
ber 13, 2000. *Depart-
ment of Defense.*

bottom
An Army medic applies
a bandage to the leg of
a Grenadian child dur-
ing Operation Urgent
Fury, November 3, 1983.
Department of Defense.

Forward surgical teams, small elements of a MASH, provided far-forward emergency trauma surgery and intensive care for brigades. Advanced Trauma Life Support (ATLS) training and skills were stressed as well as the need for combat stress detachments for mental health issues. Area support medical companies and battalions provided medical support to those units without organic medical elements.

The new concept emphasized treating and returning to duty as many soldiers as possible at the lowest level, such as company or battalion. Medical logistics were enhanced and swift patient evacuation emphasized. In the corps support area, U.S. Air Force mobile aeromedical staging facilities managed aeromedical evacuation flights.

When completed, the HSSALB combat medical support program reorganized every active and reserve component medical unit with a "go to war" mission. It was renamed Medical Force 2000 in the late 1980s.

COMBAT HOT SPOTS
Evolving Army medical capabilities were tested in the sudden mission to the Caribbean island of Grenada in October 1983. Shortcomings were observed in certain medical aspects, especially the insufficient integration and training of PROFIS clinicians with their assigned tactical medical units and the lack of a rapidly deployable surgical capability. The lessons learned were fully incorporated into HSSALB and later concepts.

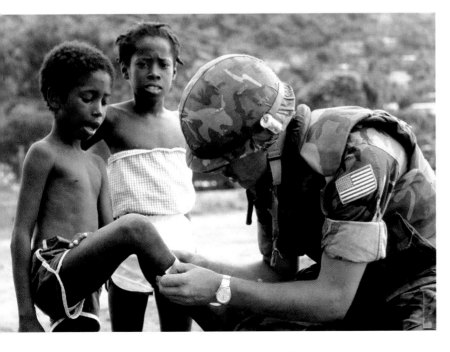

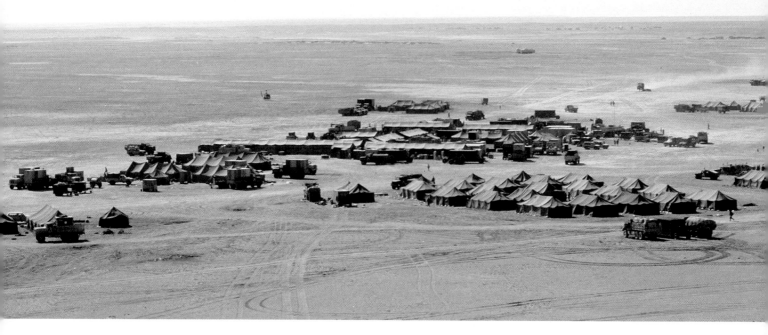

Manuel Noriega's regime in Panama had been a problem for some years before Operation Just Cause removed him in December 1989. Medical personnel jumped with the airborne units. Forward surgical teams deployed to Howard Air Force Base in the Canal Zone and provided life-saving emergency surgical care. Physicians and medics with ATLS training provided critical far-forward life-saving care. Air Force C-141 transports evacuated casualties to Army and Air Force hospitals in San Antonio, Texas. Private First Class James Maxwell, a medic from the 44th Medical Brigade, was killed in action.

Within a year, American forces would be committed halfway around the world. The Berlin Wall fell in November 1989, beginning the disintegration of the Soviet Union and the Warsaw Pact. On August 2, 1990, Iraq's Saddam Hussein invaded Kuwait and threatened Saudi Arabia. The United States and coalition allies responded immediately to the aggression.

The rapid aerial deployment of the XVIII Airborne Corps and its 44th Medical Brigade from Fort Bragg, North Carolina, to Saudi Arabia in August 1990 began a massive buildup of American and coalition forces under Operation Desert Shield under control of Central Command (CENTCOM). Forward surgical teams accompanied the early deploying Army elements, along with combat stress control detachments, preventive medicine detachments, and veterinary food inspection detachments.

From Europe, the 45th Medical Company (Air Ambulance), augmented by the 421st Medical Battalion, also deployed to Saudi Arabia in August. Between August 21 and September 2,

1990, the 45th moved in two serials of six aircraft each. The crews flew from Germany more than 3,500 miles in five days in one of the longest helicopter self-deployments in Army history. The 45th was operational with the 44th Medical Brigade at Dhahran, Saudi Arabia, on September 2.

In theater, a medical structure had to be built within the Army component of CENTCOM. As medical capacity increased to care for the expanding American forces, preventive medicine units were particularly active. Educating soldiers in coping with the desert environment and climate and proper food and water discipline was a major mission. After some initial problems, admissions to hospitals and troop clinics stabilized at remarkably low levels.

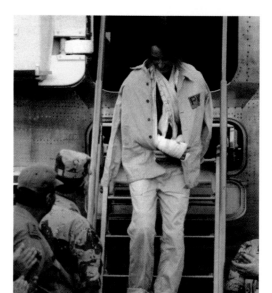

top

The 44th Medical Brigade occupies desolate terrain in southern Iraq during Operation Desert Storm. March 3, 1991. *Department of Defense.*

bottom

Major Rhonda Cornum, MC, U.S. Army, returns from Iraqi captivity after Operation Desert Storm, March 1991. Major Cornum served as a flight surgeon during the operation. Her helicopter was shot down by enemy fire while on a search and rescue mission. More than a decade later, as a colonel she commanded the Landstuhl Regional Medical Center in Germany during Operations Enduring Freedom and Iraqi Freedom. *Uniformed Services University of the Health Sciences.*

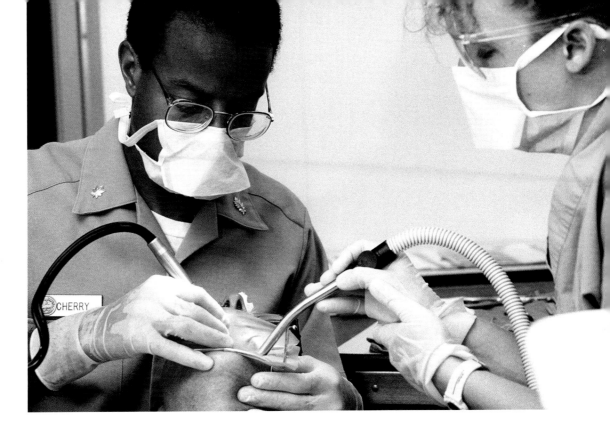

A Navy dentist and assistant work on a patient aboard the hospital ship USNS *Mercy* in the Persian Gulf region in support of Operation Desert Shield. October 1, 1990. *U.S. Navy.*

By the beginning of the ground phase of Desert Storm in late February 1991, the Army had 44 hospitals and 13,500 beds deployed in support of American forces in Saudi Arabia and the theater. Of the 44 hospitals, 16 were active Army, 11 came from the Army National Guard, and 17 were from the U.S. Army Reserve. The hospitals included new X-ray units plus laboratory and pharmaceutical packages. New technologies such as computed tomography (CT) scanners and telemedicine were available. During Operation Desert Shield and Operation Desert Storm, the Medical Department's active duty strength grew to 87,000, the largest medical force assembled since the end of World War II. Of these, 25,000 were from the Reserve components. A total of 23,493 medical personnel served in the Gulf War—with 55 percent from the Reserve components.

Army medical facilities in the theater had 192,214 outpatient visits. They admitted 18,441 inpatients, of whom 10,667 returned to duty (58 percent) and 35 died (0.02 percent). The Medical Department suffered four killed in action, 11 wounded, 13 non-battle deaths, and 28 non-battle injuries. Army battle casualties included 96 killed in action and 356 wounded. Two soldiers died of wounds, while an incredible 99.4 percent of the wounded survived. The high quality of medical support provided throughout the Army during these operations was ample proof of the successful transition of the Medical Department since Vietnam.

NAVY MEDICINE IN DESERT SHIELD AND DESERT STORM

IMMEDIATE DEPLOYMENT

Navy medicine's primary mission has always been to provide medical care to active duty Navy and Marine Corps personnel wherever they are called upon to serve. Following Iraq's invasion of Kuwait on August 2, 1990, the Navy Medical Department immediately deployed to the Middle East as part of Operation Desert Shield and Operation Desert Storm.

In support of this effort, Navy medicine mobilized two hospital ships (USNS *Mercy* and USNS *Comfort*), three fleet hospitals, and mobile medical augmentation readiness teams supporting more than 2,000 beds available in the operating theater.

USNS *Mercy* and USNS *Comfort* were sister ships, almost identical in layout. They were converted supertankers and equipped to the high standards of the largest city hospital in the United States. Each had 12 operating rooms, modern X-ray equipment, a CT scan, and trained specialists able to handle the most seriously injured patients. Although capable of being configured as 1,000-bed hospitals, neither vessel reached that number during the war due to the very low number of coalition casualties.

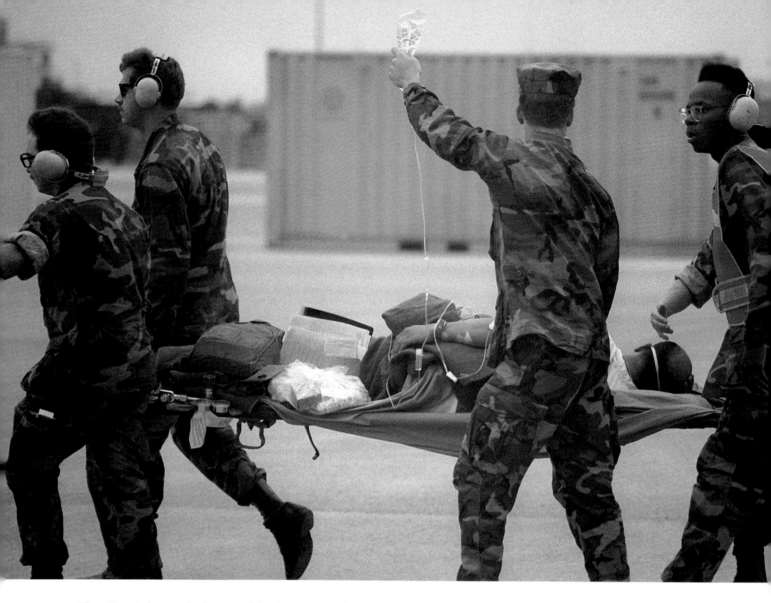

Fleet Hospital 5 was the largest of the three fleet hospitals. It was a modular 500-bed combat zone medical facility located in Al Jubail, Saudi Arabia, less than 100 miles south of the Kuwaiti border. The facility's components were deployed on September 1, 1990. Once assembled, the hospital became operational in an astounding 11 days.

The hospital consisted of 14 acute care wards, four intensive care units, several operating rooms, a complete decontamination unit, and a landing pad for helicopter evacuations. More than 900 persons staffed the facility. Throughout its seven-month deployment, nearly 600 surgeries were performed and the hospital's pharmacists filled more than 22,000 prescriptions. Together, Fleet Hospitals 5, 6, and 15 cared for 32,000 patients throughout the war.

The Marine Corps Trauma Hospital, a 270-bed facility, was deployed closer to the combat zone at Al Khanjar close to the Kuwaiti border. Staffed by Navy medical personnel, it treated 90 percent of coalition casualties plus 350–400 wounded Iraqi enemy prisoners of war.

Hostile Iraqi forces constituted only part of the perils of the desert battlefield. The threat of chemical and biological warfare was always a possibility. To help combat these hazards, the Navy attached two preventive medicine teams. One team emphasized disease prevention and control and the other concentrated on disease vector control. These medical teams, attached to the 1st Marine Expeditionary Force Service Support Group, were charged with identifying possible health hazards and minimizing or eliminating their effects if possible. The Navy also deployed the Navy Forward Laboratory, which assisted the preventive medicine teams in evaluating and assessing potential health risks.

top left
Litter bearers carry a wounded Marine across the helicopter pad at Fleet Hospital 5 during Operation Desert Storm. Saudi Arabia, February 1, 1991. *Department of Defense.*

top right
Wounded Hospital Corpsman 1st Class Conners of the 1st Reconnaissance Battalion, 1st Marine Division, is interviewed in the 1st Medical Battalion recovery room on January 18, 1991. Conners was the first combat casualty of Operation Desert Storm. *Department of Defense.*

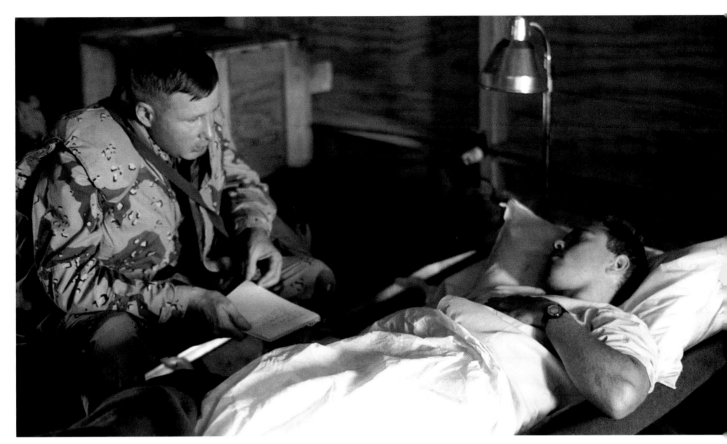

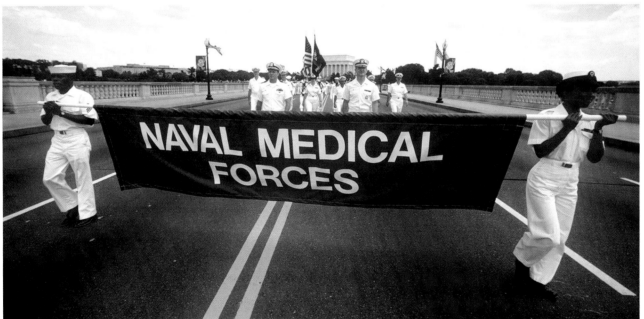

bottom
Two sailors lead a formation of Navy medical forces across Memorial Bridge in Washington, D.C., during the National Victory Celebration parade on June 8, 1991.
Department of Defense.

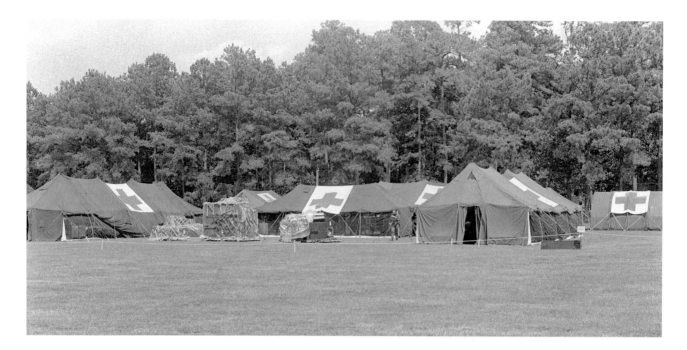

AIR FORCE MEDICINE, POST-VIETNAM

READINESS, 1979-90

Most of the Air Force's hardwall medical shelters used in the Vietnam War were converted to tents in the late 1970s. In the early 1980s, the Air Force Medical Service (AFMS) also began to pre-position several large contingency hospitals in Europe and Asia. Special reserve units were created starting in 1982 to help the active duty medical force staff these contingency hospitals in wartime.

Modernization of Air Transportable Hospitals (ATHs) continued through the 1980s. In late 1983, the AFMS began a five-year program to enlarge the standard 24-bed ATH to 50 beds. The new design was also more flexible, providing for 14, 25, or 50 beds. By mid-1990, the Air Force had more than two dozen 50-bed ATHs. Most were attached to tactical fighter wings in the Continental United States (CONUS) for rapid deployment where needed.

In 1985, the Air Force also started to develop aeromedical staging facilities to complement ATHs deploying to Europe and Asia. These facilities had up to 250 beds for holding patients awaiting evacuation by Military Airlift Command to more advanced medical treatment in other theaters. Since few host nations offered suitable buildings for allied medical units, the Air Force started developing staging facilities constructed mainly with tents. With adequate site preparation, they could be ready in five days.

By the late 1980s, the Air Force staff foresaw the scarcity of airlift for major deployments. Many equipment items, such as ambulances, were already positioned by 1990. Several complete medical treatment facilities were also stored overseas.

AFMS IN OPERATION DESERT SHIELD

On August 8, 1990, only six days after Iraq's invasion of Kuwait, the AFMS began its largest deployment since the Vietnam War, as part of Operation Desert Shield. In August and September 1990, the Air Force deployed the first U.S. medical facilities capable of both surgery and chemical decontamination. The first Air Force medical teams arrived on the Arabian Peninsula two days after the combat units. These teams were the main source of medical support to American forces until the second week in September 1990.

U.S. Air Force 354th Air Transportable Hospital set up for a medical training exercise at Seymour-Johnson Air Force Base, North Carolina, June 25, 1984. *Department of Defense.*

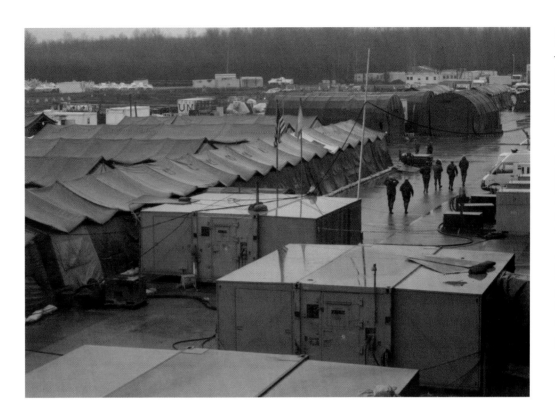

U.S. Hospital Zagreb at Camp Pleso, Zagreb, Croatia. The 74th Medical Group (Provisional) of Wright-Patterson Air Force Base, Ohio, operated the hospital. It served the United Nations Protection Force from November 1992 to December 1995. *Department of Defense.*

The overall AFMS deployment in Desert Shield went much faster than in the Vietnam War, even though 175 more hospital beds deployed (925 versus 750). Air transportable clinics and hospitals were the key to rapid mobility. The clinics deployed immediately with their flying squadrons. The first squadron medical elements and air transportable clinics left the United States only one day after their first fighter aircraft deployments. The first ATHs left on August 11 from Shaw, MacDill, and Langley Air Force bases.

Most of the air transportable medical facilities were committed to the operation by late October. In November, the Persian Gulf deployment expanded to include hospitals from 10 CONUS air bases.

AIR TRANSPORTABLE HOSPITALS

Before the start of Operation Desert Shield, the 50-bed version of the ATH, including personnel and mobility bags, was transported by six C-141 aircraft. Once on site, weather and other conditions permitting, the ATH staff and base support units could erect the hospital within 24 to 48 hours.

ATHs were the backbone of the Air Force medical treatment system in the region. The ATH could meet the medical needs of a deployed tactical fighter wing with up to 72 aircraft and about 4,000 people. The ATH also assisted the squadron medical elements, air transportable clinics, and aeromedical staging facilities that deployed with their tactical and strategic units.

A combination of hardwall shelters and modular tents, the hospital was equipped with several exterior air-conditioning units for operations in harsh climates. The hospital deployed with sophisticated medical equipment and supplies, and a competent staff of 128 medics. The three hardwall shelters of the 50-bed hospital had two surgical tables, a laboratory, an X-ray machine, and blood storage equipment. The hospital's dental chair could serve as a third operating table. In the early months of Desert Shield, the staff of the deployed hospitals found that most of their equipment worked well in the desert climate. Each ATH was equipped to function for 30 days without resupply and was supported by a 19-person decontamination team to handle chemical warfare casualties.

In Germany and England, several contingency hospitals and smaller tactical fighter wing hospitals were already in place. The Air Force contingency hospitals, containing from 500 to 1,500 beds, were "turn-key" facilities fully equipped and calibrated, needing only professional staff deployed from CONUS to begin operations. By early February 1991, these hospitals were ready for full operation.

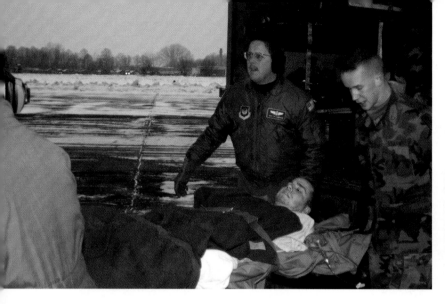

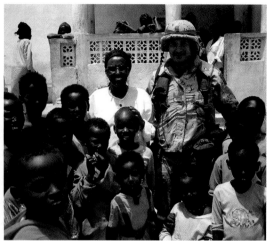

OPERATION DESERT STORM, JANUARY–FEBRUARY 1991

Most Air Force planners anticipated that the air and ground fighting during Desert Storm would not tax the medical system severely. Coalition casualties were so light that the staff at Air Force contingency hospitals in Europe, like many of their counterparts in the Arabian Peninsula, practiced little combat medicine. From August 1990 to March 1991, disease and non-battle injuries accounted for most of the patients of Desert Shield and Desert Storm who were evacuated from Southwest Asia to Europe. Aggressive preventive medicine was effective in minimizing the losses to disease. Orthopedic injuries alone accounted for about 43 percent of the evacuees from the theaters.

The 15 ATHs, with help from a 250-bed contingency hospital staffed by MAC, supplied most of the in-theater hospital beds and staff for the Air Force in Desert Storm. First-stage medical care and evaluation was available at 31 deployed air transportable clinics, a few from the Strategic Air Command. The Air Force eventually set up 925 beds in Southwest Asia staffed by 4,900 medics, almost one out of every 10 Air Force members who deployed. The Air Force also deployed 6,900 medics to staff 3,740 beds in the Air Force fixed and contingency hospitals in Europe. By the end of the Gulf War, the size of AFMS was at its highest point in history— 14,500 officers, 30,000 enlisted medics, and about 9,500 civilians. The Reserve mobilization was a key part of the operation. One-half of the Air Force medics who went to Europe and Southwest Asia by February 1991 were members of the Air National Guard and the Air Force Reserve. The Reserves accounted for 97 percent of the aeromedical evacuation cadre.

PEACEKEEPING AND HUMANITARIAN OPERATIONS IN THE 1990S

Since its creation in 1949, the AFMS has assisted United States humanitarian and peacekeeping operations around the globe, aiding victims of natural disasters and wars. The AFMS helped give aid to victims of earthquakes in Europe, to victims of hurricanes in the United States and Latin America, to Southeast Asian orphans and refugees during the Vietnam War, and to Cuban refugees fleeing to the United States.

After the collapse of the Soviet Union in the early 1990s, the AFMS began to support an increased tempo in Air Force humanitarian and peacekeeping operations. It contributed to the U.S. missions in Somalia (1993–94) and Haiti (1994–95). It was also active in supporting operations in the Balkans from 1994 to 1999.

To respond to changed conditions in the mid-1990s, the AFMS started to reengineer the size and configuration of its ATHs and aeromedical evacuation systems, making them more flexible and responsive. Improved coordination between the active duty AFMS and its Reserve components was especially important. In January 1995, the AFMS inaugurated the "Mirror Force" initiative to promote closer integration of active duty and Reserve medical components, which soon led to increased responsibilities for the Reserve medics. Starting in 1995, the AFMS also began to reengineer medical readiness units to make them smaller and more transportable.

top left
Taszar, Hungary, January 3, 1996. Members of the 86th Aeromedical Evacuation Squadron, Ramstein Air Base, Germany, load Specialist Martin Begosh of the 709th Military Police Battalion into a C-130 Hercules for evacuation. Begosh was wounded when the vehicle he was driving struck a land mine in northern Bosnia. *Department of Defense.*

top right
Lieutenant Colonel Chris Marino, MC, U.S. Army, was battalion surgeon with the Quick Reaction Force Somalia in October 1993. The force was ambushed while attempting to rescue American soldiers in Mogadishu. During the night battle, Doctor Marino provided immediate medical care for his wounded comrades. *Uniformed Services University of the Health Sciences.*

top
Suicide bombing of USS *Cole* in Yemen on October 12, 2000, killed 17 and wounded 39 among the crew of 295 and led to cooperation among military and civilian medical assets to assist the victims. *U.S. Navy Bureau of Medicine and Surgery.*

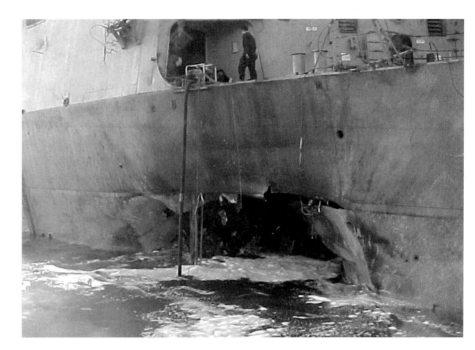

middle
USS *Cole* patients embark aboard U.S. Air Force C-9 aircraft for evacuation from Aden, Yemen, to Ramstein Air Base, Germany, October 14, 2000. Two Critical Care Air Transport Teams (CCATTs) and two C-9s deployed to Djibouti and Aden for the evacuation of 39 injured sailors, two of them in critical condition. Thanks to the teams' superb efforts, not one of the patients died en route. For their extraordinary efforts that saved several lives, the CCATTS and the C-9 crew members received the National Aeronautic Association's Clarence MacKay trophy for 2000. *U.S. Air Force.*

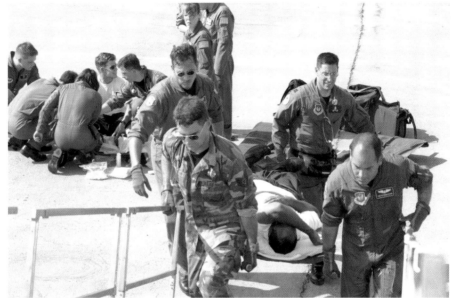

bottom
A severely injured sailor from the USS *Cole* is taken from an ambulance at Ramstein Air Base, Germany, October 15, 2000, and loaded aboard a C-141 Starlifter by medical personnel from Landstuhl Regional Medical Center. The injured sailor is being transported to the USS *Cole's* homeport at the Norfolk Naval Air Station, Virginia. *Department of Defense.*

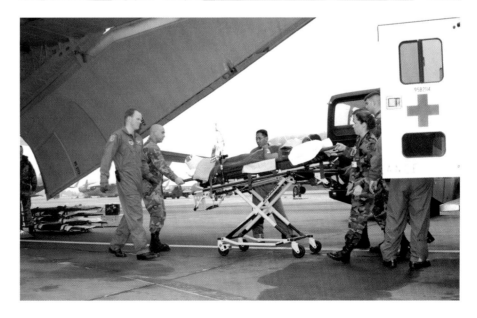

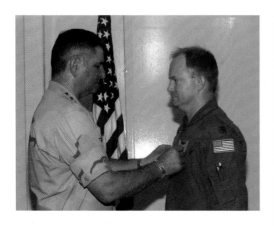

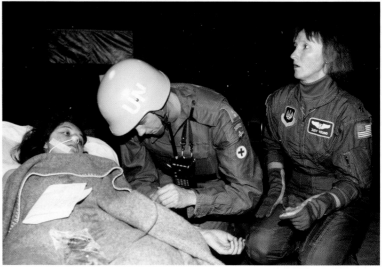

In 1997 the AFMS began to train special Critical Care Air Transport Teams (CCATTs) to reduce the need for medical facilities located near active combat fronts. These teams could transport critically ill or injured, but stabilized, patients aboard aircraft to advanced medical facilities far to the rear or even out of the combat theater. The use of CCATTs entailed a new strategy that moved most definitive medical care away from active contingency theaters to rear areas or the continental United States.

REENGINEERING AIR FORCE PEACETIME HEALTH CARE IN THE 1990S

The AFMS began to reengineer peacetime health care in 1992 with a series of internal managed care reforms. Reengineering the Air Force's base-level medical system was also necessary. In 1993, the AFMS adopted a new base-level organizational template, the Objective Medical Group, to increase medical responsiveness to the needs of line commanders. In 1994, the AFMS began to reduce its overall size and reorganize its clinics and hospitals. Originally known as "Right-Sizing," this restructuring was later renamed "Tailored Force."

In 1995 the AFMS formalized its recent reforms in a five-part Parthenon strategy. The strategy emphasized a coordination and acceleration of readiness reengineering, structural reforms, managed care innovations, customer satisfaction efforts, and disease prevention programs.

After 1995, the structural reforms of the AFMS Parthenon included the reengineering of the six Air Force medical centers. A renewed customer satisfaction program emphasized both high-quality health care and the professionalism and caring attitudes of Air Force medics. In this program the AFMS looked for ways to fulfill its historic obligations to Air Force retirees and their families. The managed care reforms of the Parthenon strategy included active support of the DOD TRICARE program, which attempted to preserve substantial medical benefits for retirees while reducing the size of the active duty health care system.

Prevention received special emphasis in the new program. In October 1994 the AFMS established the Office for Prevention and Health Services Assessment (OPHSA) at Brooks Air Force Base, Texas. In July 1995, the AFMS inaugurated a new program called Put Prevention into Practice, devised by OPHSA to increase the appropriate delivery of clinical preventive services. In January 1996, the Chief of Staff and Secretary of the Air Force directed the creation of a Health and Wellness Center at each Air Force base. Each center designated a single point of contact for fitness information, training, and testing. In a related move, in June 1996 the AFMS began to develop a suicide prevention program that significantly reduced the Air Force suicide rate and earned both DOD and civilian recognition.

top left
U.S. Air Force Chief of Staff General Ronald R. Fogleman, left, presents the Airman's Medal to Major Steven Goff, MC, United States Air Force, on July 3, 1996. Goff earned the award for the medical support he rendered to the dying and injured after the terrorist bombing of Khobar Towers in Saudi Arabia, June 25, 1996. Although injured, Dr. Goff continued to aid others. The explosion killed 19 people and injured more than 260. *Department of Defense.*

top right
Major Judy Young, flight nurse of the 2d Aeromedical Evacuation Squadron, assists a Norwegian United Nations medic to care for a patient on an aeromedical evacuation flight from Sarajevo, Bosnia, to Ramstein Air Base in Germany, February 1994. *Department of Defense.*

OPERATION DESERT SHIELD AND OPERATION DESERT STORM SERVICE AND CASUALTIES 1990–91

Total U.S. Service Members (Worldwide)	2,322,332
Deployed to Gulf	694,550
Battle Deaths	147
Other Deaths (in Theater)	235
Other Deaths in Service (Non-Theater)	914
Non-Mortal Woundings	467

Source: Department of Veterans Affairs from Department of Defense.

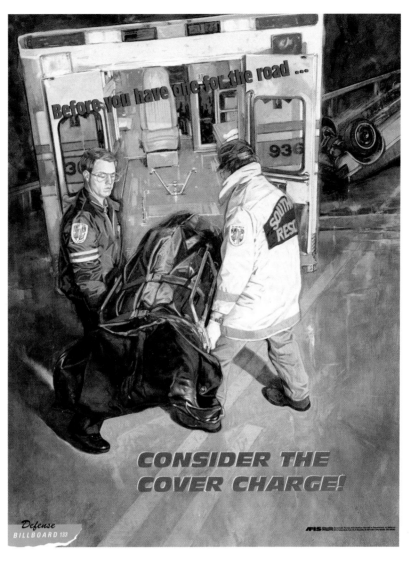

Department of Defense billboard poster cautions against misuse of alcohol. *Department of Defense.*

A key preventive program, which originated in January 1998, was known as the Preventive Health Assessment (PHA). At least once a year, the AFMS began to review each airman's health care needs and medical readiness status. The PHA pinpointed airmen who required special preventive screening and services. The most important risks targeted were smoking, alcohol abuse, and injuries.

Air Force medical facilities made sure each airman had received the recommended and required preventive care, screenings, immunizations, and assessments. In the past, only airmen assigned to flying or air controlling duty received an annual examination. Starting at age 25, each airman would receive a comprehensive physical examination every five years. Preventive Health Assessments were the equivalent of the routine inspections and preventive maintenance on aircraft.

In the summer of 1998, the recent Air Force prevention initiative became a part of a larger coordinated DOD preventive effort. The military health services selected three areas for their preventive efforts: tobacco use, alcohol abuse, and accidental injuries. The Air Force took tobacco abuse as its research focus, while the Navy looked at alcohol abuse, and the Army explored accidental injuries.

CLOSING OUT THE 20TH CENTURY
The medical departments of the armed services ended the 20th century in better shape than before. They possessed broad experience in combat and humanitarian activities blended with continuous care for a larger population of families, civilians, and retirees. The medical components of the active and Reserve forces interlocked for smooth functioning in peace and war. As the nation entered the 21st century, its military medics were practiced and ready for all eventualities. They and the nation would soon be tested severely.

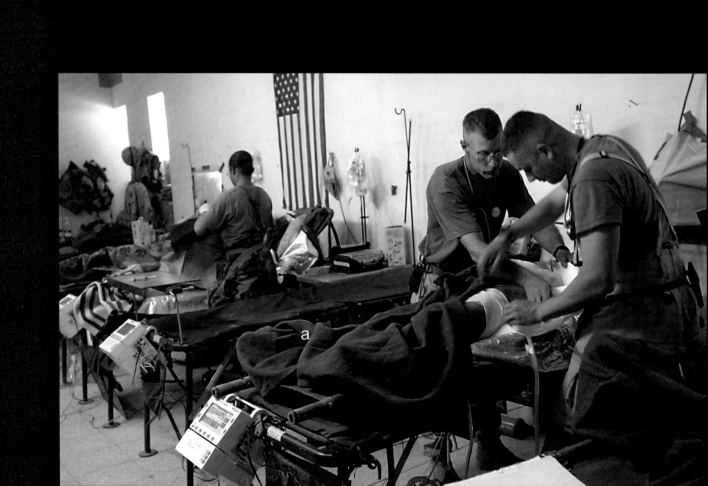

Chapter 10
Homeland Security and Recent Combat Operations, 2001-05

Members of the Army 86th Combat Support Hospital attend to a patient April 5, 2003, at Tallil Air Base in southern Iraq during Operation Iraqi Freedom. *Department of Defense.*

ENGAGING A NEW ERA OF WAR

EFFECTS OF "PEACE DIVIDEND" ON ARMY MEDICINE

The Army Medical Department emerged from Operations Desert Shield and Desert Storm with a solid record of success in caring for the deployed Army forces but not without some problems. Politicians were stimulated by the demise of the Soviet Union to harvest a "peace dividend" by slashing American defense spending. The entire Army was restructured again. Army strength dropped from 780,000 troops and 16 active divisions to 480,000 and 10 divisions.

As the Army reduced, so did the Medical Department's tactical units and its hospital structure. Active and Reserve component hospitals declined from 168 in 1990 to 47 in 2002. The number of medical personnel declined rapidly over the same period, with 20 percent of officers and 40 percent of enlisted personnel cut.

The number of fixed medical facilities followed the same trend. In 1988, the Medical Department managed 10 medical centers, 30 hospitals, and 183 clinics. Those numbers dropped by 2004 to eight medical centers, 19 hospitals, and 155 clinics. The Base Realignment and Closure process claimed Letterman Army Medical Center in San Francisco, California, in 1992–93, and Fitzsimons Army Medical Center in Aurora, Colorado, in 1996. As other Army installations closed or downsized, Army hospitals were closed or reduced to clinics. As a result of such actions, in the 20 years from 1980 to 2000 the number of operating hospital beds declined almost 80 percent, from 7,789 to 1,594.

RESERVE COMPONENTS REDUCED

The reductions of the active Army were mirrored in the Reserve components. They still accounted for more than 60 percent of personnel and units in the total Army medical force in 2004 but had also lost 38 percent of their personnel since 1994. In the years following Desert Storm, the Reserve components had significant problems recruiting and retaining critical medical, dental, physician assistant, and nurse anesthetist specialties due to the losses they had suffered in career and individual practices while on active duty.

By 1996, 25 percent of the selective Reserve officers were gone and some units were only 50 percent staffed. Across the board, only 64 percent of critical Reserve component positions were filled. A series of rotations to the Balkans in the late 1990s added to the misery when 33 percent of Reserve practitioners who deployed did not sign on again.

Action was required to reduce the drainage. Incentive pay and retention programs offered one approach; so did providing regular Army fillers to reserve component units where necessary. Another solution modified unit structures under the Medical Reengineering Initiative (MRI) force redesign. It reduced the number of critical specialties required in the Reserve medical units. While that would help in the long run, the short term was more important and personal. Thus, the Army shortened the active duty recall commitment for critical specialties to 90 days so that civilian practices would not suffer. However, with mobilization and processing time, the 90 days often stretched well beyond the 90-day "boots on the ground" obligation.

In 2004, a new Army Reserve Medical Command was established within the U.S. Army Reserve Command to address many of these problem areas and provide better planning and coordination. With 28 medical units (no hospitals) in the Army National Guard and 178 (no air ambulance units) in the Army Reserve in 2003, the reserve components were essential to Army readiness and any long-term Army operational commitments.

REORGANIZATION OF ARMY MEDICINE

After Operation Desert Storm and with the ongoing reductions, the idea of combining the Office of the Surgeon General with the Health Services Command gained general acceptance.

The major reorganization began under Lieutenant General Frank Ledford, Surgeon General (1988–92). The initial change came in July 1991, when the former Academy of Health Sciences at Fort Sam Houston became the Army Medical Department Center and School. Ledford's successor, Lieutenant General Alcide LaNoue (1992–96), continued the reorganization implantation. Lieutenant General Ronald R. Blanck (1996–2000) added the finishing details. His successor, Lieutenant General James B. Peake (2000–04), put Army medicine on an entirely new road to transformation.

On October 4, 1994, the U.S. Army Medical Command (MEDCOM) replaced the former Health Services Command. The Surgeon General now wore two hats. As the Surgeon General he was the principal advisor to the Army Secretary, Chief of Staff, and Army Staff on health matters, including coordination with the other service surgeons general and the Assistant Secretary of Defense (Health Affairs). As commander of MEDCOM, he directed the everyday activities of medical support for the entire Army.

In 1994, the new MEDCOM's subordinate organization was restructured into seven Health Service Support Areas (HSSAs) under medical center commanders in the United States, the Pacific, and Europe. The HSSAs were responsible for all Medical Department functions in their geographic areas, including close coordination with the Reserve component medical units but excluding dental and veterinary activities. A major goal of the HSSAs was to improve liaison with the Army Reserve Command and the Reserve component units in their areas to correct readiness shortcomings experienced during the Gulf War. This realignment also permitted better support for the Army's three deployable corps and the commanders of the unified warfighting commands worldwide. The HSSAs were redesignated Regional Medical Commands (RMCs) in 1996 and reduced to six in 1998.

The 1994 reorganization created separate commands for the Army's dental and veterinary activities. Dental Command was created to manage the dental activities throughout the Army, while the Veterinary Command assumed responsibility for all Army and Defense Department veterinary activities worldwide.

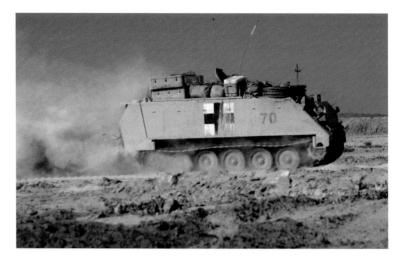

below
A medical M113 armored personnel carrier rushes wounded soldiers to timely medical attention during combat operations in Fallujah, Iraq, on November 12, 2004. The vehicle is assigned to the 7th Cavalry, 2d Brigade Combat Team, of the 1st Cavalry Division. *Department of Defense.*

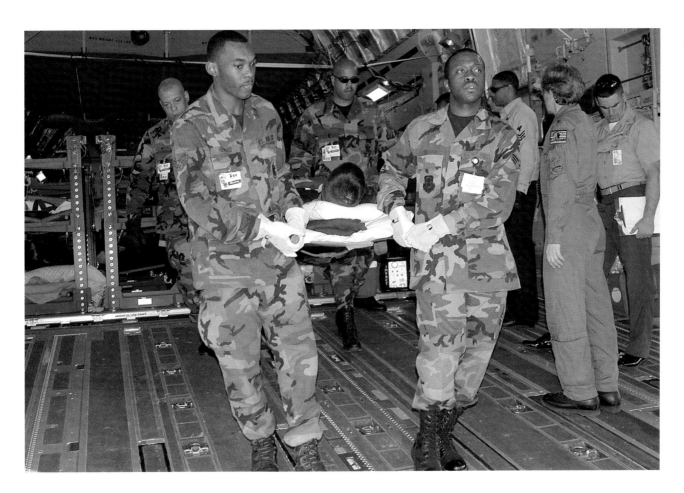

Andrews Air Force Base, Maryland, April 14, 2003. Medics from the 459th Aeromedical Evacuation Squadron carry an injured military member from a C-17 Globemaster III aircraft to a waiting medical evacuation bus. The aircraft carried injured military members from Germany to the United States. Their next stop is one of the armed services' medical centers in the Washington, D.C. area. *U.S. Air Force.*

The Medical Research and Materiel Command replaced the former Medical Research and Development Command and assumed responsibility for all medical research programs and laboratories, information management, logistics, and hospital planning and construction.

In 2003, in line with the continuing transformation of the Army, Lieutenant General Peake began advocating a basic change in the way that Army medicine supported deployed Army component commands within the Joint Commands. In his Task Force Medical concept, a medical command would support Army forces in a theater and have the capacity to reach back to the U.S. regional medical commands for any medical units or support needed. The concept was still being refined in 2005.

FORCE HEALTH PROTECTION
Protecting the health and welfare of the soldiers had been a responsibility of the Medical Department since 1775. New initiatives within both the Department of the Army and Health Affairs stressed the overall importance of health promotion, physical fitness, and preventive medicine. "Force Health Protection" became the phrase most often used to describe

these imperatives that embraced both U.S. and deployment health issues. The Army Environmental Health Agency, which had handled occupational health and safety issues for years, became the U.S. Army Center for Health Promotion and Preventive Medicine in 1994 with a much broader mission in force protection. Its Army Medical Surveillance System became the Defense Medical Surveillance System that monitored areas of potential operations for health-related problems that could affect deploying troops. The Walter Reed Army Institute of Research assumed leadership of another important new initiative, the Defense Department's Global Emerging Infections Surveillance and Response System, which tracked and responded to new and deadly diseases.

Other Army Medical Department initiatives dealt with the emerging threats of chemical and biological warfare. After Secretary of Defense William Cohen directed the vaccination of all armed forces personnel against anthrax, the Anthrax Vaccine Immunization Program began in May 1998. A smallpox vaccination program for all deploying forces was added in 2003.

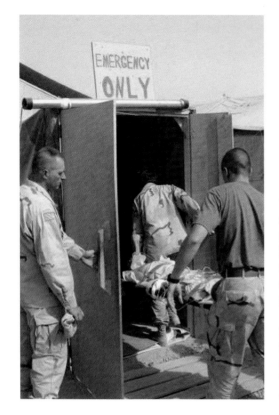

Concerns about unconventional warfare and weapons of mass destruction spurred efforts to enhance Chemical, Biological, Radiological, Nuclear and High-Explosive programs, training, and equipment. New inflatable Chemical-Biological Protective Shelters were developed to protect hospital units from such attacks. The Army and Air Force modified the standardized deployable medical systems (DEPMEDS) into the Chemically Protected DEPMEDS that protected essential elements of combat support hospitals from chemical attacks.

FORCE REDESIGN

Operation Desert Storm revealed deficiencies with a medical force essentially designed to fight a massive land war against the Soviets in Europe. All hospital units, even the supposedly mobile surgical hospitals, were large, heavy, and lacked the organic transportation needed to move with the highly maneuverable combat forces.

Combat Health Support for a new power projection Army had to be redesigned to put the medical force on the same page with the Army's evolving Force XXI. In October 1993, the Medical Department began the redesign of the entire medical structure above the division via the MRI.

The centerpiece of the new MRI was the combat support hospital for corps or echelons above corps. The 248-bed MRI combat support hospital would have 84-bed and 164-bed hospital companies that could operate separately or combined. The 84-bed company could cut out a fully capable, early-entry 44-bed slice.

MRI melded into the overall U.S. Army transformation plans. By 2004, 139 units converted or were activated to the MRI force design. Ultimately 376 medical units will be converted, with 292 to be completed by 2010.

Concurrently, forward surgical care was clearly refined with creation of the forward surgical team (FST) of 20 personnel. The FST was small, easily deployable, and fully mobile with its own transportation. Positioned with brigade combat teams and supported by forward support medical companies, the FSTs provided emergency surgery far forward on the battlefield. By 2003, there were 13 FSTs in the active Army and 23 in the Army Reserve. Personnel of the FSTs gained experience and maintained skills through regular rotations to the Army Trauma Training Center at the Ryder Trauma Center of Jackson Memorial Hospital in Miami, Florida.

During the 1990s, the Medical Department began forming small, specialized medical teams that could deploy with their personnel and equipment within hours of notification for short-term missions. These Special Medical Augmentation Response Teams provided a wide range of care from surgery to preventive medicine.

U.S. Army medics admit a casualty to the emergency room at the 21st Combat Support Hospital (CSH) in Iraq, Summer 2003. The 21st CSH is an 84-bed hospital that provides inpatient and outpatient care to troops in Iraq. The hospital also cares for civilian casualties and wounded prisoners of war. *Uniformed Services University of the Health Sciences.*

91W COMBAT MEDIC

A vital part of the Medical Department evolution was the transformation of the Army medic from the Military Occupational Specialty, series 91, into the 91W, Health Care Specialist. In the late 1990s, combat medics' training was completely redesigned to provide the enhanced skills of an emergency medical technician (EMT)-paramedic with a wide range of the most current trauma life support training to make them more versatile and valuable.

The first class of new 91Ws completed their training in February 2001. By 2009 all enlisted medics in the active Army and Reserve components will complete 16 weeks of training and the transition. All 91Ws will be EMT-certified and require annual training and recertification. The initial combat test of the 91Ws came on the battlefields of Afghanistan and Iraq where they continued the tradition of life-saving service to the soldier at the risk of their own lives.

AIR FORCE MEDICAL READINESS

At the turn of the century, the Air Force Medical Service (AFMS) improved its ability to operate from modular, portable medical facilities known as Expeditionary Medical Support (EMEDS) units. The development of EMEDS units began in August 1998. The goal was to design small, highly trained, rapidly deployable units that could be joined together quickly to meet the needs of a particular medical crisis.

The AFMS officially adopted the EMEDS concept, for use at home or abroad, in September 1999. The basic EMEDS inpatient unit was small enough to fit on only three cargo pallets, and needed a staff of only 25 medics. With just four folding beds, it provided only the emergency services of combat medicine; but it was designed to rapidly expand to 50 beds and a more capable staff of 87 personnel. Some EMEDS were equipped with special liners, ventilation, and accessories to protect against biological and chemical warfare attacks. The Air Force's

Mobile Aeromedical Staging Facilities were also redesigned on this modular pattern.

Initial EMEDS units, such as the Mobile Field Surgical Team (MFST), were successfully employed in the Balkans in Operation Allied Force in the spring of 1999. The highly trained MFST included a general surgeon, an orthopedic surgeon, an emergency medical physician, and operating room staff, including an anesthesia provider and an operating room nurse or technician. The five team members each carried a 70-pound, specially equipped backpack of medical and surgical equipment. The five backpacks contained enough medical equipment to perform 10 emergency, life-or-limb-saving surgeries without resupply.

A key medical component of the new EMEDS unit was the Small Portable Expeditionary Aeromedical Rapid Response (SPEARR) team. A SPEARR team of eight medical personnel required only one pallet (or less) and required only one C-130, C-12, or C-23 aircraft. In the spring of 2000, SPEARR teams were tested at Camp Bullis and Lackland Air Force Base, Texas; plus Elmendorf Air Force Base and King Salmon Air Force Station, Alaska. In May 2000, the AFMS made SPEARR teams available for state disasters when civilian assets were not available to respond to the emergency. Into the year 2000 the AFMS organized nearly 30 SPEARR teams as the mobility components of each new EMEDS basic unit.

At the same time, the AFMS continued to refine its aeromedical evacuation capability. The Critical Care Air Transport Team (CCATT) developed in the late 1990s offered in-flight critical care transport of three patients using a staff of one physician, one nurse, and one respiratory technician. With the addition of a second critical care nurse, a CCATT could transport five stabilized patients in critical condition. The CCATT worked alongside a standard five-member aeromedical evacuation crew.

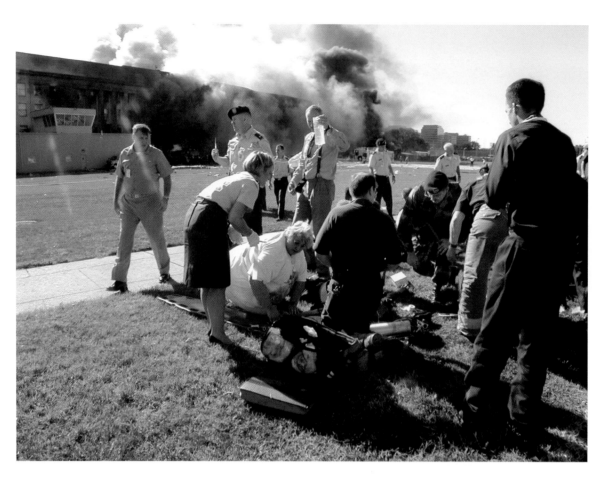

In June 2000, a disaster in Texas provided another opportunity to use the new AFMS deployable platforms. Tropical storm Allison caused severe flooding and power outages in Houston, nearly shutting down the city's hospitals and medical care system. In response, a 25-bed EMEDS deployed from Wilford Hall Medical Center, Lackland Air Force Base, to Houston from June 14–24. The 87 Air Force medics brought 22 pallets of medical equipment and supplies and treated more than 1,000 patients. The mayor of Houston, the governor of Texas, and the director of the Federal Emergency Management Agency recognized their contribution.

FIGHTING TERROR AT HOME AND ABROAD

Between 1989 and 2000, the Army Medical Department was involved in 38 major deployments. Only Operations Just Cause (1989) and Desert Shield/Desert Storm (1990–91) involved significant combat operations, but all required considerable medical support. The other missions ranged from domestic disaster relief to peacekeeping and stabilization operations in the Sinai, Bosnia, and Herzegovina after 1995, and Kosovo after 1999. The department also participated in responses to terrorist bombings of American embassies in East Africa in August 1998 and the attack on the USS *Cole*.

On September 11, 2001, terrorism struck the U.S. homeland. Muslim terrorists hijacked four U.S. commercial airliners. They flew two into the World Trade Center towers in New York City and one into the Pentagon in Washington, D.C. Passengers on the fourth hijacked airliner fought the terrorists and it crashed into a rural Pennsylvania field. Army, Navy, and Air Force medical personnel and civilian first responders dealt immediately with the Pentagon tragedy.

Medical personnel and volunteers work the first medical triage area set up outside the Pentagon after a hijacked commercial airliner crashed into the southwest corner of the building, September 11, 2001. *U.S. Navy.*

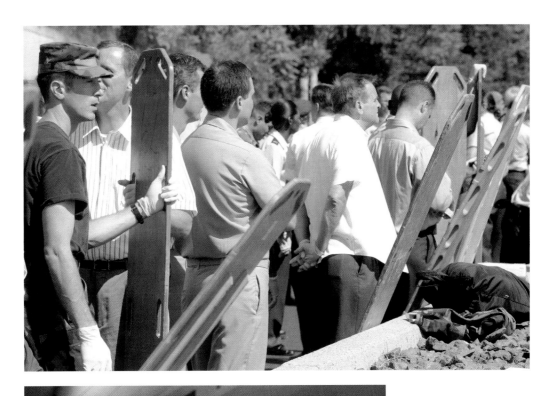

top
Stretcher crews and Pentagon employees stand ready to carry injured people to waiting ambulances, September 11, 2001. *U.S. Air Force.*

below
A U.S. Marine keeps watch over USNS *Comfort* at the pier on Manhattan's West Side, September 18, 2001. *U.S. Navy.*

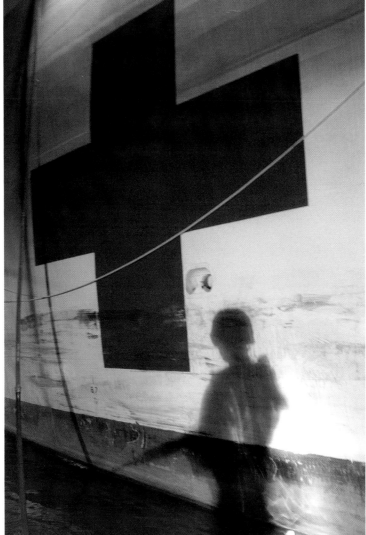

Personnel from the DiLorenzo TRICARE Health Clinic on the other side of the Pentagon from the impact point responded immediately. Army medics also responded right away from the Rader Army Health Clinic at Fort Myer, Virginia; the DeWitt Army Hospital at Fort Belvoir, Virginia; and the Walter Reed Army Medical Center in Washington. They strove to save those who could be saved and care for those who were injured. Colleagues of the other services joined without delay.

When American Airlines Flight 77 crashed into the building, Air Force Surgeon General, Lieutenant General Paul K. Carlton, Jr., USAF, MC, and several members of his staff pitched in at once. They were working in the Pentagon that day, rather than at his office on Bolling Air Force Base in Washington, D.C. General Carlton and his staff helped other medics and Pentagon personnel pull victims from the burning rubble and carry them to safety and medical care. Assisted by 70 additional Air Force medical personnel from Andrews Air Force Base, Maryland, they helped organize emergency medical treatment on the scene. For their courageous efforts, General Carlton and several other airmen were awarded the Airman's Medal.

Within hours of the terrorist attacks, Navy personnel readied the hospital ship USNS *Comfort* for deployment to New York City to help care for the survivors of the World Trade Center. Sadly, its mission changed when it was learned that few victims had survived. Nevertheless, the great white ship became a presence on lower Manhattan's West Side waterfront providing a refuge for thousands of firefighters and other rescue workers.

In the immediate aftermath of the 9/11 attacks, the Air Force sent special medical units as backup to the medical system of New York City. Four EMEDS units from Langley, Lackland, Keesler, and Travis Air Force bases, plus several

CCATT aeromedical evacuation teams, were dispatched. More than 500 Air Force medics deployed to nearby McGuire Air Force Base, New Jersey, within 24 hours, and remained there until September 14. The units stood ready to provide relief to strained civilian medical facilities if needed.

Several weeks later, working with the U.S. Navy, the AFMS sent environmental sampling teams to New York City and the U.S. Capitol to assist civilian medical experts and local authorities in testing for anthrax. The Air Force biological augmentation teams identified pathogenic agents using a commercial product called a Ruggedized Advanced Pathogen Identification System (RAPIDS). RAPIDS could quickly and accurately identify a variety of pathogens, including conventional biological agents; it could accomplish the tests in less than two hours, a marked improvement over former pathogen identifiers that required as long as 48 hours for results.

The 9/11 attacks changed Americans' perception of the world forever. The institution of Navy medicine had also changed. On September 27, 2001, by order of Navy Surgeon General Michael Cowan, new signal flags, "Charlie Papa: Steaming to Assist" began flying above all Navy medical activities. As Vice Admiral Cowan explained, "The men and women of Navy Medicine were among the first to respond, providing aid to the injured at the Pentagon and comfort and care for thousands of rescue workers who worked around the clock in the desperate race to find survivors beneath the rubble that was the World Trade Center. [Similarly] we are no longer standing by to help when a Sailor or Marine is sick or injured. We are out in front of the problem, providing preventive care, promoting wellness, and anticipating crises before they occur."

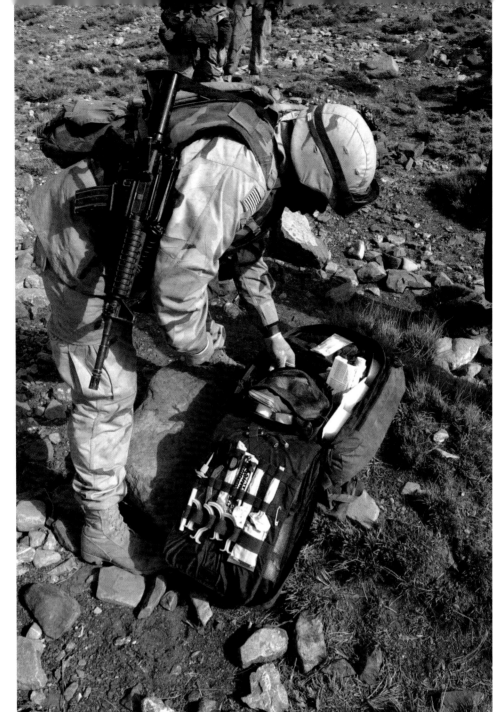

U.S. Army Specialist Estevan Garcia, a medic assigned to the 1st Battalion, 505th Parachute Infantry Regiment, prepares his medical bag during a medical assistance mission conducted in a village located near Keyki, Afghanistan, July 29, 2002. *Department of Defense.*

In this climate of preparedness, the Navy Medical Department created its own Office of Homeland Security to develop and execute a comprehensive strategy in support of civilian-military disaster preparedness and to respond to and recover from threats and attacks that would involve the Navy. The new office was quick to conduct an assessment of more than 75 Navy medical treatment facilities to see if they were prepared to respond to a chemical, biological, radiological, or nuclear event. The office concluded that there should be an emphasis on medical surveillance for potential bioterrorism and education in the diagnosis and management of chemical and biological casualties.

STRIKING BACK IN AFGHANISTAN

Afghanistan was identified as the breeding ground for the 9/11 attacks. The Taliban regime harbored Osama bin Laden and his al Qaeda network and training centers. Operation Enduring Freedom began on October 7, 2001, and initiated the global war on terror. Military operations by U.S. forces and coalition partners struck forcefully to overthrow the Taliban and eliminate bin Laden and his followers.

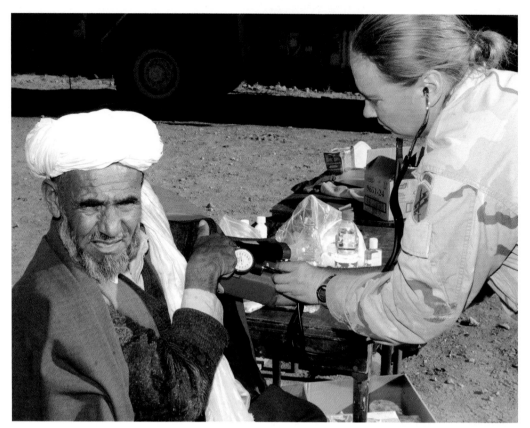

left
U.S. Army Specialist Amy Popke checks the blood pressure of an Afghan man during a medical assistance operation conducted by U.S. Army medical personnel in Khargar, Afghanistan, on December 15, 2004. Popke is assigned to the Task Force Victory surgeon cell. *Department of Defense.*

Organic medical support accompanied the Army Ranger and Special Forces units that first moved into the country to join the Northern Alliance forces. Elements of a combat support hospital set up at air staging bases in Uzbekistan for medical support until facilities could be gained in Afghanistan. Medevac helicopters transported the wounded and sick Americans and Afghan freedom fighters to airfields for Air Force air evacuation flights back to Ramstein Air Base and on to its next-door neighbor, the Landstuhl Regional Medical Center (LRMC). LRMC, jointly staffed by the Army and the Air Force, became the primary overseas hospital for casualties coming out of Afghanistan. They remained at LRMC until returned to duty or moved on to the United States for additional specialized care.

After defeating the Taliban and terrorist organizations, Army medical units continued to serve American and coalition forces in Afghanistan. Much of the post-combat medical support focused on assisting the Afghans to rebuild their national medical system. Medical, dental, and veterinary civic action programs (MEDCAP, DENCAP, and VETCAP) helped to reestablish health care in many isolated towns and villages. Veterinary assistance programs were particularly important in a rural country dependent on animals for farming, food, and transportation.

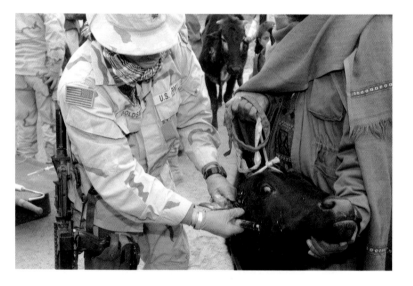

AIR FORCE AND NAVY MEDICS IN OPERATION ENDURING FREEDOM

Using the EMEDS configuration, the AFMS was among the first functional specialties to deploy to Southwest Asia in Operation Enduring Freedom. The portable EMEDS units fit into a small space on the first deploying aircraft. By 2002, each 25-bed EMEDS was one-third the weight and size of the typical 25-bed Air Transportable Hospital of the Gulf War era. A single C-130 aircraft transported a comprehensive field emergency medical and surgical unit—an entire EMEDS basic package, including personnel, equipment and shelters. To achieve

above
U.S. Army Major Steven Goldsmith, a veterinarian, treats a cow in the small village of Aroki, Afghanistan, January 21, 2003, while conducting a Veterinarian Civic Action Program. *U.S. Army.*

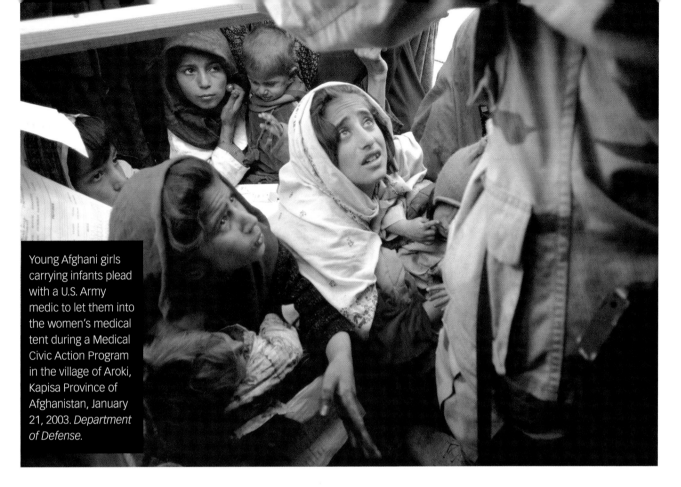

Young Afghani girls carrying infants plead with a U.S. Army medic to let them into the women's medical tent during a Medical Civic Action Program in the village of Aroki, Kapisa Province of Afghanistan, January 21, 2003. *Department of Defense.*

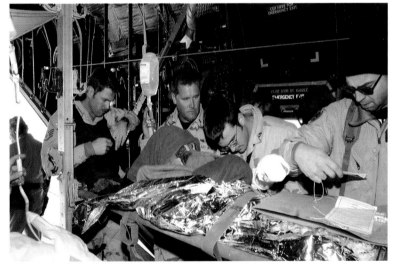

bottom
In the mid-1990s, the Air Force Medical Service developed Critical Care Air Transport Teams. They revolutionized both peacetime and wartime care by allowing critically ill patients to be flown to advanced medical facilities. *U.S. Air Force.*

this reduction in weight and size, the AFMS reengineered tents and medical equipment and also reduced the size of the basic EMEDS supply package. The basic EMEDS units were also designed as flexible "force modules," whose equipment and personnel might be stationed at different places before deployment.

Aeromedical evacuation was altered in Operation Enduring Freedom. Because of the small-scale dispersed nature of the combat operations in Afghanistan, the AFMS was able to station many of its new aeromedical teams and patient support equipment far forward in the operating theater. The immediate availability of these aeromedical resources created a minimal evacuation delay and optimum usage of returning aircraft. Rapid evacuation reduced the theater medical footprint but placed more stress on the aeromedical evacuation system. By dispersing aeromedical evacuation assets to forward locations, more aeromedical evacuation forces were required.

In addition to supporting Marine Corps forces in Operation Enduring Freedom in Afghanistan, U.S. Navy medical personnel were deployed to the southern Philippine islands of Basilan and Mindanao, long a stronghold for Abu Sayyaf and the Moro Islamic Liberation Front. Working with the multi-service Joint Task Force, Navy medicine fought terrorism through kindness—assisting in the rebuilding of villages and providing medical aid to a needy populace.

PREPARATION FOR COMBAT IN IRAQ

Medical planning for the possibility of combat operations against Saddam Hussein's Iraq began in 2002. The large forces for the campaign (dubbed Operation Iraqi Freedom) required considerable medical support split between a northern attack from Turkey (which never took place) and a southern force from Kuwait.

The medical force dedicated to Operation Iraqi Freedom was much smaller than previous combat operations. It represented approximately 5 percent of the deployed forces versus 14 percent for the 1990–91 Gulf War. A major reason for this was the decision laid out in Joint Health Services Support Vision 2010 in 1997 and in joint medical planning that only essential care would be provided in theater sufficient to stabilize patients for evacuation. Seven days was established as a normal baseline for evacuation to the next echelon of care along the line of communications or in the U.S.

For operations in Iraq, the Air Force would now evacuate patients to Landstuhl for definitive care, which reduced the number of hospital units and the Medical Department presence in theater.

When operations began on March 19, 2003, organic medical assets, including the new 91W medics, supported the frontline combat units. Forward Surgical Teams assigned to the brigade combat teams provided far-forward surgery. Medevac duties were handled by air ambulance units, including the 507th Medical Company (Air Ambulance) with 12 modern HH-60L Black Hawks. The 498th Medical Company (Air Ambulance) supported the

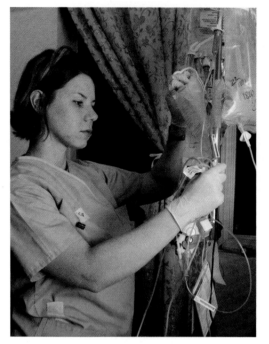

Marine Expeditionary Force—the first time that dedicated Army medevac resources were attached to the Marines for this mission. The 86th and 21st Combat Support Hospitals and the Army's sole surviving mobile army surgical hospital (MASH), the 212th from Germany, provided the hospital support in the initial thrust under the overall direction of the 30th Medical Brigade of the V Corps from Europe. The 212th proved the "mobile" in its designation by accompanying the spearhead of the V Corps, 3d Infantry Division, on a 78-hour, 270-mile thrust to the area of Najaf. There it set up its hospital, survived a monster sandstorm, and soon was handling both American and Iraqi casualties.

left
First Lieutenant Sarah Grivicic, an intensive care nurse assigned to the Army's 28th Combat Support Hospital, hangs a tube feed for her patient in Baghdad, November 24, 2003. *Department of Defense.*

right
Crew members of an HH-60L air ambulance from the 82d Medical Company (Aviation), 82d Airborne Division, unload their aircraft to prepare for another mission April 4, 2003, at a forward deployed location in southern Iraq. *U.S. Army.*

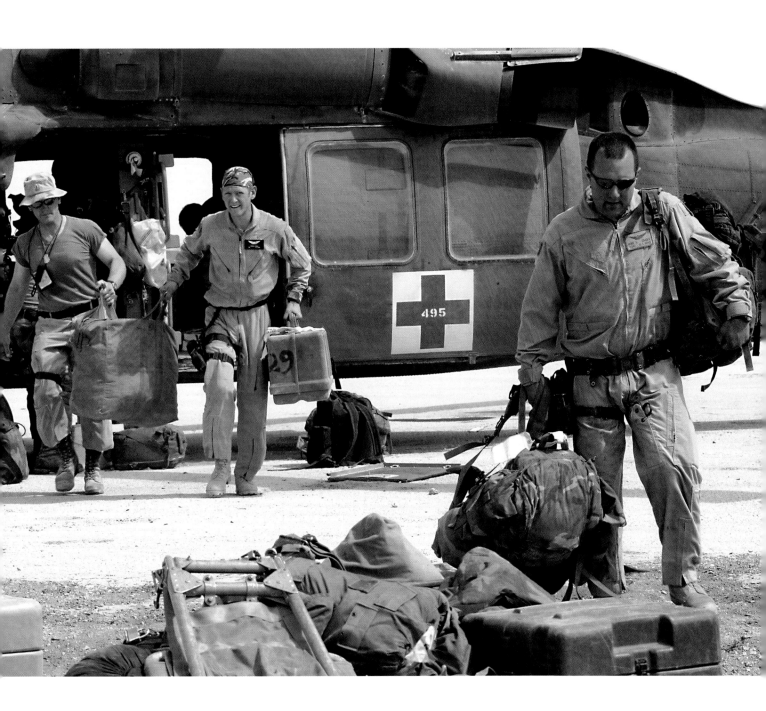

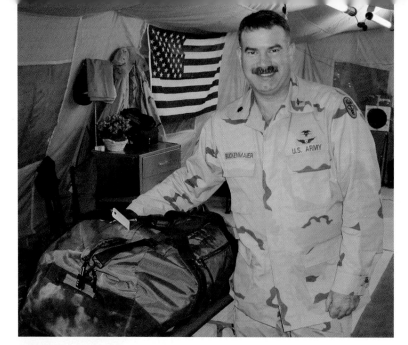

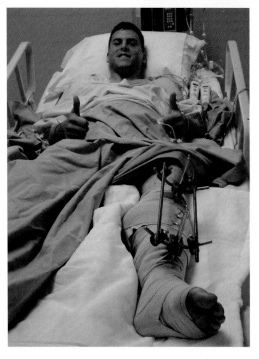

The upsurge in insurgent and terrorist activities and the use of improvised explosive devices (IEDs) and car bombs against American convoys and soldiers took a significant toll as terrorist activities developed within Iraq. More coalition casualties were generated in this phase than in the initial fighting that overthrew Saddam Hussein.

New personal protective equipment for soldiers, especially the improved ceramic body armor, reduced wounds of the thorax and abdomen which, in the past, were often the most life threatening. The IED weapons caused numerous severe head and extremity wounds, the latter requiring many amputations.

Working closely with the Department of Veterans' Affairs, Lieutenant General Peake established the Military Amputee Patient Care Program, or Amputee Center, at Walter Reed Army Medical Center in 2003 and another at Brooke Army Medical Center in San Antonio, Texas, in 2004. This program ensured the finest care of the amputees and their rehabilitation and adjustment to new prosthetic devices and, in some cases, even their return to active duty service.

The military's commitment to refining emergency medicine has enabled many soldiers and Marines who would not have survived their wounds in previous wars to stay alive, albeit with terrible injuries. Life-threatening injuries are fewer with the chest and abdominal protection provided by advanced Kevlar™ body armor, but head and extremity wounds are plentiful. Unfortunately, so are amputations and the non-physical but no less incapacitating psychological injuries.

After the fall of Saddam Hussein's regime and President George W. Bush's announcement of the end of major ground combat operations on May 1, 2003, Army hospital units continued to support the American and coalition forces stationed in Iraq. They included the 10th, 21st, 28th, 31st, 47th, 67th, 86th, and 228th Combat Support Hospitals plus the 212th MASH. Army medical and dental personnel assisted the new Iraqi Ministry of Health in restoring the Iraqi health care system, reopening hospitals and neighborhood clinics, and training Iraqis.

top
Lieutenant Colonel (Dr.) Chester C. Buckenmaier III is chief of the regional anesthesia section at Walter Reed Army Medical Center. *Uniformed Services University of the Health Sciences.*

bottom
U.S. Army Specialist Brian Wilhelm was the first combat casualty to benefit from a peripheral nerve block on the battlefield. On October 7, 2003, he sustained a severe wound from a rocket-propelled grenade that blew off the hamstrings of his left leg. Lieutenant Colonel (Dr.) Chester C. Buckenmaier III performed the battlefield regional anesthesia procedure. The regional anesthesia pain management technique improves battlefield pain control from first care through the entire evacuation chain. *Uniformed Services University of the Health Sciences.*

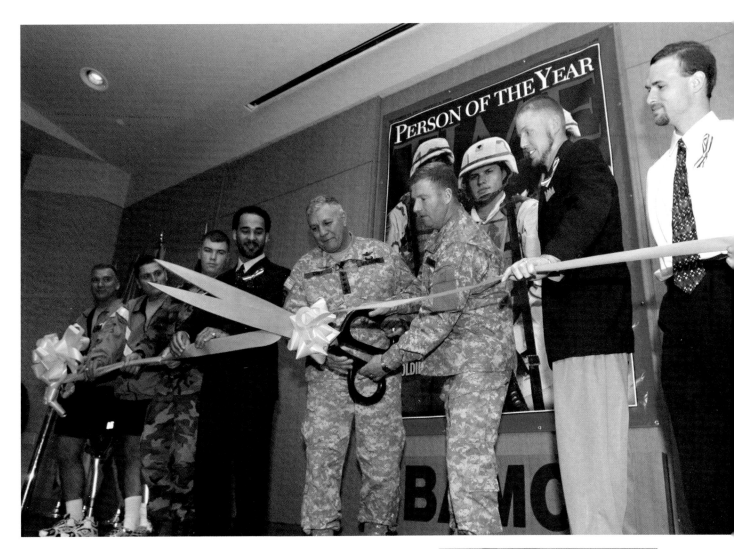

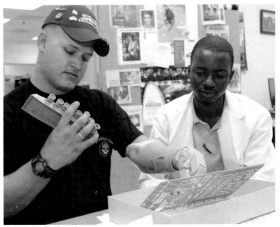

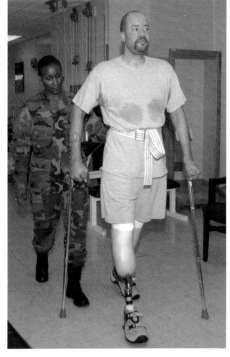

top
U.S. Army Vice Chief of Staff General Richard A. Cody, center left, and Sergeant Major of the Army Kenneth O. Preston cut the ribbon to open the Army's second Amputee Center at Brooke Army Medical Center, Fort Sam Houston, Texas, January 14, 2005, as amputee patients hold the ribbon. *U.S. Army.*

bottom left
Occupational therapy at Walter Reed Army Medical Center. *U.S. Army photo by Paul Haring.*

bottom right
Physical therapy at Walter Reed Army Medical Center. *U.S. Army Photo by Bobby Jones.*

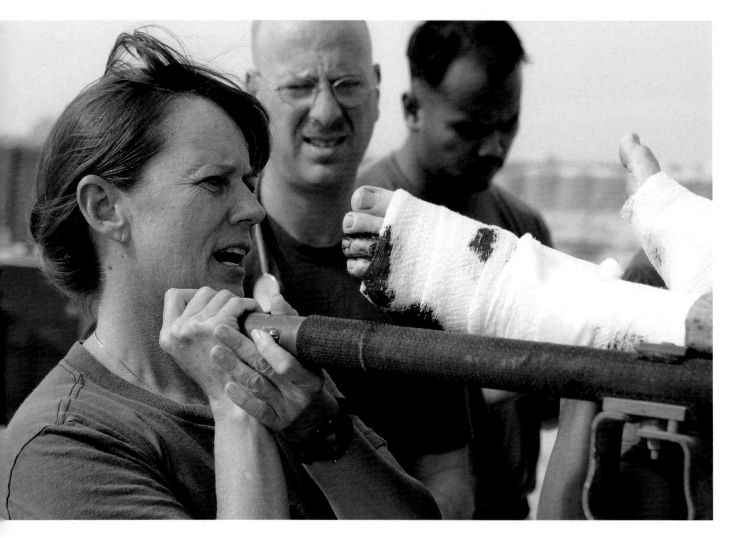

NAVY MEDICINE IN OPERATION IRAQI FREEDOM

From March 19, 2003, as the Marines fought their way from Kuwait to Baghdad, Navy physicians, corpsmen, and critical care nurses accompanied them. The Navy medics stabilized the critically wounded and coordinated their evacuation to facilities better equipped to provide further care. Some of these facilities were the Forward Resuscitative Surgery Systems (FRSS). These highly mobile, rapidly deployable trauma surgical units provided emergency surgery to stabilize critically injured casualties before moving them on to other care. Each unit consisted of an eight-person team: two surgeons, an anesthesiologist, a critical care nurse, an independent duty corpsman or a physician's assistant to run preoperative triage and advanced trauma life support surveys, two operating room technicians, and a general duty Fleet Marine Force corpsman. The system weighed about 6,400 pounds including food, water, shelter, generators, and all the equipment needed to handle 18 surgical patients for 48 hours. Six such FRSS teams saw action during the first phase of the war.

The hospital ship USNS *Comfort* cruised offshore to provide definitive care for casualties. As events unfolded, the hospital ship cared more for injured Iraqi civilians and enemy prisoners of war (EPW) than for coalition casualties. During the 56 days the vessel was in the northern Persian Gulf, medical staff performed more than 600 surgeries, including 350 inpatients. Seventy percent of the surgeries were orthopedic in nature and almost three quarters of all patients treated were Iraqis, both civilian and EPWs.

The second phase of the conflict, after May 1, 2003, continued in 2005. It was characterized by escalating and increasingly violent insurgent activity. This combat in a largely urban environment placed continuing demand on the Navy medical personnel deployed with the Marines.

U.S. Navy Chief Hospital Corpsman Suzette Dugger, assigned to the Surgical/Shock Trauma Platoon at Camp Taqaddum, Iraq, helps offload a patient from an ambulance, November 17, 2004. *U.S. Marine Corps.*

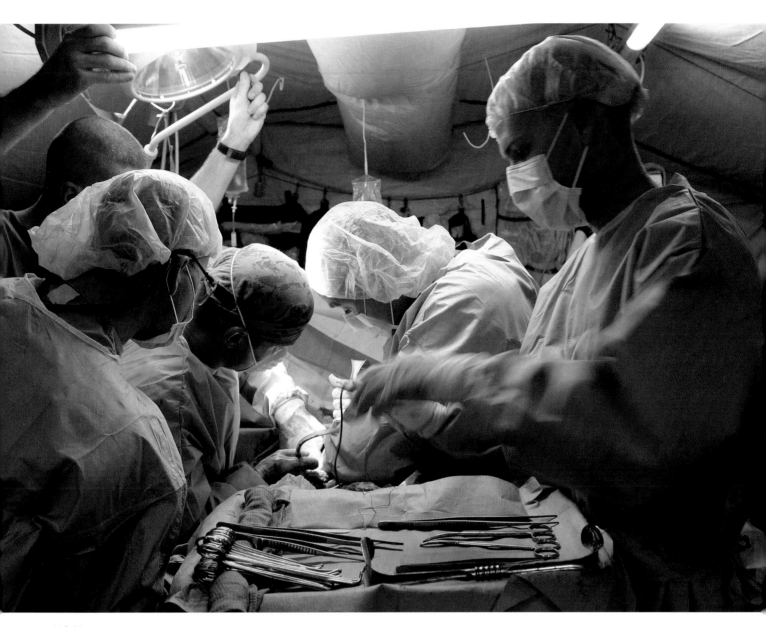

U.S. Navy surgeons and hospital corpsman assigned to the Surgical/Shock Trauma Platoon at Camp Taqaddum in Iraq operate on a Marine injured by an improvised explosive device on November 17, 2004. The shock trauma platoon is one of three major immediate surgical and trauma care teams assigned to Marine forces operating in Iraq. *Department of Defense.*

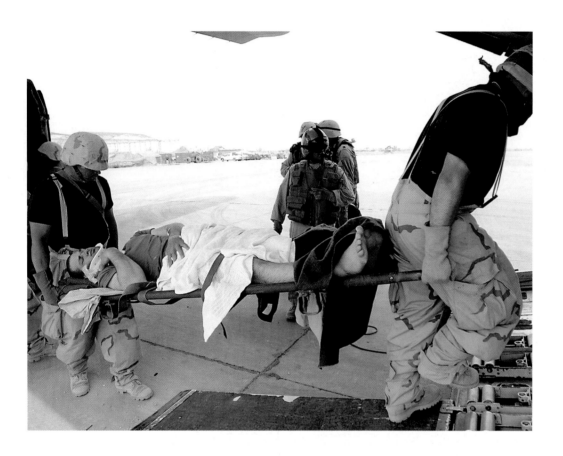

U.S. AIR FORCE MEDICAL SERVICE IN
OPERATION IRAQI FREEDOM

The major combat in Iraq between March and May 2003 resulted in nearly 2,000 aeromedical evacuations, including 640 battle casualties. At the peak of Operation Iraqi Freedom, 3,300 personnel of the AFMS supported the 75,000 deployed Air Force personnel.

By September 30, 2003, nearly 10,000 patients had been moved from the theater of operations. This aeromedical evacuation effort was the largest since the Vietnam War. In a major system change, the Air Force began to fly 50 percent to 60 percent of patients back to the United States on commercial rather than military aircraft, partly because this reduced the transit time to home.

Aeromedical evacuation was lighter, more adaptable, and able to use the best available airframe at any particular time and place. The Air Force moved away from dedicated airframes, such as the C-9 or C-141, and began to use the best airframe in the flow. The AFMS also moved towards lighter, more adaptable aeromedical evacuation equipment, such as patient support pallets, that could be moved easily from one aircraft to the next. The pallets were built on a standard frame that could fit all Air Force cargo and transport aircraft, from the C-130 to the C-5.

Members of the 86th Combat Support Hospital from Fort Campbell, Kentucky, load injured U.S. soldiers onto a C-130 aircraft for medical evacuation on April 4, 2003, at Talil Air Base, Iraq. *Department of Defense.*

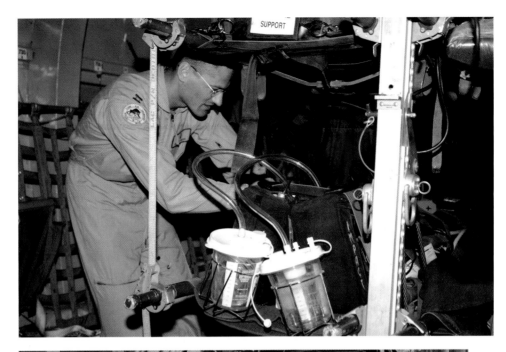

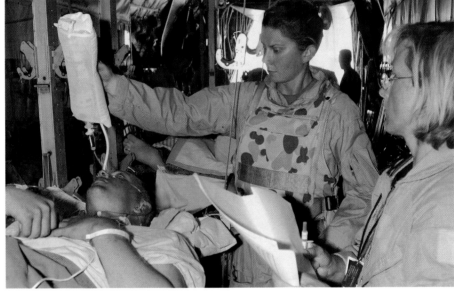

top
U.S. Air Force Captain Rocky Hosie, a Registered Nurse with the Critical Care Air Transport Team from Keesler Air Force Base, Mississippi, transports a patient from Prince Sultan Air Base, Saudi Arabia, on a U.S. Air Force C-141 Starlifter back to Ramstein Air Base, Germany. *Department of Defense.*

bottom
Australian medic Leading Aircraft Woman Megan Sellars, center, and U.S. Air Force Major Kate Flarity care for wounded and injured coalition troops aboard an Australian C-130 aircraft at Baghdad Airport for a flight to Kuwait. *Courtesy of Australian Ministry of Defence.*

In contrast to its efforts in the 1990–91 Gulf War, the Air Force could track its patients in the evacuation chain and make sure the right people were moving at the right time. To do this, the Air Force started to use a system called the TRANSCOM (U.S. Transportation Command) Regulating and C2 Evacuation System (TRAC2ES) that came into the aeromedical evacuation inventory just before September 11, 2001.

TRAC2ES was a joint Defense Department enterprise that allowed medical planners to decide which patients should fly out on what aircraft, what equipment was needed to support each patient, and to which hospital they should fly. TRAC2ES was also not dependent on any particular type of aircraft. This assured its success if a national emergency required activation of the DOD's Civil Reserve Air Fleet (CRAF) of up to 78 commercial aircraft—both cargo and passenger—provided to DOD by civilian airline companies. The CRAF would be used to transport material and people into the theater of operations, and, if necessary, evacuate sick or injured troops out of a combat theater.

PEACETIME HEALTH CARE AND HOMELAND SECURITY

After September 11, 2001, the AFMS also continued to pursue improvements in the peacetime, stateside medical system. One focus was on finding less expensive ways to provide traditional, high-quality care. A promising change that also entailed health benefits was to establish nurse-run clinics to handle the prevention and treatment of diabetics, asthmatics, and others with chronic conditions. Such clinics focused heavily on prevention. For example, a clinic in Little Rock, Arkansas, warned asthmatics when air-quality levels were unhealthy.

The Air Force Nurse Corps also explored ways to make its personnel structure more responsive to particular medical needs. In the past, Air Force nurses had to serve as commissioned officers, and therefore they sometimes were not the ideal nurse for the patient. The Nurse Corps explored ways to establish a multi-level nurse career field, with nurse assistants, licensed vocational nurses, and registered nurses, which would allow some personnel positions to be moved to the enlisted ranks or even to the civilian side.

Increased cooperation with civilian institutions was another promising approach to cost optimization. For example, the Air Force explored ways to send Air Force patients to two graduate medical institutions in the San Antonio area at no extra cost to the Air Force. From the Air Force standpoint, providing increased access to off-base medical facilities at no extra cost could help the AFMS attract more 65-year-old and over retirees back into the Air Force system.

The need to strengthen homeland security led the AFMS to improve its medical training for homeland disasters and medical emergencies. For instance, in January 2002, the first Center for Sustainment of Trauma and Readiness Skills (CSTARS) opened at the University of Maryland's Shock Trauma Center in Baltimore. This program gave Air Force medics valuable hands-on clinical experience covering the full spectrum of acute trauma care: from the first emergency response to transport of the patient, trauma unit reception, operating room intervention, and intensive care treatment.

The three-week CSTARS session also had an advanced trauma care course for nurses and a pre-hospital trauma life support course for medical technicians. Building on the success of this first site, the Air Force opened two new CSTARS programs, one at St. Louis University primarily for Air National Guard team training, and the other at the University Hospital of Cincinnati for Reserve teams.

In January 2004, recognizing the increased physical demands of Operation Iraqi Freedom, the Air Force began to require a new fitness test that emphasized aerobic and muscular fitness rather than body weight and fat percentage. Fitness testing now focused on four metrics: a 1.5-mile run time, measurement of waist circumference, and the number of sit-ups and push-ups accomplished in one minute.

Airmen earning scores of excellent and good were retested in one year. Marginal scores were retested in six months, and poor in 90 days. Airmen with poor scores also had to enter a monitored exercise program. The bicycle ergometry test of aerobic capacity that the Air Force required in the 1990s was abandoned, except for those airmen who were medically disqualified from making the 1.5-mile run.

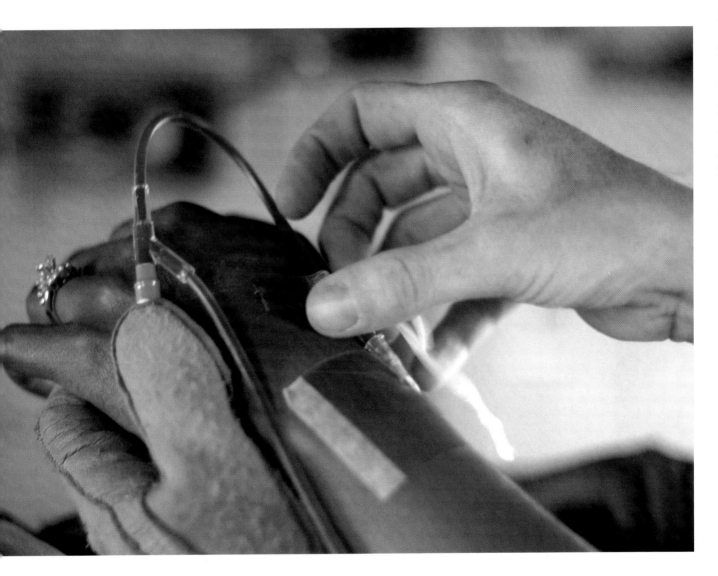

A U.S. Army flight medical technician checks a soldier's pulse during the helicopter medevac flight to a Combat Support Hospital in Baghdad, Iraq, August 26, 2004. *U.S. Air Force.*

Improvements in field medicine were also evident in Operation Iraqi Freedom. The EMEDS concept continued to work well. And because of unprecedented commander support of force health protection, the disease, non-battle injury rate was at an all-time historical low. There were, however, a few persistent difficulties. For instance, the AFMS still lacked the ability to transport contagious patients safely. Communications equipment was not interoperable among the different medical components in theater, and the joint medical logistics system was sometimes unresponsive to urgent AFMS needs. But the successes of the AFMS in Operation Iraqi Freedom far overshadowed these problems.

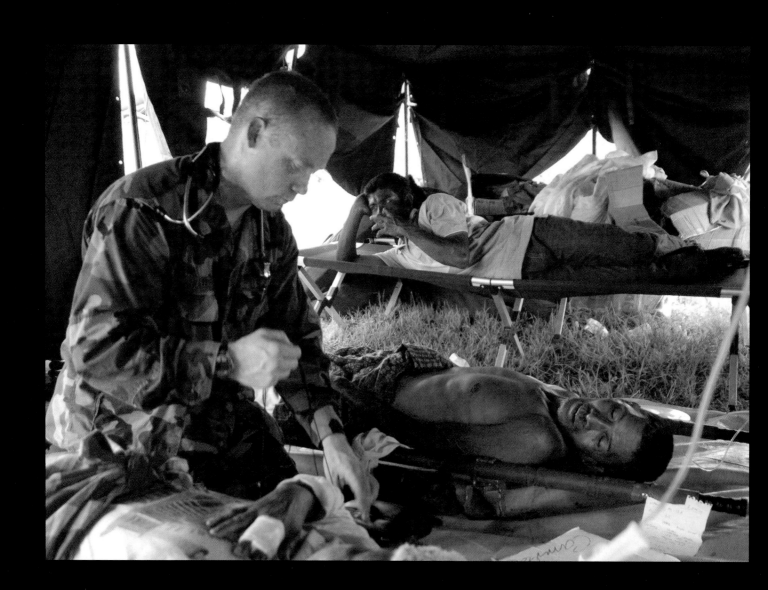

Chapter 11
Global Activities and Looking Ahead

A U.S. Navy doctor treats patients from tsunami-devastated villages in Banda Aceh, Sumatra, Indonesia, on January 6, 2005. Helicopters from the USS *Abraham Lincoln* Carrier Strike Group are providing humanitarian assistance to areas devastated by the December 26, 2004, Indian Ocean tsunami. *Department of Defense.*

PREPARING FOR THE FUTURE

ARMY MEDICINE: QUEST FOR EXCELLENCE

If history teaches anything, the lesson is that the past is usually a good indicator of the future. For 230 years the Army Medical Department has been responsible for the health and welfare of the American soldier upon which an effective fighting force has depended. To carry out this mission successfully, it must always maintain the most advanced health care in the world, both on the battlefield and in its military treatment facilities from troop clinics to the most modern medical centers.

Army battlefield medicine has constantly evolved from its first trials at Breed's Hill in Boston on June 17, 1775, to its latest challenges in Afghanistan and Iraq in 2005. The underlying theme across these years has always been to save the wounded soldier through application of the most modern medical and surgical techniques by trained and ready medical personnel. Leaders of the Medical Department have relentlessly studied and changed the field medical organization to take advantage of the latest medical advances better to serve the soldier. The cumulative effect of those changes across 230 years has yielded a medical structure that provides superlative medical and surgical care, often under enemy fire and at the cost of the providers' own lives.

That quest to serve the soldier continues today as the Medical Department lays out an entirely new approach to providing medical support for the transforming Army. The ongoing work of Task Force Medical that began under Surgeon General James Peake envisions a seamless medical structure from the Medical Command's (MEDCOM) regional entities in the United States to the deployed tactical units anywhere in the world. These changes will improve the integration of the medical support throughout the Army while remaking the medical command and control structure within Army and theater Army commands.

Readiness of the Reserve component medical units will improve through closer coordination with the new Army Reserve Medical Command (AR-MEDCOM) and the Army National Guard. To manage the readiness and training of Reserve medical units, the AR-MEDCOM will organize its own regional medical commands and medical area support groups that parallel the MEDCOM's regional organization.

With these changes in place, the Army MEDCOM will become the Army's single medical force provider. This will eliminate many of the inefficiencies of the past caused by often conflicting lines of command and control.

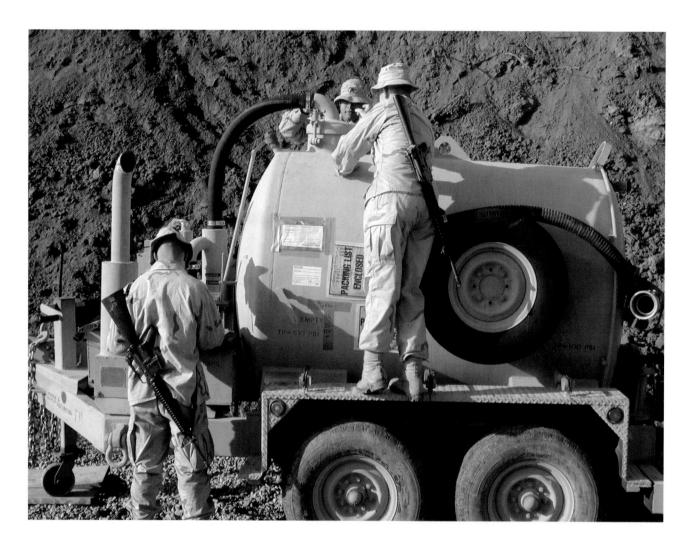

REALIGNING COMMAND AND CONTROL

As this process moves along, a remodeling of the medical command and control system will take place. Medical deployment support commands will replace theater medical commands and medical support commands will replace corps medical commands and brigades. A new multi-functional medical battalion will be created to replace the present-day medical logistics, area support, and evacuation battalions. Army, MEDCOM, and joint planners and commanders will have a wider range of choices and more flexibility in crafting the medical support packages and command and control structures to accompany deploying forces.

The key to the success of the command and control changes will be the ongoing and programmed changes in the field medical force. As the Medical Reengineering Initiative (MRI) program has evolved since the mid-1990s, constant refinement has been a major factor in maintaining alignment with the Army's overall transformation. With 50 percent of the units now activated or converted, a new approach

to MRI design, called the Adaptive Medical Increments (AMI), has been added. The AMI is updating the MRI design to reduce the size of deployable modular increments of each MRI unit. Medical units will now be subdivided into smaller packages that can fit better with whatever size force is deployed. The increased modularity created with AMI allows greater flexibility in mixing and matching capabilities to meet the medical requirements of a wide spectrum of potential operations from major theater combat to small humanitarian and disaster relief missions.

The success of these changes depends heavily upon continued integration of new equipment, medicines, and techniques. Much of the Medical Department's history has been marked with significant advances in medical research and development. Today the frontiers of medical research are being pushed every day in laboratories and research institutes throughout the Medical Department.

At a U.S. base in Uzbekistan, U.S. Army preventive medicine personnel inspect a "water buffalo," a mobile trailer used to store and transport safe drinking water to deployed soldiers. *U.S. Army.*

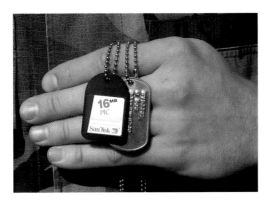

top
The Personal Information Carrier enables service members to carry their complete medical record at all times. *U.S. Army Medical Department.*

bottom
The Personal Information Carrier transports medical encounters from one echelon of care to another via the patient. The care provider will have a legible, easily accessed history of previous encounters and a waterproof medium on which to record new information. *U.S. Army Medical Department.*

Work continues at the Institute of Surgical Research on the care and treatment of burn victims, while the Walter Reed Army Institute of Research works on new approaches to the age-old problems of malaria and other tropical diseases that afflict soldiers. The Medical Research Institute for Infectious Diseases is at the forefront of research on the newest and most virulent and deadly diseases from Hanta to Ebola as well as on some of the oldest from anthrax to smallpox. The development of effective protection for American soldiers and citizens from such diseases remains a critical priority. Only constant work on new ideas and technologies has produced advances such as the fibrin sealant bandage or the various blood products now in use. While many avenues of research do not produce usable results, many others yield significant advances. Just as Major Frederick Russell's work on a typhoid vaccine in the early 20th century helped rid the Army and the country of that scourge, Army medical researchers continue their efforts to improve or develop a wide range of vaccines to protect soldiers from emerging new disease threats and maintain a healthy fighting force.

NEW TECHNOLOGY

The Medical Department seeks out and applies new technologies continuously. From patient information to logistics and real-time data on environmental and disease threats, medical personnel worldwide have virtually instantaneous awareness and communications. Developments in telemedicine already allow consultations and transfer of vital patient information between physicians in remote theaters and specialists in Army medical centers in the United States. Systems are under development that will provide remote personnel monitoring of soldiers to determine not only their location on the battlefield but also their physiological condition and allow medics to intervene if necessary.

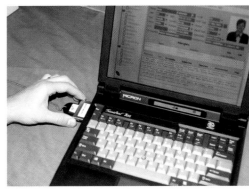

The Personal Information Carrier (PIC) offers the potential for soldiers to carry their complete medical record at all times. It is a small electronic device that carries demographic and medical information about the soldier who carries it. The PIC is about the size of a soldier's dog tag. A medic caring for the soldier can pull up the records via a laptop computer or other device.

Medics can also make use of the Battlefield Medical Information System-Telemedicine (BMIS-T). It was designed by the Theater and Advanced Technology Research Center at Fort Detrick, Maryland. BMIS-T is programmed with health care reference manuals and can provide medical personnel with suggested diagnosis and treatment plans.

The BMIS-T and the new Medical Communications for Combat Casualty Care computer network linked to the Theater Medical Information Program also provide a new level of information sharing and medical communications.

New bandages, such as the fibrin sealant and chitosan bandages, and blood clotting compounds, such as QuikClot™, can stop bleeding and control hemorrhaging, a major cause of battlefield deaths in the past. A one-handed tourniquet that a soldier can use to stop bleeding in an arm or leg has also been developed and distributed. These new technologies are especially important for Rangers and Special Forces personnel who often operate in isolated areas and away from access to medical care.

New medical evacuation helicopters are being assigned to air ambulance companies. Two are noteworthy: the advanced HH-60L with advanced life support equipment and full medical monitoring and care during evacuation flights; and the UH-60Q, which is an upgraded UH-60A with the medical equipment of the HH-60L.

For ground evacuation and battlefield care, the Surgeon General sought replacements for the aged armored M577 medical treatment vehicle and the M113 evacuation vehicle, more than four decades old. The medical companies of the new Initial Brigade Combat Teams that are part of the Army transformation initiative deployed to Iraq in 2003 with the new wheeled, armored Stryker medical evacuation vehicle.

The transformational world of the 21st century Army medic would have been as unimaginable to a medic in the jungles of Vietnam as the medevac helicopter would have been to the stretcher bearer in the trenches of World War I or a vaccine to prevent typhoid to a physician of the Civil War. All of the advances of Army medicine over the years have resulted from the ideas, hard work, and selfless sacrifices of thousands of Army medical personnel: from physicians, dentists, nurses, and veterinarians to laboratory technicians and wardmasters to frontline medics and medevac crews. They have served their fellow soldiers unstintingly since 1775. They all have remained true to the

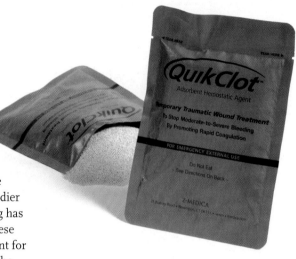

Medical Department's motto "To Conserve Fighting Strength."

AIR FORCE MEDICAL SERVICE INNOVATIONS

In the last few years, the Air Force Medical Service (AFMS) has partnered with frontline elements of the Air Force to explore essential aspects of fatigue and human performance under stress. Air Force medics looked at the schedule, dietary, and biorhythmic challenges for each scenario or deployment. They used this information to devise ways to mitigate in-flight fatigue. Counter-fatigue medicines were used as a last resort. Written, well-publicized policy statements regulated the issuance of these medicines. Their use involved the line

top
QuikClot™ hemostatic agent stops blood loss and hastens clotting. It was tested through cooperation among the Office of Naval Research, the Uniformed Services University of the Health Sciences, and the Henry M. Jackson Foundation for the Advancement of Military Medicine. Z-Medica Company produces QuikClot™. *Courtesy of Z-Medica Company.*

bottom
Medical improvements of the HH-60L medevac helicopter include an on-board oxygen-generating system, an infrared radar system that helps locate patients on the battlefield, an externally mounted rescue hoist, and improved litter lift and medic seating. *U.S. Army Medical Department.*

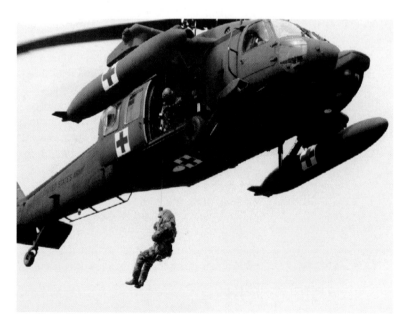

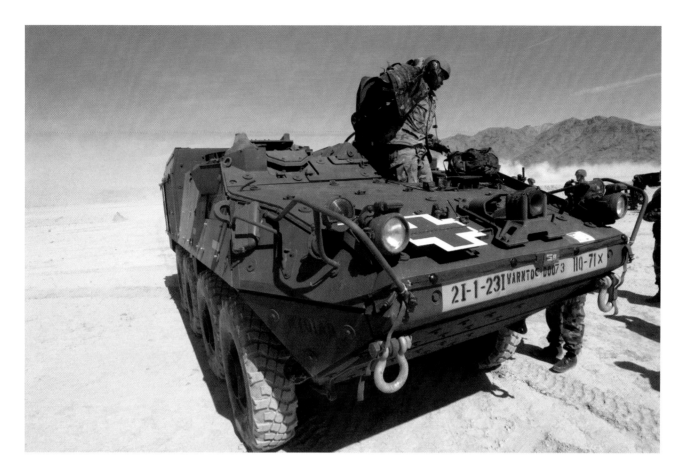

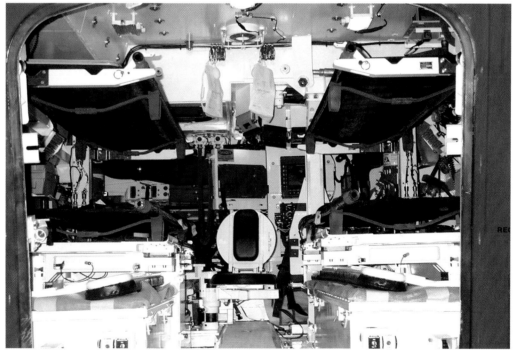

top
The Stryker medical evacuation vehicle can evacuate four litter patients or six ambulatory patients while its crew of three medics provides basic medical care. *U.S. Army Medical Department.*

bottom
Interior of the Stryker medical evacuation vehicle shows its centrally located medical attendant seat and high roof. *U.S. Army Medical Department.*

commander, the flight surgeon, and ultimately the pilot flying a mission. Everything was appropriately considered before a pilot was issued the medication. Even then, use of the medication on each flight was still a voluntary decision of the pilot.

Another AFMS research program in the new millennium was "super vision." Its goal was to enhance or optimize vision through refractive surgery and advanced designs in night vision and interactive helmet visors.

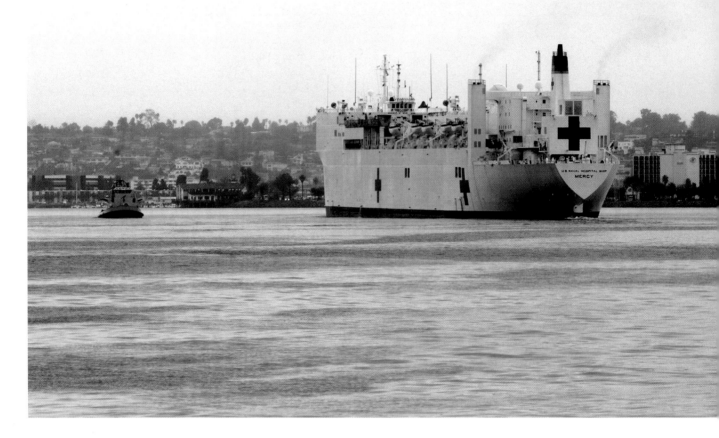

In the realm of countermeasures to chemical agents, the AFMS improved its personal protective gear, medical shelters, and patient decontamination capability. For instance, the AFMS gradually began to harden many of its EMEDS shelters. These hardened facilities enable medics to treat patients and operate safely even under chemical attack.

Flight nurse researchers at Wilford Hall Medical Center in Texas have studied ways to improve the care of critically ill or injured patients in stressful military conditions, such as excess heat or cold in cargo aircraft used for aeromedical evacuation. Another flight nurse study identified previously unrecognized limitations in accurate measurement of patient oxygenation during flight.

NAVY MEDICINE AND GLOBAL ACTIVITIES

Since the creation of the Navy Medical Department more than 200 years ago, Navy medical personnel have cared for the fighting forces with dedication and skill in peace and war. On land, on and beneath the sea, in the air, and in the vacuum of space, Navy medics have performed superbly. They have also practiced their healing arts with allied militaries, and with foreign governments and civilian populations.

In recent years, Navy medical personnel have steamed to assist almost anywhere with an urgent need for health care. Navy doctors, nurses, dentists, Medical Service Corps officers, and hospital corpsmen have deployed worldwide on those missions. Here is a short listing of the recent range of locations:

- Albania, Bosnia, and Kosovo in the Balkans in humanitarian activities;
- Cambodia and Sri Lanka to provide care to land mine victims;
- Djibouti to conduct an industrial health survey;
- Iraq as part of the Coalition Provisional Authority to assist in training the newly formed Iraqi army in combat lifesaver skills;
- Zambia to conduct an HIV/AIDS research project and provide HIV lectures to Zambian military personnel;
- Ghana to provide humanitarian aid, civic assistance, and medical peacetime support;
- Honduras for a humanitarian support mission; and
- Vietnam, Laos, and Cambodia with the Joint POW/MIA Accounting Command providing medical support for teams searching for, recovering, and identifying U.S. service member remains.

U.S. Navy hospital ship USNS *Mercy* gets under way from San Diego, California, before deploying to Southeast Asia. The *Mercy* is steaming to assist U.S. service men and women, to deliver humanitarian relief supplies, and provide medical assistance to the tsunami-stricken countries as part of Operation Unified Assistance. *Department of Defense.*

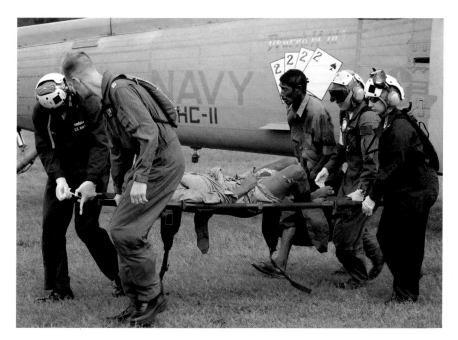

U.S. Navy personnel rush to carry an injured Indonesian from a Navy helicopter to a triage site located on an Indonesian air base in Banda Aceh, Sumatra, January 7, 2005. Medical teams from the USS *Abraham Lincoln* Carrier Strike Group and Carrier Air Wing Two worked with the International Organization for Migration and the Australian Air Force to provide initial medical care to victims of the tsunami-stricken coastal regions. *U.S. Navy.*

At the end of 2004 and start of 2005, the Navy dealt with another urgent need for health care. The magnitude-9 earthquake on December 26, 2004, resulted in the massive tsunami waves that wrought devastation in coastal areas throughout the Indian Ocean. Navy resources responded immediately. The effort focused on Indonesia's hard-hit Aceh Province. Medical teams with the aircraft carriers USS *Bonhomme Richard*, USS *Abraham Lincoln*, and Carrier Air Wing Two worked tirelessly to reinforce the worldwide relief effort. Helicopters lifted from carrier decks with food, water, and medical supplies. Medical personnel flew ashore and immediately began providing medical care to injured and homeless survivors.

Wherever and however America's interests lie in the future, Navy medicine is ready and will always be "Steaming to Assist."

Military medics are always aware of their two primary missions—readiness to support their forces anywhere in the world at any time and the provision of health care to their families and all other beneficiaries at all times. In many ways, military medicine is similar to a civilian health maintenance organization (HMO), except that, as Lieutenant General Ronald R. Blanck, Army Surgeon General from 1996 to 2000, often said, it was "an HMO that had to go to war."

NAVY MEDICINE'S ASTRONAUTS

In 1973, the National Aeronautics and Space Administration (NASA) selected Commander Joseph Kerwin, MC, USN, to be a part of the first crew of the Skylab spacecraft. As a scientist-astronaut, Kerwin monitored the crew's health and conducted a series of medical experiments. The experiments investigated several significant areas. They evaluated the effect of weightlessness on man's ability to perform mechanical tasks; assessed the effects of long exposure to zero gravity on the cardiovascular system; determined whether normal sleep rhythms such as sleep and wakefulness are influenced by zero gravity and a rapid day-night cycle; and studied nutritional requirements. Since the early 1970s, seven Navy physicians have served as NASA scientist-astronauts. One, Jerry M. Linenger, flew a space shuttle mission before spending 132 days orbiting the earth as a scientist/crew member of the Russian Space Station Mir. Their names:

CHARLES E. BRADY, JR.

DAVID M. BROWN

MANLEY L. "SONNY" CARTER
(DIED IN A CIVILIAN AIRCRAFT ACCIDENT)

LAUREL BLAIR SALTON CLARK

JOSEPH KERWIN

JERRY M. LINENGER

LEE M.E. MORIN

Tragically, two of these astronauts—Captain David Brown and Captain Laurel Clark—died February 1, 2003, on board the space shuttle Columbia when it disintegrated during reentry.

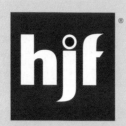

The Henry M. Jackson Foundation
for the Advancement of Military Medicine

The Henry M. Jackson Foundation for the Advancement of Military Medicine, Inc. (HJF) is a private, not-for-profit organization dedicated to improving military medicine and public health. We accomplish this by helping researchers at the Uniformed Services University of the Health Sciences (USU) and others in the military medical community conduct quality medical research and education programs.

FOSTERING MILITARY MEDICAL RESEARCH
Over the Foundation's 20-year history, we have established a responsive and focused infrastructure that supports researchers within the military medical community. This unique approach provides the military with the flexibility to accomplish its research goals quickly and cost-effectively, and removes administrative burdens so researchers may maintain their scientific focus.

The research conducted and our list of sponsors continues to grow in scope and diversity. Over the last five years, the Foundation and USU have ranked in the top 10 percent of all institutions receiving National Institutes of Health research grants.

In addition to investigator-initiated research at USU, the Foundation has helped establish several large military research and clinical programs. The Foundation has been an active partner in the U.S. Military HIV Research Program since its inception in 1988. Other collaborative programs include the Center for Prostate Disease Research, the Clinical Breast Care Program, and the Center for Deployment Health Care.

PROMOTING PRIVATE-PUBLIC PARTNERSHIPS
Congress chartered the Foundation, in part, to foster cooperative relationships between military medicine and the private sector. We work with military investigators on research projects sponsored by private industry, including clinical trials. Another important goal of the Foundation is to facilitate the transfer of useful new technologies developed at USU to the marketplace to improve public health. We patent and license medical technologies and foster collaborative research and development efforts with private industry.

SUPPORTING MILITARY MEDICAL EDUCATION
A key part of the Foundation's mission is to support graduate and continuing medical education at USU and throughout the military medical community. We provide this support by soliciting, securing, and administering funds from private donors, which help bring under-funded educational opportunities within reach of military personnel. They are used to support visiting speakers, seminars, and conferences.

HJF also provides support to USU graduate students through its annual Fellowship Program, which provides stipend and travel support for three USU graduate students entering the fifth year of study.

Now in its third decade of service, the Foundation remains committed to providing solutions to improve the health of our military and the quality of life around the world.

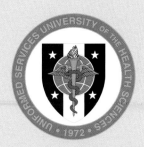

Uniformed Services University of the Health Sciences

Established by Congress in 1972, and graduating its first class in 1980, the Uniformed Services University of the Health Sciences (USU) is the nation's fully accredited federal school of medicine and graduate school of nursing. Its education, research, and consultation programs are unique, relating directly to military medicine, tropical diseases, disaster medicine, military medical readiness, and adaptation to extreme environments.

The F. Edward Hébert School of Medicine, in the top 25 percent (class size) of accredited American medical schools, has a year-round, four-year curriculum. This curriculum is nearly 700 hours—or about 20 weeks—longer than those found at other U.S. medical schools. In these extra hours, students focus on epidemiology, health promotion, disease prevention, tropical medicine, leadership and field exercises, and other subjects that relate to the unique requirements of career-oriented military physicians.

USU offers 14 graduate degrees in the biomedical sciences and public health. Doctor of philosophy degrees are offered in nine areas that range from clinical psychology to emerging infectious diseases. The university also offers a doctor of public health degree, and has a new physician-scientist program. The university's continuing education program is unique and extensive, serving the professional and readiness requirements of the Defense Department's worldwide military health care community through on-site and distance education.

The fully accredited Graduate School of Nursing offers a master of science in nursing degree in the following specialty areas: nurse anesthesia, family nurse practitioner, and perioperative nursing (clinical nurse specialist). In 2003, the school was expanded to include a Ph.D. program in nursing science.

MEDICAL RESEARCH

In cooperation with The Henry M. Jackson Foundation for the Advancement of Military Medicine, the National Institutes of Health, the military services, and other government and private institutions, the university's nationally ranked military and civilian faculty provide cutting-edge research and development in the biomedical sciences, and in areas specific to the Defense Department's health care mission, such as combat casualty care and infectious diseases. The university also holds more than 65 U.S. patents and additional foreign patents.

A UNIQUE MEDICAL EDUCATION

The university specializes in military medicine, which is more than practicing medicine in the military, and differs significantly from civilian medicine. Military medicine requires a solid background in tropical medicine and hygiene, parasitology, and a full understanding of epidemiologic methods and preventive medicine. Knowledge in areas of military medical intelligence, the psychological stresses of combat and trauma, and the medical effects of extreme environments, whether in aerospace, undersea, tropics, or desert conditions, are essential to properly advising a military commander on how to best keep troops fit. Also critical to a military physician's focus is disease prevention and health promotion in a wide variety of venues. USU provides this type of unique education. Simply put, we help students learn how to care for those in harm's way.

Bibliography

Adams, George W. *Doctors in Blue. The Medical History of the Union Army in the Civil War.* Baton Rouge, Louisiana: Louisiana State University Press, 1952.

Amberson, Julius M. "Operation Passage to Freedom: 17 August 1954–19 May 1955." Lecture, U.S. Navy Medical School, June 1, 1955, Amberson Biography File, Bureau of Medicine and Surgery Archives, Washington, D.C.

Armstrong, Blanche B. *Organization and Administration in World War II.* Washington, D.C.: Office of the Surgeon General, Department of the Army, 1963.

Ashburn, Percy M. *A History of the Medical Department of the United States Army.* Boston, Massachusetts: Houghton Mifflin Company, 1929.

Bayne-Jones, Stanhope. *The Evolution of Preventive Medicine in the United States Army, 1607–1939.* Washington, D.C.: Office of the Surgeon General, Department of the Army, 1968.

Beebe, Gilbert W., and DeBakey, Michael E. *Battle Casualties: Incidence, Mortality, and Logistic Considerations.* Springfield, Illinois: Charles C. Thomas, 1952.

Bispham, William N. *The Medical Department of the United States Army in the World War.* Vol. VII: *Training.* Washington, D.C.: U.S. Government Printing Office, 1927.

Brown, Harvey E. *The Medical Department of the United States Army from 1775 to 1873.* Washington, D.C.: The Surgeon General's Office, 1873.

Cash, Philip. *Medical Men at the Siege of Boston. April, 1775–April, 1776. Problems of the Massachusetts and Continental Armies.* Philadelphia, Pennsylvania: American Philosophical Society, 1973.

Condon-Rall, Mary Ellen, and Cowdrey, Albert E. *The Medical Department: Medical Service in the War against Japan.* Washington, D.C.: U.S. Army Center of Military History, 1998.

Cosmas, Graham A., and Cowdrey, Albert E. *The Medical Department: Medical Service in the European Theater of Operations.* Washington, D.C.: U.S. Army Center of Military History, 1992.

Cowdrey, Albert E. *Fighting for Life. American Military Medicine in World War II.* New York: The Free Press, 1994.

_____. *The Medics' War.* Washington, D.C.: U.S. Army Center of Military History, 1987.

Crile, Grace (ed.). *George Crile: An Autobiography.* 2 vols. Philadelphia, Pennsylvania: J.B. Lippincott Company, 1947.

Crosby, Nancy J. *Journal* (January 1952–September 1953). Nancy J. Crosby Collection, Women in Military Service for America Memorial Foundation, Inc., Arlington, Virginia.

Dorland, Peter, and Nanney, James. *Dust Off: Army Aeromedical Evacuation in Vietnam.* Washington, D.C.: U.S. Army Center of Military History, 1984.

Duncan, Louis C. *Medical Men in the American Revolution, 1775–1783.* Washington, D.C.: Army Medical Field Service School, 1931.

_____. *The Medical Department of the United States Army in the Civil War.* Reprint. Gaithersburg, Maryland: Olde Soldier Books, n.d.

Engelman, Rose C. *A Decade of Progress. The U. S. Army Medical Department, 1959–1969.* Washington, D.C.: Office of the Surgeon General, U.S. Army, 1971.

Ford, Joseph H. *The Medical Department of the United States Army in the World War.* Vol. II: *Administration American Expeditionary Forces.* Washington, D.C.: U.S. Government Printing Office, 1927.

Foster, Gaines M. *The Demands of Humanity: Army Medical Disaster Relief.* Washington, D.C.: U.S Army Center of Military History, 1983.

Futrell, Robert. *Development of Aeromedical Evacuation in the United States Air Force, 1909–1960.* USAF Historical Study No. 23. Maxwell AFB, Alabama: USAF Historical Division, Aerospace Studies Institute, November 1961.

Garrison, Fielding H. *John Shaw Billings: A Memoir.* New York: G. P. Putnam's Sons, 1915.

Gibson, John M. *Physician to the World: The Life of General William C. Gorgas.* Durham, North Carolina: Duke University Press, 1950.

Gillett, Mary C. *The Army Medical Department, 1775–1818.* Washington, D.C.: U.S. Army Center of Military History, 1981.

_____. *The Army Medical Department, 1818–1865.* Washington, D.C.: U.S. Army Center of Military History, 1987.

_____. *The Army Medical Department, 1865–1917.* Washington, D.C.: U.S. Army Center of Military History, 1995.

Ginn, Richard V. N. *The History of the U.S. Army Medical Service Corps.* Washington, D.C.: Office of the Surgeon General, U.S. Army, and U.S. Army Center of Military History, 1997.

Hering, Eugene R. "Combat Medical Practice." *The Military Surgeon, Journal of the Association of Military Surgeons of the United States.* Ed. James M. Phalen. Washington, D.C., 1952. *AMSUS* Vol. 110 (January–June 1952): 102-106.

Herman, Jan K. *Battle Station Sick Bay: Navy Medicine in World War II.* Annapolis: Naval Institute Press, 1997.

_____. *A Hilltop in Foggy Bottom: Home of the Old Naval Observatory and the Navy Medical Department.* Washington, D.C.: U.S. Government Printing Office, 1991.

_____. "Hospital Ships are Back." *Navy Medicine* (January–February 1985): 14-21.

_____. "Welcome Back BUMED." *Navy Medicine* (July–August 1989): 10-15.

_____. "Field Medical Service School: Training a Different Kind of Corpsman." *Navy Medicine* (January–February 1988): 13-21.

The History of the Medical Department of the United States Navy, 1945–1955. NAVMED P-5057. Washington, D.C.: Bureau of Medicine and Surgery, 1955.

Hooper, Edwin B., Allard, Dean C., Fitzgerald, Oscar P. *The United States Navy and the Vietnam Conflict: The Setting of the Stage to 1959,* Volume 1. Washington, D.C.: Naval History Division, Department of the Navy, 1976.

"Hospital Corps, U.S. Navy," *Hospital Corps Quarterly* 19, (August 1946): 1-12.

Hume, Edgar Erskine. *Victories of Army Medicine: Scientific Accomplishments of the Medical Department of the United States Army.* Philadelphia, Pennsylvania: J.B. Lippincott Company, 1943.

Jones, David R., and Marsh, Royden W. *Flight Surgeon Support to United States Air Force Fliers in Combat.* Report No A710224. Brooks AFB, Texas. U.S. Air Force School of Aerospace Medicine, May 2003.

Langley, Harold D. *A History of Medicine in the Early U.S. Navy.* Baltimore: The Johns Hopkins University Press, 1995.

Letterman, Jonathan. *Medical Recollections of the Army of the Potomac.* New York: D. Appleton & Company, 1866.

Love, Albert G. *The Medical Department of the United States Army in the World War.* Vol. XV, Part 2: *Medical and Casualty Statistics.* Washington, D.C.: U.S. Government Printing Office, 1925.

Love, Albert G., Hamilton, Eugene L., and Hellman, Ida Levin. *Tabulating Equipment and Army Medical Statistics.* Washington, D.C.: Office of the Surgeon General, Department of the Army, 1958.

Link, Mae Mills, and Coleman, Hubert A. *Medical Support of the Army Air Forces in World War II.* Washington, D.C.: Office of the Surgeon General, U.S. Air Force, 1955.

Lynch, Charles, Weed, Frank W., and McAfee, Loy. *The Medical Department of the United States Army in the World War.* Vol. I: *The Surgeon General's Office.* Washington, D.C.: U.S. Government Printing Office, 1923.

Lynch, Charles, Ford, Joseph H., and Weed, Frank W. *The Medical Department of the United States Army in the World War.* Vol. VIII: *Field Operations.* Washington, D.C.: U.S. Government Printing Office, 1925.

Medical Department of the United States Navy With the Army and Marine Corps in France in World War I. Washington, D.C.: Bureau of Medicine and Surgery, 1947.

Medical Support in Operations Desert Shield and Desert Storm: Special issues, *The Journal of the U.S. Army Medical Department*, January–February 1992, March–April 1992, September–October 1992, November–December 1992.

Nanney, James S. *Army Air Forces Medical Services in World War II*. Washington, D.C.: Air Force History and Museums Program, 1998.

_____. *The Air Force Medical Service, 1949–1999: A Commemorative History*. Washington, D.C.: Office of the Surgeon General, USAF, 1999.

Neel, Spurgeon. *Medical Support of the U. S. Army in Vietnam, 1965–1970*. Washington, D.C.: Department of the Army, 1991.

Parks, Robert J. (ed.). *Medical Training in World War II*. Washington, D.C.: Office of the Surgeon General, Department of the Army, 1974.

Peyton, Green. *Fifty Years of Aerospace Medicine: Its Evolution since the Founding of the United States Air Force School of Aerospace Medicine in January 1918*. Brooks Air Force Base, Texas: U. S. Air Force School of Aerospace Medicine, 1968.

Phalen, James M. *Chiefs of the Medical Department of the United States Army, 1775–1940*. Carlisle Barracks, Pennsylvania: Army Medical Field Service School, 1940.

Redmond, Daniel. "Reminiscences of Passage to Freedom," *Navy Medicine* (January–February/March–April 1989): 33-36.

Reiss, Oscar. *Medicine and the American Revolution. How Diseases and Their Treatments Affected the Colonial Army*. Jefferson, North Carolina: McFarland and Company, Inc., 1998.

Reister, Frank A. (ed.). *Medical Statistics in World War II*. Washington, D.C.: Office of the Surgeon General, Department of the Army, 1975.

_____. *Battle Casualties and Medical Statistics: U.S. Army Experience in the Korean War*. Washington, D.C.: Office of the Surgeon General, Department of the Army, 1973.

Roddis, Louis H. "The Bureau of Medicine and Surgery, a Brief History." *U.S. Naval Institute Proceedings*, 75 (April 1949).

Sarnecky, Mary T. *A History of the U.S. Army Nurse Corps*. Philadelphia, Pennsylvania: University of Pennsylvania Press, 1999.

Siler, Joseph F. *The Medical Department of the United States Army in the World War*. Vol. IX: *Communicable and Other Diseases*. Washington, D.C.: U.S. Government Printing Office, 1928.

Sobocinski, André B. "A Little Engagement at Vera Cruz." *Navy Medicine* (May–June 2004): 16-18.

_____. "Widow's Island: The Forgotten Naval Hospital," *Navy Medicine* (March–April 2002): 11-13.

Sternberg, Martha L. *George Miller Sternberg: A Biography*. Chicago, Illinois: American Medical Association, 1920.

U.S. Navy Medical Department Administrative History, 1941–1945: Narrative History. Vol. 2, chapters 9-18, and chapter 17. Unpublished typescript in the BUMED Archives.

Washington, D.C.War Department, Surgeon General's Office. *Annual Reports of The Surgeon General, 1818–1980*.

_____. *Manual for the Medical Department*. 1899, 1906, 1916, 1916 Corrected to June 1918. Washington, D.C.: U.S. Government Printing Office, 1899, 1906, 1916, 1918.

_____. *Medical and Surgical History of the War of the Rebellion*. 6 vols. Washington, D.C.: U.S. Government Printing Office, 1870–88.

Weed, Frank W. *The Medical Department of the United States Army in the World War*. Vol. V: *Military Hospitals in the United States*. Washington, D.C.: U.S. Government Printing Office, 1923.

Wiltse, Charles M. *The Medical Department: Medical Service in the Mediterranean and Minor Theaters*. Washington, D.C.: Office of the Chief of Military History, 1965.

Index

Italics indicate photographs or illustrations.